's are to be returned on or before

THE PEOPLE'S HEALTH
1830-1910

THE PEOPLE'S HEALTH 1830-1910

F.B. SMITH

Weidenfeld and Nicolson
LONDON

Copyright © F. B. Smith, 1979, 1990
First published 1979
Paperback edition (with corrections) 1990
First published in Australia in 1979 by the
Australia National University Press, Canberra

Paperback edition first published in Great Britain
in 1990 by
George Weidenfeld and Nicolson Ltd,
91 Clapham High St, London SW4 7TA

British Library Cataloguing in Publication Data
is available upon request.

ISBN 0 297 82047.8

Printed and bound in Great Britain by
Butler & Tanner Ltd, Frome and London

CONTENTS

For my mother

ABBREVIATIONS

BMJ	*British Medical Journal*
COS	The Charity Organization Society
GMJ	*Glasgow Medical Journal*
JSS	*Journal of the Statistical Society*
JRSS	*Journal of the Royal Statistical Society* (from 1887)
L	*The Lancet*
PP	*Parliamentary Papers*
RC	Royal Commission

PREFACE

I owe much to my colleagues in the Research School of Social Sciences who helped when I ventured into fields unfamiliar to me during the preparation of this book. Professor W.D. Borrie and Dr Lincoln Day instructed me in demography and silently corrected my bad arithmetic. Dr Ian Maddocks, a former visitor to the School and presently Director in South Australia of the Family Medical Programme of the Royal Australian College of General Practitioners, read successive drafts and patiently rectified my blunders in medical matters. Another visitor, Professor J.F.C. Harrison, from the University of Sussex, read the early chapters to my great profit. Professor A.M. McBriar of Monash University supplied me with information about the Royal Commission on the Poor Law.

My friends in the Department of History have typed and checked my drafts, read and criticised them, and supplied me with quotations and references from their reading. Mr Derek Abbott, Miss Janice Aldridge, Mrs Jean Dillon, Mrs Elspeth Douglas, Dr G.C.L. Hazlehurst, Professor K.S. Inglis, Professor Oliver MacDonagh, Dr A.W. Martin and Mrs Lois Simms have each of them been marvellously helpful, and cheerfully tolerant at morning tea of my ghoulish anecdotes.

The nature of this book is such that I must emphasise my responsibility for such errors of fact and opinion as remain in it. Occasionally I have persisted with dubious arguments and speculations against excellent advice.

Canberra, 1978

PREFACE TO THE PAPERBACK EDITION

The radical form of this book has puzzled some readers. I realize that I did not sufficiently explain my intentions. I broke with the unspecific, triumphant sequential structure of traditional medical history in order to define the changing risks over time to human beings at various stages of the life cycle. Infants received a lot of attention because they comprised the major part of society at immediate risk and they constituted the largest group whose life chances were determined by their circumstances.

My arrangement of the material rests on three assumptions. The first is that sick persons and patients should predominate. They embody the illness which, for many of them, controls their lives. Their condition attracts notice and is the *raison d'être* for the medical and nursing providers. The sick also represent the environment in which their sickness arose and was transmitted. From this view the history of well-being and ill-being must incorporate societal and economic issues beyond the standard descriptions of medical attendance, therapeutic forays, professional attainments and relations with the governing classes. Equally, the contextual issues are inextricably involved with individual experiences of immunity, pain, suffering, coping and relief. I do not find that these questions have been clarified by recent abstruse discussions about what a 'patient' was or what 'illness' signified, with small regard to historical evidence.

The second assumption is that a patient-oriented, environmental approach entails a concentration on endemic, chronic, unspectacular sources of morbidity and morality – infant diarrhoea, childhood measles and scarlet fever, industrial accidents, sexually transmitted diseases, influenza after 1890, cardiac disorders, rheumatisms, malnutrition and deprivation – rather than a focus on epidemics of cholera or smallpox which were relatively unimportant in their demographic and economic consequences.

The patterns of endemic, chronic illness provoke investigations into the structural elements which conduce to well-being: safe water supplies, effective waste disposal, easier working conditions in the home and factory, rising real wages, improved nutrition. These relate to the third assumption, that unequal access to these goods profoundly affects unequal life chances. I hope this book will prompt the reader to ask 'who got what' out of the system, expressed as survival opportunities, self-esteem, material comforts and reasonable healthiness.

I have corrected errors in the original edition and have taken the opportunity to supply a better index.

Canberra 1989

INTRODUCTION

Patients loom small in medical history. They are the off-stage army in the drama of medical advance: the necessary adjuncts as clinical material and sources of income to the heroes and heroines of the story, doctors, administrators and nurses, but otherwise irrelevant to the curative process and therefore unworthy of differentiation. A fortunate few retain their names because their treatments made the reputations of their doctors and signal triumphs in the march of medicine. James Phipps, the boy successfully inoculated with cowpox by Edward Jenner in 1796; Anarcha, the black slave, the subject, after 30 attempts, of the finally successful operation for vesico-vaginal fistula by Dr Marion Sims in 1848; Francis Smith, the bill-poster, whose fractured patella was the first to be operated upon and wired by Joseph Lister in 1878, demonstrating that antiseptic methods could extend the range of surgery.

Yet Phipps, Anarcha and Smith remain but names, *sans* life story, *sans* family, *sans* everything – missing even from the indexes of the treatises which mention them – lost to history once 'they walked out of the hospital', their curative procedure completed to their doctors' satisfaction, the very impact of the cure upon their lives untraced. Beyond these, the hundreds of nameless failures have passed unrecorded. Doctors name diseases after the first man among them to describe the symptoms in print (as with Pott's disease, Parkinson's disease and Leiner's disease), never after the patient whose condition led them to try to understand the malady. Beyond these, the multitudes of untreated sick, the self-medicators and those who resorted to unorthodox treatments remain practically unknown.

This perspective on the subject is not surprising, given that most medical history has been compiled by medically trained men and published by medical publishers seemingly only for medical men. Economic and social historians, with the notable exception of Professor M.W. Flinn, have tended to keep clear of the area. They have been both intimidated by the technical knowledge that appeared to be required and repelled by the crudity of a historiography that is still enmeshed in celebratory 'great man' antiquarianism. It followed from the historians' lack of interest that archivists did little to collect such records of everyday medical attendance as might have survived. Moves to gather such material are beginning only now. Even when the health of the people

9

was a central component of the historians' subject, they contrived to evade its difficulties by concentrating upon the kinds of sources and causative explanations they were accustomed to, census and demographic materials in tracing the increase of population from the late eighteenth century, details of wages and food prices in the controversy about the standard of living after 1780, the administrative procedures of the Poor Law Commissioners, or the political repercussions of cholera outbreaks. In the event, the people at the receiving end of these developments, or more accurately the human beings who endured, indeed constituted, these 'developments', have slipped from view.

We have thus two fronts to explore. On the management of sickness side, there is much to be discovered about the contribution of patients to diagnosis and choice of treatment, and the outcome from the patient's point of view. On the general historical side, information, however patchy and circumstantial, about the well-being and ill-being of the people can enlarge our understanding of the transformation of British society during the industrial age.

The evidence is patchy and inconclusive for several reasons. The overwhelming bulk of reports of patient-doctor relationships and treatments come from the doctors. A few biographers of aristocrats and middle-class literary people report occasional dealings with doctors from their subjects' papers and letters, but only Queen Victoria, who is hardly typical, has in print a case-history that goes beyond the briefest mention. The parliamentary committees of inquiry into the Poor Law, medical education and the aged poor hardly ever took evidence on the medical aspects from patients or inmates. There are scraps of information about sick members of the middle classes and their doctors in the reports of court proceedings about disputed doctors' bills, and a rather larger amount of information about sufferers in the lower classes in evidence taken at coroners' inquests. But then as now, patients and their friends were inarticulate or guarded about what they revealed publicly of their health-care dealings. In the result the historian is constrained to approach the patient through the doctors' versions, as an historian of Africa, before the advent of oral history, had to use travellers' and missionaries' tales to reconstruct the life of preliterate peoples and their view of the white interlopers.

The doctors' writings and newspaper reports enable us to describe the various choices available to people through the century when they believed themselves to be sick; to learn whom they turned to for solace or treatment, and when and how often; to discover what they paid for such services and to estimate whether the service was worth the outlay.

Ideally, this study ought to begin in the later eighteenth century, contemporaneously with the rise of clinical medicine. But until the 1830s, when specialist medical journalism started to flourish and relevant parliamentary inquiries began, the paucity of evidence restricts the historian to dubious anecdotage from physicians' recollections, accounts of the treatment of royalty and of some sophisticated patients in their letters and journals, and hospital histories. This book therefore commences in the later 1820s, when reasonably consecutive sets of evidence can be found. The terminal date is about 1906, when the infant mortality rate finally fell decisively towards its present level. This turning-point provides an opportunity to weigh the various claims made for medical care, public health procedures and nutritional improvement in accounting for the diminution of death from disease and longer expectations of life in nineteenth-century Britain. Excellent books by Dr Ruth Hodgkinson, Professor B.B. Gilbert and Dr J.L. Brand also carry the story on into the twentieth century.[1]

Other omissions must also be explained. Ireland appears in this narrative only as a source of sick poor, accident victims and medical practitioners in Great Britain. The distinctive system of medical provision in Ireland, especially the state-supported dispensary network, and first the absence and then the strikingly different pattern of Poor Law services, demand a separate book. Scotland, too, for want of evidence, is treated more sketchily than its importance warrants. The mentally ill and handicapped also do not appear. The handling of the large body of official evidence about them and their treatment would distend this book unmanageably and they have already received attention from historians, notably Professor Kathleen Jones, Dr Ida Macalpine and Dr Richard Hunter, and Dr W.L. Parry-Jones.[2]

Many of the generalisations made in this book will be refined and altered by detailed scrutiny of particular suburbs, towns and regions, social ranks and medical procedures over time. None the less my object will be achieved if I can persuade the reader to look more sceptically at the older literature and see medical history as the history of social relations, with the patient as client, mostly but not always passive, and the medical practitioner as only another of the forces, albeit in many transactions the dominant and crucial one, shaping the well-being and ill-being of men and women during their seven ages.

Notes
1. Ruth G. Hodgkinson, *The Origins Of The National Health Service*

(London, 1967); B.B. Gilbert, *The Evolution of National Insurance in Great Britain* (London, 1966); Jeanne L. Brand, *Doctors and the State: the British Medical Profession and Government Action in Health, 1870-1912* (Baltimore, 1965).

2. Kathleen Jones, *Mental Health and Social Policy, 1845-1959* (London, 1972); Richard Hunter and Ida Macalpine, see especially *Psychiatry for the poor: Colney Hatch Asylum – Friern Hospital 1973: a medical and social history* (London, 1974); W.L. Parry-Jones, *The Trade in Lunacy: a study of private mad houses in England in the eighteenth and nineteenth centuries* (London, 1972).

1 CHILDBIRTH

Despite progress in public health and medical science during the nineteenth century childbirth remained dangerous to women and infancy precarious for their children.

The anxious rituals associated with Victorian childbirth become more understandable when we begin to count the numbers of deaths. In 1847, the first year for which we have reasonably firm figures, over 3,200 childbirth deaths in England and Wales were reported to the Registrar-General, nearly 3,000 in 1861, nearly 4,000 in 1871, 4,200 in 1881, 4,400 in 1901, and 3,800 in 1903, the year when the incidence of maternal mortality began decisively, though still slowly, to decline. Measured against each 1,000 live births, these figures represent rates of 6 per 1,000 in 1847, 4.3 in 1861, 4.9 in 1871, 4.8 in 1881, 4.7 in 1891 to 4.8 in 1901, to 4.03 per 1,000 in 1903. The maternal death rate did not fall below 1 per 1,000 births until 1944-5.[1]

This general rate can be divided into two categories, 'puerperal fever' and 'accidents', which indicate broadly the cause of death. Between 1847 and 1854 deaths reported as the consequence of 'puerperal fever' amounted to 1.72 per 1,000 and 'accidents' to 3.01 per 1,000.[2] During the period 1855-94 reported 'puerperal fever' deaths increased to 2.53 per 1,000, while 'accidents' declined steadily if slowly to 2.41 per 1,000. In 1903, the turning-point, 'sepsis' fell to 1.73 (from 2.13 in the preceding year) and 'Other Causes' accounted for 2.31.[3]

These rates are bad enough in terms of preventible deaths, broken families and orphaned children, but before we interpret them we must measure their limitations. They under-represent the numbers. Deaths in childbed were under-reported throughout the period: probably grossly so until the 1880s. Doctors, midwives, officials of lying-in hospitals and Poor Law guardians all had an interest in keeping the numbers down. Neither 'puerperal fever' nor 'accident' was defined for the purpose of registration throughout the century. 'Puerperal fever' meant at various times a single comprehensive disease covering diverse kinds of inflammation and symptoms, or congeries of differing forms of infection, or specific streptococcal infections, and also included excessive bleeding and paralysis of the limbs. 'Accident' was normally believed to cover ectopic pregnancies (the foetus developed outside the uterus in the uterine tubes) leading to abortion and sepsis, eclampsia (convulsions and coma associated with high blood pressure and fluid retention in late pregnancy) and 'exhaustion'. Only very rarely, after an unavoidable coroner's inquest, did 'accident' as a cause of death apparently include negligence by the *accoucheur*. Conveniently, then, until the 1880s when reporting procedures were tightened, women deceased in childbed who had shown symptoms of heart disease, dysentery or 'peritonitis' were entered under that particular heading, irrespective of whether they had also displayed more proximate causes of death, such as extensive infection or haemorrhage.[4] Even after 1881, when the regulations were first improved, infections which set in ten days or more after delivery were also reported as causes of death independent of childbirth.[5] Doctors, midwives and officials in some towns, notably Birmingham, simply refused to specify deaths in childbirth or from puerperal fever.[6] In 1895, after an investigation of 4,000 deaths among women, the Registrar-General estimated that between 1885 and 1890 one-half of the deaths ascribed to 'metria' among women of child-bearing age, one-third of the 'blood poisoning, pyaemia etc.', and one-quarter of those reported as 'haemorrhage' were actually 'connected with childbirth', thereby indicating that, even allowing for yet worse earlier under-registration, the incidence of 'puerperal fever' held up throughout the later nineteenth century.[7]

Under-registration was probably greatest in regions of high maternal mortality and it would heighten what we already know of regional variations through the period. In general, as for example the decade 1881-90, maternal death rates for both 'puerperal fever' and 'accidents' were reported as lowest in London, where registration was effective, and the Home Counties, and highest in manufacturing, mining and rural districts, where registration was often poor. 'Puerperal fever' was the dominant ascribed cause of death in urban places, 'accidents' in rural and mining areas.

The general death rate of the south-west of England was below the national average, although its reported 'accident' rate was higher. The pattern indicated in Table 1.1 is related to social class and thereby to the kinds of attendance to be had, but not in any simple way. Within London, for example, wealthy parishes such as Hampstead and St George's, Hanover Square, had higher puerperal fever and general maternal mortality rates than wretched St Giles and St George in the East. Wrexham, a small manufacturing, semi-rural town, had the same reported incidence of puerperal fever deaths as Swansea and a higher maternal mortality.[8]

Table 1.1: Mean Annual Death Rate per 1000, 1881-90

	'Puerperal fever'	'Accidents'	Total
England and Wales	2.59	2.13	4.73
London	2.44	1.53	3.91
Manchester	3.13	2.06	5.20
North Wales — counties	3.25	3.47	6.73
South-west England — counties	2.05	2.32	4.36

Source: Dr Thursfield, *Lancet*, 7 January 1893, p. 21; *Parliamentary Papers*, 1884-5, vol. XVII, p. lxxiv.

Ante-Natal Procedures

Women in the upper and middle classes ought to have had the easiest passage. They could afford the best ante-natal preparation and the best *accoucheurs*. Their role was that of a patient moving towards the crisis of her illness. From the time the baby quickened, during the fourth month, and the pregnancy was confirmed, their possession of servants enabled them to increase their amount of rest each day. Their dwelling in a large house allowed them to stay indoors in quiet, cool rooms in order to keep their sensibilities calm, lest the baby become imprinted with harsh passions or disfigurements. Until the 1870s, when more physical exercise and strengthening foods began to be ordered by the doctors, popular manuals such as the *The Ladies' Friend*, or Dr Thomas Andrew's *Cyclopaedia of Domestic Medicine and Surgery* advised them to live tranquilly and take enough nourishment to gratify the appetite 'without overloading the stomach'. Beef, mutton and veal were allowable provided they were plain-cooked, preferably boiled, without injurious spices or coarse vegetables. Fish was permissible, but without sauces. Jellies and chicken broth and, later in the century, beef broth were authorised as snacks, but excessive use of wines, spirits, tea, coffee and chocolate, vegetables and fruit, was forbidden, while wine diluted with water was the usual recommendation.[9] In the light of modern knowledge the diet was sensible.

The pregnant lady's dealings with her doctor began during the fourth or fifth month. In the first half of the century her chosen doctor would be the local gentlemanly practitioner calling himself a 'pure' surgeon, or a surgeon apothecary like Mr Perry of Highbury in *Emma*, rather than the local general practitioner apothecary, and after the 1850s the local fashionable *accoucheur*, parading his qualifications as surgeon and physician. Sometimes he might have been summoned earlier to prescribe a course of purgatives and opiates for costiveness and morning sickness. At his first examination, he would confirm the pregnancy by laying his hand on the lady's abdomen to feel for the foetus, inspect the raised umbilicus or, if the lady was fastidious, feel it under the bed-clothes, and, after the mid-1840s, occasionally resort to a rather fallible urine nitric acid test, to establish that the pregnancy was not simply a case of dropsy. If the woman had previously been healthy, if this was not her first baby, and if she continued lively with a good colour, the surgeon normally would not examine his patient again until the seventh month. Until the 1870s the drift of medical opinion was against 'meddlesome midwifery'. Moreover, there was little he could do to help. He could prepare for the worst if he discovered an anomalous pregnancy or frequent haemorrhaging, but, until the end of the century, unless he were a great fashionable obstetric surgeon, he had no effective means of intervention to save the woman. His ignorance was profound, his education had not provided him with an understanding of the living functions of menstruation, conception, foetal growth and birth. In the intervening weeks he would call at intervals, varying with what the family looked likely to pay, and do all he really could do in the nineteenth century, that is, supply pills and purges and manage the patient's daily regimen.[10]

During the seventh month he would make his first vaginal examination. With the patient on her back or side, and legs doubled up, lying on the special red leather underlayer the doctor carried about with him, he inserted two fingers well covered with lard and with nails trimmed, to feel for the enlargement of the uterus, and for the weight of the head of the foetus. (Finger stalls and rubber gloves were not commonly used until after 1906. The rubber was thick and opaque and impaired the doctor's 'touch'.[11]) Unduly modest patients and sensitive doctors preferred the examination to be conducted under a sheet covering the patient, but as she was doped with opiates, had usually been extensively bled, until the 1850s at least, and had had her labia rubbed with opium tincture and softened with linseed or starch fomentations, she often neglected to keep the sheet about her when the time came. The examination completed, the doctor washed his hands. Unless serious trouble was apprehended, surgeons, excepting the race of dominating fashionable *accoucheurs* after the 1850s such as Dr Robert Lee, hesitated to use the vaginal speculum on wealthy private patients. This was an instrument mostly reserved for use when the doctor was reluctant to handle the noisome pudenda of the poor.[12]

The stethoscope became known in Britain in the 1820s, but was little used in pregnancy cases until the 1830s, and then but rarely. Patients, especially lower-class ones, liked it because they were, as Dr Ryland noticed, 'gratified by the appearance of additional attention'. But doctors, modish-scientific and conservative rule-of-thumb men alike, eschewed it: they feared 'its appearance of quackery'.[13] In part, they were right in this. The foetal heart is difficult to hear and the stethoscope is difficult to use for unambiguous signs.

The woman and her family meanwhile proceeded with the recruitment of a 'monthly' nurse, to assist at the confinement and stay on for some weeks to help with the infant. The advice Mrs Beeton's tame surgeon proffered in the *Book of Household Management* is representative of that in most manuals: the nurse ought to be strong, free of encumbrances, between 30 and 40 and not addicted to snuff or spirituous liquors. If the lady was one of the apparent minority who did not intend to try to feed the infant herself, the search also began for a suitable wet-nurse.[14]

Birth Procedures

The paucity of examination before the birth process began often meant that an abnormal presentation or still birth came as a surprise and provoked a crisis. If the patient began to haemorrhage the medical man would help apply manual pressure and administer tincture (i.e. 1 in 4 proof spirit) of ergot, until the 1840s or 1850s, by the 'spoonful' (i.e. presumably, containing about one drachm), and after this, the age of heroic dosage, more moderately (i.e. by the 1880s, about 30 minims). He would also intervene if the expulsion of the placenta seemed unduly delayed, that is, beyond forty minutes or so. In this situation he would give 'large' (i.e. about one drachm) doses of tincture (about 1 in 8 proof spirit) of digitalis and again, routinely until the 1850s for most practitioners and till the 1890s for old-fashioned ones, bleed the patient to syncope.

During the thirty years after the late 1840s, he would administer tincture (1 in 6 proof spirit) of cannabis indicus, again in large doses (i.e. 20 or more minims) if the patient's pain seemed unusually bad.[15] Until the gradual spread of chloroform anaesthesia after 1847, most prudent doctors did not use instruments to hasten labour. On the other hand, whenever the mother's life was in jeopardy, in cases of pelvic obstruction for example, Protestant and Catholic doctors alike did not hesitate to destroy the child to save the mother. Dr Alexander Miller, looking back to the 1860s, estimated that instruments were used in private practice in only about 8 to 10 per cent of cases. Medical opinion changed during the early 1870s. Some medical teachers returned to the well-founded traditional belief that the faster the delivery, the less the susceptibility to puerperal fever, although, by a sad irony, they hastened delivery with instruments that commonly were poorly cleaned. Others, filled with antiseptic zeal, found their aspirations fulfilled with carbolic acid spray, washings, endless new-fangled forceps and other implements, hot baths, tartar emetics.[16] By 1899 doctors were estimated to employ instruments in over 25 per cent of all cases, and the rate was thought to be increasing. Doctors with 'large practices' in obstetrics, that is, 200 or more deliveries a year, were finding it 'very trying' 'to wait patiently on so many women'. The forceps, observers alleged, were being used earlier and more often. There is one curious set of data and reasoning which shows an enormous increase in the use of instruments, coinciding with the increased resort to antiseptic methods. Professor Jardine of Glasgow argued, to his satisfaction, that birth weights had increased through the nineteenth century. He quoted an average for both sexes of 7 lbs in 1826. He had taken the average weight of 100 full-term infants – gender unspecified – born in the Glasgow Maternity Hospital in 1866: the average had been 7 lb 3½oz. In 1904 he took a similar sample: this time the average was 7 lb 9 1/3oz. (The average weight of full-term boys born in the 1970s in Britain is about 7 lb and girls somewhat less.) Jardine concluded that infants were not deteriorating prior to birth. Yet everybody knew there was national deterioration. This, Jardine argued, resulted from the rickets which set in after birth. Rickets, he asserted, must have increased dramatically since 1850. The proof was the increase in instrumental deliveries among Glasgow Maternity Hospital cases as shown in Table 1.2.

Some practitioners cannot even have had time to do this; in 1877 one *accoucheur* 'attended' 12 confinements each week, for a grand total of over 600 a year. Meanwhile, as I suggested earlier, the puerperal fever and accident rate held its own. 'Antisepsis', the retiring president of the Gynaecological Association lamented in 1897, 'was still little used in private midwifery practice.' He confessed to believing that the death rate in private practice was higher than in the hospitals, and that the gap had widened since 1870.[17] The promise of the earlier nineteenth century, when medical men greatly extended midwifery practice among the classes who could pay, was being fulfilled. By 1849 one-eighth of all admissions to Bethlehem Hospital were 'puerperal mania' sufferers. Dr John Webster confessed himself baffled by the fact that they included more patients from 'the upper classes than the lower'.[18]

Ether anaesthesia, within months of the announcement of its rediscovery in January 1847, succeeded by the announcement of chloroform in November, was rapidly and generally accepted into amputation and other surgical procedures. The spread of ether and chloroform anaesthesia in childbirth was slower. Chloroform was justifiably (in retrospect, it was the methods of administering chloroform, rather than the drug itself) thought dangerous, particularly with delicate women — especially when we recall that until the 1870s and 1880s doctors thought it fussy to use a stethoscope in maternity cases. During the rest of the century about one death annually was reported as directly attributable to chloroform anaesthesia, all of them, as it happened, associated with surgical or dental procedures. In many of these cases it is clear that the patient suffered a death from heart failure more merciful than that he would have endured under the same operation under opiates. The real point is that, given the ignorant, rough and ready dosage and handling of anaesthetics throughout the century, the reported deaths are so few. The under-use of chloroform during childbirth has probably been exaggerated, for there are reports of its application throughout England from mid-1848. Dr Hearne of Southampton argued in August 1847 that the cessation of pain often made the difference between life and death in weak patients undergoing protracted labours, and that ether anaesthesia removed the need for opiates and alcohol. Dr Protheroe Smith agreed, adding that anaesthesia reduced the danger because it allowed doctors to turn babies more easily and deal more decisively with haemorrhages.[19] But its acceptance by the profession was hindered by the style of propaganda of its first advocate.

J.Y. Simpson in Edinburgh and I.B. Brown in London first reported successful applications of chloroform during childbirth in November 1847. Coming soon after the exploding of the medical mesmerism fraud surrounding Dr John Elliotson, and rows over the appointment of Scots to London teaching hospitals, Simpson's announcement appeared as the work of yet another 'bragging Scot', according to one English practitioner. Even the great Dr John Snow, who, among other contributions, invented a controlled inhaler which made safe ether or chloroform application possible, thought that Simpson's bravura with handkerchiefs and pads and his boldness in public controversy had made his disciples arrogant and careless.[20] It was Simpson, the T.H. Huxley of medical advance, who first traversed the religious and ethical arguments about chloroform anaesthesia during childbirth and who antagonised both aspiring professional *accoucheurs* and conservative oldsters by declaring that patients would demand the final say in the matter.

Table 1.2: Instrumental Deliveries at Glasgow Maternity Hospital, 1869-98

1869-78	Outdoor cases	— 4 craniotomies	(1:2,138 cases)
1869-78	Indoor cases	— 4 craniotomies	(1:1,480 cases)
1869-78	Indoor cases	— 2 inductions of labour	(1:1,480 cases)
1879-88	Outdoor cases	— 20 craniotomies	(1:620 cases)
1879-88	Indoor cases	— 38 craniotomies	(1:76 cases)
1879-88	Indoor cases	— 10 inductions of labour	(1:296 cases)
1879-88	Indoor cases	— 3 Caesarian sections	(1:987 cases)
1889-98	Outdoor cases	— 16 craniotomies	(1:1,260 cases)
1889-98	Outdoor cases	— 3 inductions of labour	(1:6,718 cases [sic])
1889-98	Indoor cases	— 112 craniotomies	(1:39 cases)
1889-98	Indoor cases	— 91 inductions of labour	(1:48 cases)
1889-98	Indoor cases	— 56 Caesarian sections	(1:77 cases)

Source: Alexander Miller, 'Twenty Years' Obstetric Practice', *Glasgow Medical Journal*, vol. LI (1899), p. 225.

Opponents of chloroform during childbirth and gynaecology always gave their arguments a medical veneer. They never stopped trying to associate deaths in other procedures with special dangers in childbirth. Their chagrined reports of failures to find deaths directly linked with chloroform and portentous analyses of near-misses recall current contributions to debates about abortion and the pill. From the radical, experimental side, Dr Tyler Smith demonstrated with guinea pigs the truth of the proposition that chloroform was dangerous to weakly parturient women because, like the old opiates, it relaxed the uterine muscles and prolonged labour.[21] His view was shared by Dr Robert Lee, FRS, Lumleian, Croonian and Harveian lecturer, who in 1853 produced a list of 17 childbirth cases in which chloroform had produced pernicious results. In two cases, contractions of the uterus were arrested by the chloroform and, Lee alleged, delivery was completed by craniotomy; in seven cases, 'insanity and great disturbance of the brain' followed its use; in five, it 'made the use of forceps necessary'; in four, 'fatal peritonitis followed'; one case was followed by 'epilepsy'; and the last by 'dangerous fits of syncope'.[22] A representative conservative, Dr Samuel Ashwell, formerly obstetrical physician at Guy's Hospital, simply asserted that old methods were best: leeches and blood-letting relaxed the uterus better than artificial interference with a 'natural process . . . of integrity and perfection'.[23]

Dr George Gream was more direct, as befitted his standing as one of the most fashionable *accoucheurs* in London between the 1850s and 1870s, and physician-*accoucheur* to the Princess of Wales in the 1860s.

His objection was that 'women used obscene language under chloroform'. Dr Tanner, his ally, fellow and secretary of the Obstetrical Society 1858-63, another fashionable *accoucheur*, also admitted to a disturbing experience in King's College Hospital when operating on the vagina of a prostitute: the 'ether produced lascivious dreams', presumably in the prostitute.[24]

Tyler Smith elaborated this with the assertion, which some psychoanalysts still proclaim, that anaesthesia stopped the 'benign and salutary' effects of pain on the emotions and instead produced

> excitement of sexual passion . . . pain in fact metamorphosed into its antitheses . . . To the women of this country the bare possibility of having feelings of such a kind excited and manifested in outward uncontrollable action, would be more shocking even, to anticipate, than the last extremity of physical pain . . . the human female [would exchange] . . . the pangs of travail for the sensation of coitus and so [sink] to the level of the brute creation.

One might expect Dr Robert Lee to have concluded his list with remarks on the clinical lessons of the seventeen cases. Instead, with a doctor's instinctive facility for making moral decisions for his patients, he moved into a new muddle of physiology and Old Testament morality:

> The exhibition of chloroform in labour . . . [was] contrary to the sound principles of physiology and morality. 'In sorrow shalt thou bring forth children', was an established law of nature — an ordinance of the Almighty, as stated in the Bible, and it was in vain to attempt to abrogate that law. There could not be a doubt that it was a most unnatural practice to destroy the consciousness of women during labour, the pains and sorrows of which exerted a most powerful and salutary influence upon their religious and moral character, and upon all their future relations in life. But he might put aside all these physiological and moral considerations, and rest his objection to the use of chloroform in labour upon the danger of introducing a subtle narcotic poison into the system at such a time.[25]

The opposition from such leaders of the profession as Gream, Lee and Tanner, the fear of causing death, and in practice among the poor, the cost of anaesthesia and its associated delays (chloroform was already worth adulterating with alcohol by early 1848) served to inhibit its full

use until the 1870s.[26] Queen Victoria's recourse to chloroform for her
confinement in April 1853 certainly did not decide the issue, but in
the provinces beyond Lee's command and among middle- and lower-
class women whom Gream and Lee as *accoucheurs* did not treat,
Simpson's prediction that 'patients will demand it' was borne out, with
the Queen's example a powerful reinforcement to his case; although her
confinement also produced the strong reaction and fierce debate in the
profession in the latter half of 1853. When Dr Snow successfully
delivered the Queen under chloroform in April 1857 there was much
less medical outcry. Although the *Lancet* remarked in 1858 that the
'great majority' of *accoucheurs* still did not resort to chloroform, Dr
Gream was lamenting at the end of 1860 that the 'squeamish upper
classes' were demanding chloroform in childbirth and that it was
'almost universally employed'.[27] This could be the date when the
fashionable old guard in London finally gave way. Beyond this outline,
the mapping, dating and results of the introduction throughout the
United Kingdom of chloroform anaesthesia in childbirth, one of the
great benisons in the history of women, must await detailed local
research.

The superfluity of the doctor in the childbirth room resulted from
the simplicity of the process when things were going well and the limitations of his arts when things were going badly. For reasons which I
shall discuss later he was trained and imprisoned in a conceptual framework which precluded the notion of the body as a dynamic system.
There was very little research in the nineteenth century into the physiology, that is, the relation of functions in gynaecology and childbirth.
This incuriosity shaped the training of medical students throughout the
period. They came to the body through morbid anatomy, resting upon
the view that structure equalled function, as ordained by God. Their
knowledge of gynaecology and obstetrics was assembled from lectures,
bottled or pemmican-like sample oddities in pathology museums, and
idealised diagrams of the womb and birth process.[28] Many students
skimped on the lectures or ignored them altogether: until the 1850s
midwifery was excluded from the general teaching courses offered by
the English hospitals and Scottish universities and was available only
if extra fees were paid to the physician-*accoucheur* in charge.[29] Occasionally this had the presumably undesired result that the *accoucheurs*
abandoned the promised lecture programme if the number of takers
proved too few, as happened at the Manchester School of Medicine in
1842.[30] Only Dublin-trained doctors had any guaranteed expertise, but
they were rarely fashionable in England.[31] The Royal College of Sur-

geons began to offer an examination in obstetrics in 1853, and from the 1870s onwards 'midwifery, and diseases of women and children' became obligatory examinations at most British medical schools, notably excepting Oxford and Cambridge.[32]

As always with qualifying institutions, the regulations promised quality higher than was actually turned out. The rules in England generally required 'attendance' at lectures on midwifery for three months, and the Scottish and Irish rules, lectures for six months. Most institutions throughout the kingdom also required students 'to be present' at at least six deliveries in a recognised maternity hospital. This requirement was always thwarted in practice because there were never enough confinements to allot among the students. In Edinburgh, for example, there were over 1,000 students in the 1870s, but only about 7,000 births in 'the rank of life' that made them available to undergraduates.[33] The General Medical Council, which after 1858 governed medical education, turned a blind eye to the situation. Mere obstetricians were not co-opted to the GMC and its members were more concerned to block proposals to make midwifery teaching effective by allowing training in the labour wards of workhouses, where there were ample subjects. The great physicians and surgeons who comprised the GMC saw workhouse practice as compromising the gentlemanly aspirations of the profession. For many of them the urgent question was the defence of Latin as a medical examination requirement.[34]

In this pursuit the GMC, whose membership overlapped with that of the councils of the Royal Colleges, was continuing the Colleges' old policies. Before the 1840s the Royal College of Physicians, an exclusive institution consisting mainly of Oxford and Cambridge MDs centred on the London voluntary hospitals, would not admit 'Obstetricians' and forbade its fellows to practise as such. As the President, Sir Henry Halford, remarked in 1841, 'midwifery was an occupation degrading to a gentleman'.[35] The Royal College of Surgeons, also centred on the London hospitals, but partially reformed during the 1830s, required for admission evidence of attendance at lectures on midwifery, but precluded practitioners of 'the *manual* branch of the . . . art' from serving on its council or on its court of examiners. It was a practice suited only to apothecary-general practitioners and therefore 'derogatory to surgeons and physicians to require examination, and proofs of skill in that subject'. The more lowly Society of Apothecaries allowed its licentiates to practise obstetrics but proudly refused to teach it or require evidence of learning in it.[36] Even in 1868, after twenty years of piecemeal reforms, the examination in midwifery consisted of a viva lasting under four minutes.

By the 1890s reformers had pressed the Conjoint Board of the Royal Colleges to require that the students 'be present' at twelve deliveries and that three 'be done personally'. But as Dr Rentoul lamented in 1897, there were still too few women to go around and medical graduates throughout the country were still learning their midwifery on the job from midwives, just as Dr B.W. Richardson, fresh from St Andrews fifty years earlier, admitted that he had begun.[37]

The neglect of the GMC and contempt for the subject in the great teaching hospitals is revealed in the confessions of 'Medicus', describing his experience in a large London hospital in the early 1890s. He did one week's practical work for his Certificate in Obstetrics. He attended one labour in that week, but was not permitted to touch the patient. After the child was delivered and the patient taken away, he never saw her or the child again. He and his colleagues asked to be shown the obstetrics instruments: the consultant refused, saying that their request 'was most irregular'; he sent them to obtain 'special permission', which was refused. 'Medicus' and his friends at the end of the week were certified as having attended the whole number of deliveries that occurred in the hospital during that week. He was thereby fully qualified in the words of his certificate 'to undertake anything required in obstetrics'.[38] However, 'Medicus' was slightly better equipped than his compeers from Oxford and Cambridge who also had a certificate, but with no experience of obstetrics whatever, even after the Conjoint Board had reinforced midwifery requirements in 1896. Twenty-three of the 37 teaching hospitals of Great Britain in 1907 were so organised that students attended deliveries before they had had any lectures or instruction on the subject. There was no bedside teaching and most students relievedly ended their 'practical' week as bored and uncomprehending as when they started.[39] Medical schools were already set in the pattern of diverting the students' concern from the conditions they were most likely to encounter in future practice.

The most dangerous part of the delivery for many mothers came with the expulsion of the placenta. The doctor and midwife had little in their armoury to enable them to stop extensive haemorrhaging.

Dr Hayden's report of a successful case in Anglesey in 1832 illustrates the range of expedients, short of operating, available to an experienced conscientious country practitioner during the first half of the century. The foetus had been born dead, but the placenta had not been expelled and the uterus remained flaccid and uncontracted. The woman was in 'agony and sinking'. 'Wine and burnt whiskey were administered with an unsparing hand, but they had not at all the effect of rousing the system', so the 'binder' (a roller of cloth usually applied to prevent flooding or haemorrhaging and the entry of 'contaminated air' often, as was likely in this case, even before labour began) on the patient's abdomen was tightened further. In desperation Hayden sprinkled cold water on her from a hearth brush dipped in a bucket. Sal volatile was held to her nostrils, while more whisky and mulled ale were forced into her mouth. Eight hours later the uterus was still not contracted. Finally, after about twelve hours, Hayden got the placenta out, he does not tell how, the uterus contracted and Hayden congratulated himself. 'The after treatment of this case did not present any peculiarity', he concluded. 'The patient was kept on a low regimen for some days and the bowels were freely acted upon by the compound rhubarb pill and the ordinary black mixture' (probably the 'black dose' compound of senna and Epsom salts).[40]

Crippled by their ignorance in an emergency, doctors sometimes panicked. William Gaches, licentiate of the Apothecaries Company, was delivering a woman at Costessey in Norfolk in 1845. She had previously borne nine children without difficulties. This time, presumably, she was well into her thirties and less resilient. The child was born after a labour of many hours; the mother was screaming in agony as Gaches thrust repeatedly in her womb for the delayed afterbirth. At last he pulled out 'something' which he hid from the midwife assisting him. The post-mortem showed that he had pulled out several pounds of womb and lower intestine. Gaches was acquitted of a charge of manslaughter by direction of Mr Justice Patteson, the presiding judge, who quoted Lord Ellenborough to the effect that no medical man would be safe to use his skill to the utmost 'and no persons of honour . . . would enter into the profession . . . with such an apprehension continually hanging over their heads'.[41]

In another typical case Mr Dickenson, surgeon at Bilston, was summoned to Mrs Hickman, the wife of a respectable farmer, who had unexpectedly begun labour. An old midwife, who had not been engaged to attend, was also summoned and had delivered the child and stopped the haemorrhage with wet cloths before Dickenson arrived. But the old woman had failed to get the placenta out. Dickenson pulled out 'most but not all' of what he thought was the placenta. Now Dr Best, a physician, arrived. He was shown a vessel with a bloody mass in it, and said, ' "You do not call that the after-birth, do you?" ' Dickenson replied, ' "Yes, it is!" '. Best retorted, ' "Now I will show you the after-birth" ', whereupon he hauled out 'a sanguineous mass', ' "There is the after-birth!" ' The patient shrieked and, one hour later, died. There was no post-mortem, the neighbouring medical men being averse to that proceeding. Like Mr Justice Patteson, Baron Platt directed the jury to acquit Dickenson. (Best was not charged.) Medical men had to be permitted 'to act with boldness', otherwise 'we should none of us, gentlemen, . . . have the benefit, in a variety of emergencies, of the services of that profession to which we are so often indebted'.[42] This legal sheltering of negligence allowed education in midwifery to languish throughout the century.

After the delivery, sensible doctors sought to let their patients rest, but midwives and grandmothers, until late in the century at least, held to the traditional practice of keeping up the perspiration with a blazing fire, lots of blankets and large draughts of ale and stout. This probably harmed the mother and infant less than the 'depletion', or blood-letting, and 'low diet' imposed by old-fashioned practitioners on patients 'tending to inflammation' (that is, sepsis).[43] Dr Blundell, whose lectures as published in the *Lancet* in the later 1820s set the pattern for a generation, advised that once inflammation set in after parturition,

> violent practices are uncalled for . . . Do not confound the disease with puerperal fever; 30 or 40 leeches, say 30 on an average, should be applied to the symphysis pubis. Now and then . . . blood to the amount of 16 ounces may be abstracted from the arm; laxatives, refrigerants, and the antiphlogistic regimen for four or five days, will commonly be found to overcome the symptoms.[44]

This system of management was changing during the 1850s, when young doctors were more reluctant to give purgatives and take blood, preferring to keep the patient drowsy with strong opiates; but the grandmother and the midwife were keen to get the patient up early, within 24 hours, to help clear the lochia from the uterus. Medical opinion throughout the century was against the custom. The doctors liked to keep the patient horizontal for at least three or four days, and much longer with delicate ones, for fear of straining the ligaments of the uterus. In one way they were right: there appears to have been a high incidence of various kinds of prolapse of the womb in the nine-teenth century, although this probably ensued rather from having too many labours than from getting out of bed too quickly. But the doctor's ancillary argument, against getting the patient on her feet, that strain of the ligaments induced 'inflammation', appears now as bitter irony.[45]

Even with wealthy cases the doctor ceased to visit the patient after about ten days, if the milk was flowing freely, the nipples were softened and there was no evidence of puerperal fever. Upon his leaving the patient he usually ordered the continuance for some weeks of a strong purgative each day, and opium to assuage pain in the loins and the breasts.[46]

Medical Costs

His bill, until the 1860s, would have ranged, if the patient's family was in 'moderate circumstances', from one guinea for the delivery, plus 5s. or 7s. 6d. per visit including medicines, plus 6d. or 1s. per mile if the journey extended beyond a couple of miles, the total amounting to around three or four guineas payable, as much as possible, immediately in cash. For patients in 'good circumstances' the bill could go above 100 guineas for the confinement, with charges for visits and mileage at a comparable rate. The attending midwife got about one-quarter of the delivery fee as 'poundage'. Members of the Royal College of Physicians, who were not supposed to deliver infants, purported to charge only for 'advice', but their bills came to much the same as a surgeon's, or a little more. The more 'ethical' among the *accoucheurs* refused to pay 'poundage', so the midwife received her half guinea or so from the family *ex gratia* and separately [47]

From the 1860s the various local medico-ethical associations moved to raise fees by fixing new schedules every few years, and by attempting to relate changes more closely to ability to pay. In 1865 the Manchester Association, for instance, ranged houses by the estimated annual rental (guessed from the appearance of the house and the neighbourhood) into four classes, from £10-£25 per year, presumably the lowest rental at which an occupier could be expected to seek regular private attendance, through class II at £25-£50, class III at £50-£100 to class IV at £100 and above. The recommended minimal charges for midwifery were one guinea for class I, one to three guineas for class II, that is, doubling the old rate for people in 'moderate circumstances', two to four guineas for class III, and five guineas and upwards for class IV. Consultants, who hitherto had shared the *accoucheur*'s fee on a basis akin to 'poundage', were recommended to charge separately, beginning at one guinea per visit.[48] A few months after this price list appeared, a parliamentary investigation revealed that many thousands of occupiers of £10 houses, especially in the Midlands and the north, were working men at the top of the working-class pyramid, receiving about 26s. to 28s. per week. At the recommended rates, a bill for one confinement almost equalled one week's wages. Working men could save for medical attention through sick clubs and benefit societies, although midwifery fees were often excluded from the benefit. The class which probably had its income really devoured by medical fees was the clerkly, schoolmaster, self-employed group in the upper range of class I.[49] They were less likely to join mutual benefit societies. Once again, only detailed local research will show the impact of medical costs on particular kinds of families. But two points stand out. First, medical fees were high in relation to wages and salaries throughout the nineteenth century. How often the doctors actually got their money is another matter, especially as fees probably rose faster than wages during the latter part of the century. Second, patients in a family below the level of a reasonably regularly employed artisan or reasonably secure small farmer could not expect to have medical attention on the basis of the idealised private professional-client relationship.

As the local medico-ethical societies and the British Medical Association strengthened their grip through the 1860s and the decade following, fees were gradually edged up. By the late 1870s Mr Jay, a surgeon-GP in the countryside at Chippenham, was considered by his fellow practitioners to be charging the 'normal' fees at a minimum of three guineas per confinement and 5s. to 8s. per visit. By 1890 consultants in Birmingham were demanding three guineas per 'attendance' at a confinement and the general practitioner's minimum charge for a bottle of medicine was 3s. 6d. (the patient usually supplied the bottle).[50]

Hospital Midwifery

Women who could not afford the tariff but who were keen to be delivered by an *accoucheur* could make themselves objects of his charity. They were especially keen if the confinement was to be their first, or if they expected a difficult labour. About twice as many women were said to have died during their first confinement as died during subsequent ones.[51]

In the towns women could use the out-patients' departments of the hospitals, or dispensaries, apply at a charity lying-in hospital, or simply wait until labour started, summon the doctor and have the baby delivered in the full knowledge that either he would not bother to ask for his money or that he would soon give up dunning the family.[52] In country villages and towns it was common for local GPs to attend confinements and not charge for them. Dr John McVail, an experienced and level-headed investigator for the Royal Commission on the Poor Laws, concluded that in Edwardian times many country GPs provided about £50 of treatment a year, much of it midwifery, without seeking payment. This came about not only because the doctors were generous but also because country doctors still did not regularly keep case-records, especially of poor patients.[53]

If doctors liked charity because it conferred absolute control, suppliants were rendered more obsequious and anxious by its un-certainty. There is evidence that not all doctors were charitable at all times. In 1871 at Dymock, near Ledbury in Gloucestershire, a girl died while giving birth to illegitimate twins. The midwife engaged by the girl's father found the case difficult through the night and at 7.30 a.m. the girl's father went to fetch the parish Poor Law medical officer, Mr Cooke, who lived about three miles away. The father had no poor relief order and no means of paying privately. Cooke refused to come. At 5 p.m. the father persuaded Mr Wood of Ledbury, four miles away, to attend his girl. When Wood arrived the mother and twins were dead. Cooke told the coroner he had frequently attended cases without pay-ment or a relief order. The *Lancet* concluded that

> Mr Cooke is a gentleman who has been more than 40 years in prac-tice, and who has reached a period of life at which he cannot be expected to be at the beck and call of every girl who has the mis-fortune to have an illegitimate child . . . The fact is, medical men are far too fearful of claptrap charges of inhumanity.[54]

At Mortlake in Surrey in 1897, Dr Macintosh was awakened at 2 a.m. to attend a dying 3-day-old boy and his mother, described at the subse-quent inquest as 'half-starved'. The child weighed 2 lb 2 oz at the post-mortem. After learning that the father could not pay, Macintosh went back to bed. Like Mr Cooke and numerous other doctors in similar situations at inquests, Macintosh told the coroner that he 'had attended 40 or 50 such cases and never received a penny', but he produced no corroborative details and as usual, the coroner did not press the matter.[55]

For admission to the books of a general hospital, a pregnant woman needed letters of recommendation from one or more governors of the hospital. This requirement, with exceptions such as the London Royal Free Hospital and the Edinburgh Royal Infirmary, lasted until the 1880s when hospital authorities began increasingly to dispense with 'lines'. To obtain the 'lines' the woman or her friends had to discover who the governors were and their addresses; some hospitals supplied lists, others did not; apparently the woman worked by local hearsay, with the consequence that some governors complained of being plagued and others chose to give out-of-town addresses. Whatever the outcome, the woman could not escape much walking and humble waiting.[56] Evidence about what happened next is skimpy. The midwifery out-patients were uninteresting to hospital men at the time and historians of hospitals ignore them. Normally the woman had to go to the out-patients' department to show her 'lines' and give the porter her name and the address where she was to be confined; if she expected a troublesome labour she might seek to be examined by one of the junior house surgeons on duty. If the surgeon agreed, she had to wait an average of about four hours and, at some hospitals, such as the Glasgow Royal Infirmary until well into the 1880s at least, until all other out-patients were dealt with and the students departed, at 4 p.m. The authorities thought it improper that students should observe the examinations of women.[57]

If the woman went to one of the few hospitals to admit pregnant women, such as the London (after 1853), Guy's or the Dumfries and Galloway Infirmary, made her plea and proved an 'interesting' case, she might be admitted as an in-patient, up to one month before delivery.

Three things are clear about general hospital midwifery. First, the woman was almost invariably delivered at home; most hospitals excluded pregnant women, at least until the 1890s. If a woman admitted with illness was found also to be pregnant, she was promptly turned out. In 1844 a young woman was admitted with fever to the Westminster Hospital. Upon being washed and examined, she was discovered to be seven months pregnant, and was promptly sent home. Next day she died after a premature birth.[58] Second, the woman was delivered by the *accoucheur*-lecturer with students attending, or apparently more commonly, by a gaggle of students, sometimes with a midwife, unsupervised. Presumably the woman sent to the hospital for help when labour commenced. Third, the number of women delivered as out-patients was very large and the women were poor: in 1857 over 400 out-patients were confined by students from the London Hospital; between 1854 and 1860 Guy's accepted 12,000 maternity cases from within a half-mile radius of the hospital, with a reported total of 36 deaths, or 1 in 333, a rate better than the national average. This reported rate is especially impressive because over 2,500 of the women were in their seventh or later confinements; one was up to her 22nd.[59] Dr Hicks, the physician-*accoucheur*, banned students in the early 1860s from attending confinements on the same day as they dissected. Guy's also dispensed with sponges in childbirth: flannels were used instead and then either burnt or washed in chloride of lime.[60] The maternity department of St George's Hospital also had a good record: a death rate of 1 in every 284 deliveries between 1864 and 1876, and then 1 in 594 between 1869 and 1876.[61] In the early 1890s the West End Branch of the Glasgow Maternity Hospital was handling over 500 out-patient deliveries annually, and losing only five mothers a year.[62] The mother and her child were isolated from some of the infections endemic in hospitals and were delivered among friends and in familiar surroundings, however wretched. Their status, contemporaries remarked, ranged from the respectable artisan rank to the very poor. Most, given the usual hospital rules, had to claim to be married, at least.

Dispensaries

Dispensaries had existed in London and Edinburgh since the seventeenth century. Originally created to supply cheap prescriptions and medicines, by the nineteenth century they had proliferated and had begun to provide a range of cheap or free treatments, including midwifery. The proliferation mainly resulted from efforts by medical men to create institutional buffers against bad debts. At least thirty provident institutions were operating in London in the 1840s and fifteen more were established between 1852 and 1890 and most large towns had at least one.[63] The doctor sought to guarantee his income in two main ways. Mr J. Baker Brown, FRCS, who created the Metropolitan Provident Dispensary in 1869 at 1 Osnaburgh Place, opened his dispensary 'to all, without letters of recommendation, every day from 12 to 2, for women and children: and from 7 to 9 p.m. for men ... For the benefit of all persons, without incomes, in every station of life'. Midwifery, like all the services, was payable in advance by weekly instalments of 6*d*. or 1*s*. It cost 10*s*. 6*d*. within half a mile, 15*s*. for one mile, one guinea for two miles. Baker Brown solicited wealthy 'subscribers', but his dispensary had no committee of management or board of governors. The actual work of the dispensary, including confinements, was done by two unregistered assistants.[64] In the 1840s the work of the Aldersgate dispensary, which named three surgeons on its letterhead when seeking donations, was done by a local GP part-time, and an apothecary and his untrained assistant. One of the surgeons lived in the West End and had not been seen in Aldersgate for years.[65] The Northampton Dispensary, founded in the 1840s, was run as a profit-sharing partnership by its four doctor founders. Midwifery, at 10*s*. a job, was a prime source of income. It had two classes of patients:

servants of donors and subscribers, 'free' members, that is 'working persons', paying one penny per week if they were over 14 and otherwise one halfpenny. In 1849 Mr Faircloth, the senior partner, who performed 70 deliveries for the year and handled 2,800 other cases, received a dividend of over £130.[66] In the 1870s the Salop Medical Aid Association, run by one surgeon, Mr Thomas Piddock, on a subscription of 4*s*. 4*d*. per person per year 'for members of the working classes', was, Mr Piddock boasted, 'entirely self-supporting' and therefore did not need donors' subscriptions and the interference this usually entailed. The doctor made £200 a year, and the 'Association' paid for his house and coals.[67]

'Free' dispensaries were established by doctors with the backing of philanthropic donors, who retained the right to recommend deserving patients. Often free dispensaries were linked with missions, especially among Wesleyans and evangelical Anglicans. The Surrey Dispensary, Union Street, Borough, was an Anglican institution. The nearly 200,000 cases its managers claimed to have relieved between 1778 and 1840 included over 31,000 confinements.[68] These institutions (though not the Surrey Dispensary itself) seem to have been readier to employ midwives and only to summon *accoucheurs* in awkward cases. This may have been because, in general, the incomes of such institutions as the Queen Street Cheapside Dispensary and the South London Dispensary were lower, and the clergy on the committees exerted themselves to limit the doctors' share. Possibly, too, they had the best success rates: the committee would have recruited only clean, experienced midwives and reasonably earnest doctors. The East London Dispensary for Women, near Stepney railway station, was founded in a former sailmaker's dilapidated warehouse in the 1860s, by a Dissenting surgeon, Mr Heckford and his wife, a trained nurse. Bereft of wealthy patrons, they nursed about eight women at a time, and were loved and trusted in the neighbourhood.[69]

In the great towns free dispensaries were also frequently the basis of private medical schools, until the latter faded out in the 1850s. We have no figures for the number of women delivered, or for successes, complications or deaths. Probably these proprietary schools were the least auspicious from the patient's point of view. Mr Laidlaw's Dispensary in Warwick Street, Golden Square, opened for business about 1830. Its advertised object was to afford 'gratuitous assistance to poor lying-in women at their own houses, and for the diseases of children'. Its real object was the training of medical students, who paid fees to Mr Laidlaw. A neighbourhood doctor alleged:

These gentlemen he sends to the poor females to learn the obstetric art as best they may, but whenever a patient requests the attendance of 'the master Accoucheur himself', that gentleman informs them he is never in the habit of affording it unless he is paid . . . although he is always willing to 'book the patient'.

A woman, who a fortnight previously was attended by a student, thought at the time that she had been unscientifically delivered. The child had died, and she became unwilling to be again placed under the hands of a pupil. She sent, therefore, for Mr Laidlaw, requiring him to visit her, at the same time stating that she would pay him for so doing, if he made a moderate charge. Mr Laidlaw, upon this promise, attended and repaired the mischief which had been previously done, and a few days after *sent in his Bill.*[70]

In Liverpool in 1831 Mary Spencer died after delivering herself of a male child and bleeding for seven hours afterwards. When labour started prematurely, she walked to the door of the North Liverpool Dispensary, which was also a medical school, but was refused attention 'on the ground of informality'. She had not obtained any 'lines' from the Ladies' Committee, presumably because she was unmarried. Mary Spencer pressed her case but a young doctor told her 'she had received her answer, and that patients could only be visited in their regular turns'. She then went to several doctors' homes but they, on learning she was 'indigent and living in a cellar' refused 'from some cause or another' to treat her. Finally she dragged herself back to the cellar, bore the child, and bled to death. When the local radical doctor, Weatherill, arrived, the child was also dead, and the bed and floor awash with blood. Weatherill sought an inquest. The coroner refused: it would only 'bring odium' on the Dispensary. The Dispensary committee of management decided that the death was a midwifery one 'outside' the institution and therefore terminated discussion on it.[71]

After the profession became ultra-respectable during the 1850s, the *Lancet* and *BMJ* virtually ceased to print details of manslaughter trials and charges of negligence. Possibly, as members of the profession gained in self-esteem, they did become more conscientious and the number of callous and brutal incidents diminished, but I doubt this, because the weekly toll of inquests and nasty stories in the daily press continues through the century. The case histories given here are representative, often of dozens of similar events; examples of humane behaviour, though probably more numerous, are harder to find because they did not come into the public legal process. The dispensary situation was still bad enough in 1886 to move Mr McMillan to explain to the Glasgow Southern Medical Society that the dispensaries accepted so many patients

> that each individual case cannot obtain the attention it deserves. If
> . . . the staff gave that sufficient time to the examination of each
> case which it demanded, the sum of time expended would be so
> great that no medical man could spare it; what he thought ought to
> be put before the public very strongly, they had no right to expect
> it.[72]

Here, as elsewhere in this book, it is worth reminding ourselves that it is easier to find evidence of failure than of success: after all, women would have ceased going to dispensaries if they destroyed more than a small minority of patients. In this line of history, survivors don't tell tales. What is indubitable is that there were a lot of them. If we take as a rough indicator the proportion of midwifery cases at the Surrey Dispensary, that is about one-sixth, and apply it over all for the London dispensaries in the 1840s, we have about 18,000 women being delivered under dispensaries' auspices each year. The London dispensaries between them then had about 100,000 patients. This figure was kept low, it was said, because of competition from the out-patients' services of the voluntary hospitals. In the provinces, up to half the population enrolled at dispensaries. By 1910 the Charity Organization Society claimed that dispensaries in England and Wales treated over 800,000 people a year. The rules about provision for midwifery had been tightened, but even if we make a conservative guess that 10 per cent of the 800,000 were maternity cases, we still have 80,000 mothers involved.[73]

The Lying-in Hospitals

The lying-in hospitals began, like the dispensaries, as charities in the eighteenth century, and proliferated during the nineteenth century as teaching and proselytising institutions. The more famous of them, Queen Charlotte's and the Royal Belgrave, for instance, figure as names at least in the medical histories and in general histories when explaining the increase of population. In terms of numbers of patients and probably numbers of students trained, they are much less important than the unsung dispensaries. By 1843 London had more than 20 small lying-in hospitals.[74] The hospitals were sly with their statistics throughout the century and it is difficult to find out how many women they delivered, and with what results. In 1848 the Islington Maternity Charity claimed to have handled 200 patients.[75] Allowing for exaggeration for the benefit of subscribers, the Islington Charity seems to be typical. On this basis we have a figure of about 4,000 women assisted each year by the London hospitals during the 1840s. The York Road Lambeth Lying-in Hospital claimed to have delivered about 208 women per year.[76] The British Lying-in Hospital, between the 1830s and 1860s, delivered about 130 women a year, and Queen Charlotte's 7,700 between 1828 and 1863, that is about 220 a year.[77] Most of the hospitals were rebuilt and enlarged in the late 1860s and their numbers of patients approximately doubled until the early years of the twentieth century, when the totals of patients at the bigger hospitals, Queen Charlotte's for example, rose more than 400 per cent.[78]

The ladies' committees and the clergymen sponsoring the lying-in hospitals were zealous that the care provided should not only be charitable, but should be seen to be so. Childbirth was beset by impurity and obscenity and it was important for their peace of mind and that of potential donors that the impure should get no bonus. Nearly all lying-in hospitals excluded unmarried women, with the notable exception of Queen Charlotte's which admitted single women for their first delivery only, as did a few small charities in the provinces.[79] Even under the pressure of the need for 'national efficiency' and the call for more fit babies for the Empire, the ladies moved slowly to lower the moral barrier. In 1899, the Liverpool Ladies' Charity and Lying-in Hospital decided by a narrow majority: 'That single women in exceptional circumstances who, after careful investigation by the ladies' committee, are found to be deserving objects of charity, shall be eligible for admission into the hospital for their first confinement'. The City of London Hospital had similarly altered its rules some weeks earlier. In Liverpool the motion had been strenuously opposed by Monsignor Nugent and the Countess of Derby, but the motion survived after a compromise addendum was carried that 'only women otherwise respectable, such as shop assistants and domestic servants' would be admitted and 'none of the profligate class'. But as Mrs Henry Tate, the mover of the motion, implied, the ladies were in danger of losing their charity: the Hospital had 15 beds, yet never more than 3 were occupied; the women preferred to be delivered by general hospital students and midwives in their own homes. Yet 200 unmarried girls were delivered annually in local workhouses.[80]

The moral exclusion rule had the extra advantage that the inevitable high infant mortality rate among illegitimates could not be attached to the hospital. A second rule of nearly all lying-in hospitals excluded married women pregnant for the first time. There was a danger that they had been impure before a hasty marriage, and again there was the advantage that the very high maternal mortality rate belonging to primi-parae could not be attributed to the hospital. Women with no child living, or a child deformed or diseased were also excluded. This situa-tion revealed culpable neglect, the authorities believed, and the rule helped keep 'constitutional' diseases out of the hospital.[81] The York Road Hospital had a grand front entrance, where subscribers in their carriages were received by the matron. Patients, even in labour, had to enter at the back door after a walk of nearly 100 yards, for there was no carriageway to the back.[82] In 1840 Ann Griffin arrived in a cab at the front door of this hospital in labour. The house surgeon, Mr Tawke, went specially to the door to confirm the porter's finding that she had no letter of recommendation. Mr Tawke did not examine her, but directed the cabby to take her to a workhouse. The child was born while they were speaking. The cabman exclaimed, 'Its a damned shame', and drove Griffin to the Westminster Hospital. There he encountered a medical student who refused to look at Griffin, but directed the cab-man to the lying-in hospital in Queen's Square; he should have said Queen *Street*. After failing to find the hospital, the cabman took his charge to Lambeth Workhouse, but it emerged that Ann Griffin was from St Anne's parish, and the matron directed her there, remarking that 'they could not have any further encumbrances'. The cabman then took Griffin to the newly opened workhouse in St James's, Poland Square. Again they were refused. The porter directed them to the Strand Workhouse. By mistake the cabman went to King's College Hospital, and was refused. The cabman now asked a policeman where to try next. The policeman advised taking Griffin to Bow Street Police Station. There the inspector wrote an order that the woman be admit-ted at St Giles' Workhouse and sent a constable with the cab. The inspector and policeman also offered to reimburse the cabby for his journey. Ann Griffin was duly admitted. The child was found to be dead.[83]

Fanny N— was 33 and pregnant with her sixth child when she ob-tained her letter for the Christ-Church St Pancras Lying-in Charity for the Delivery of Poor Married Lying-in Women at their own Habitations, in 1840. Her husband, a shoemaker, was out of work and the family 'were in the greatest poverty'. When the pains started at 4 p.m. on 10 November her neighbour, who was nursing her, went to the Society's *accoucheur* to tell him to come. He arrived at 6 p.m., and found great fault with the apartment. 'Halloa! I thought you would have had the place ready. My time is precious. As for you (to the husband) you must go.' The patient was very weak and the nurse described her as being frightened by the doctor's remarks. He examined her for 20 minutes and then went to tea. Forty-five minutes later he returned and 'gave her no time whatever, but forced the labour [by hand] and in a quarter of an hour the child was born'. He remained for 20 minutes, and then left his patient, 'much exhausted and . . . flooding'. The flooding continued throughout the night and the next day. Despite pleas, the doctor did not return until 8 p.m. He did nothing to stop the bleeding: it was not normal for the smaller religious societies to supply drugs. Besides, as he remarked, 'it was no use giving medicine to a poor woman who had not proper food'. He left and never returned, despite repeated calls. Once he despatched a bottle of opium mixture with the messenger. Then the nurse herself went to plead with him, on 4 December. He refused to return with her: 'the patient's time was up.' Attendance at a confinement only ran for 9-10 days. She would have to obtain a fresh letter of recommendation before he would consider it. Finally, another man, Dr Pitman, visited her, voluntarily. Upon the woman's death, five days later, the husband, apparently egged on by the neighbour, sought and obtained a coroner's inquest. It emerged that the *accoucheur* was not paid by the Society, but was permitted to charge for the medicines he prescribed for patients. The want of cash in the N— household explains why he did not supply ergot and opium for the flooding. The Rev. Mr W—, the president of the Society, told the coroner's jury that the *accoucheur* 'had the strong approval of the . . . charity', and succeeded in having his name suppressed. The jury brought in a verdict of 'natural death from inflammation of the lungs'.[84]

Mrs N—'s fate helps justify the sarcasm by general hospital *accoucheurs*, lecturers and neighbourhood GPs that the lying-in hospitals were staffed by 'raw country boys' and uncouth apothecaries, and that they were dangerous places for mothers. Lying-in charities creamed off students' fees from the general hospital teachers and undercut the local GPs.[85] The allegations about the mortality rates of the hospitals are difficult to prove because the hospital statistics are so slippery. In addition to the moral rules excluding risky patients, women were normally required to leave the hospital's books, as in Fanny N—'s case, within nine or ten days and there was no after-care. The hospitals commonly ignored the Registrar-General's requirement that deaths occurring within 30 days of parturition be registered as associated with childbirth.[86] Finally, confined women in hospital who showed symptoms of fever or sepsis were promptly removed to fever or general hospitals.[87] The hospital authorities claimed huge successes throughout the century. Their claims have been swallowed by historians and built into influential explanations of the increase of population which ascribe importance to alleged improvements in medical practice.[88] The Royal Maternity Charity, which reported to its donors that it dealt among the 'most destitute' in London, claimed 18,751 deliveries up to 1862, with only 56 deaths, or 1 in 335.[89] York Road claimed to have had no deaths in 1861-2; but did not reveal that it was closed for the year because of the preceding epidemic of sepsis and puerperal fever. Nearly all the hospitals had to close periodically to arrest epidemics and each seems to have used the gap to improve its reported mortality rate.[90]

The in-patient death rate at Queen Charlotte's Hospital was justifiably high, explained Dr Blakely Brown, the senior physician, because they admitted single primiparae women. They were 'depressed when they came in'; they were 'often of superior station in society', but they had been 'thrown out by the family', and were starving. Many entered with complications after unsuccessful attempts at abortion. Of 369 deliveries in 1861, 154 were married, and 215 single women. Three died among the 154 married, that is 1:51, but 15 of the 215 single women died, or 1:14.[91] The figures allegedly quoted from 'records' for the British lying-in hospitals, which run at 1 death in 938 for 1799-1800 and 1 in 216 deliveries for 1799-1808, and 1 in 143 for 1849-61 are simply unbelievable in the light of the Queen Charlotte figures.[92]

There is some evidence that women delivered at home survived much better than those delivered in hospital. St Mary's Hospital Manchester claimed over 7,600 out-patient deliveries during 1878, 1879 and 1881 with only 20 deaths, or 1 in 381. (1880 is missing, rather ominously.) The Newcastle-upon-Tyne Lying-in Hospital, again almost entirely an out-patient charity, in 1879-81 inclusive, helped 1,259 cases, with only 2 deaths. Both charities depended heavily on midwives.[93] At the British Lying-in Hospital in 1881: of 160 women delivered in the hospital, including 32 primiparae, there was 1 death; of 460 delivered at home, mostly by midwives, there was also one death. This report suggests that the authorities admitted women likely to have a difficult labour, and left the others at home. A much higher proportion of in-patients needed 'operative interference' than out-patients; but again this might also indicate that in-patients were more readily accessible clinical material.[94] The clearest evidence of all comes from the Birmingham Lying-in Charity in 1868. There, after years of endemic puerperal fever and high mortality rates, the authorities decided to deliver all patients at their homes, using midwives and summoning the doctors only in emergencies. After 156 cases and no deaths and only four 'needing the calling in of doctors', the Charity decided to remain an out-patient institution.[95] By 1878 the Registrar-General was confident enough to report that in London, where the general maternal death rate was 5 in 1,000 live births, a woman increased her chances of death in childbirth sixfold by entering a London lying-in hospital, where he estimated the over-all rate at 25.7 per 1,000.[96]

The ladies' committees, the uncouth apothecaries, raw country boys and midwives did not adopt antiseptic procedures until the 1880s, when the death rate began to fall. York Road Hospital reported only 1 death among 334 in-patient deliveries and none among 741 out-patients. 'Strict antisepsis' prevailed in the hospital. Each patient was douched night and morning in 'antiseptic solution of perichloride of mercury', 1 in 2,000 parts at 110°F. Nurses and doctors 'must regularly wash their hands'.[97]

But many institutions continued unregenerate. In 1873 the first resident physician was appointed at the Royal London Lying-in Hospital. He set about introducing paid trained nurses, redistributing the 60 to 90 mothers and infants huddled indiscriminately in the wards, and ordering some rudimentary cleansing such as whitewashing the walls. In 1875 the ladies' committee dismissed him.[98] The City of London Lying-in Hospital occupied a building 124 years old in 1897. Only the matron and a midwife lived in. In 1870 there had been 12 deaths among 227 deliveries, or 1 in 19. The hospital had been closed, as had often happened before, for the three summer months, the worst period for infection. The old wooden bedsteads with curtains were replaced by iron ones without curtains, and straw palliasses and hair mattresses were introduced instead of the old feather beds. The drains were capped, the cesspools filled with concrete and new water-closets installed. Then the building was fumigated with chlorine gas. In 1871 there were only 103 confinements, with 1 death reported. Pyaemia swept the wards again in 1877 and the hospital was closed in December. The drainage was again improved, at a cost of £4,500. In 1880 there were again 12 deaths among 382 deliveries and £600 was spent on improvements during 1881. In 1882 the medical staff recommended that the hospital be demolished and rebuilt. The governors rejected the proposal and instead voted £1,000 for renovations and whitewash. Next year, 1883, the hospital closed again when the death rate rose to 1 in 23 confinements. It was discovered that the soiled linen chutes had never been cleansed:

hitherto the pervasive odour of the hospital had disguised the fault. In 1886 the hospital had to close again, with a death rate of 1:44 and worse threatening. Only after the reopening in late 1886 were antiseptic methods introduced, under protest at the expense from the governors. The chosen antiseptic for the next decade was fierce corrosive sublimate (mercuric chloride — an acid poison): probably its cost fortunately led to its being much diluted. Thereafter the reported death rate fell to 1 in 419. The story of the York Road (by the 1870s commonly called the General Lying-in) Hospital is very similar.[99]

Sixpenny Doctors

Women who disliked charity or who could not obtain 'lines' and yet had insufficient money for a regular doctor could turn to a 'sixpenny doctor' or a midwife. The 'sixpenny', who gained his name because he was both cheap and allowed payment by instalment, was likely to be uncertificated and totally untrained. Many were druggists. Yet, as with the scarcely better equipped regulars, most of their patients survived their ministrations. Medical men were assiduous in hunting down and prosecuting bad cases among their non-professional competitors, but the total number of scandalous deaths appears no greater among irregulars than regulars.

A confinement attended by a sixpenny doctor cost about 3s. to 7s. 6d., and the price remained stable throughout the century.[100] Many poorer women preferred them because they knew them as neighbourhood purveyors of cheap medicines and advice. They dressed and talked like their own menfolk; which also meant that they were probably rougher and dirtier in their person, if not more callous, than the local regular GP. The sixpennys were notorious for being quick and unrelenting with the dilators and the forceps and very unforthcoming with the chloroform.[101] But the women were stoical and the use of instruments proved to them and the neighbours that the 'doctor' had tried his best. Many of the women must have been weak, anaemic and exhausted long before their labour began and an instrument delivery was inevitable. In Liverpool in 1841 Mary Sheridan, aged 27, had 'suffered from severe privation during the winter' and could produce only feeble contractions when her time came. The uterus never dilated more than a half-crown piece. After 48 hours the sixpenny tore the foetus out, with Sheridan screaming, 'Oh, your nails are killing me.' He could not get the child's head out, and left to attend another patient. Sheridan died 20 minutes later.[102] Patients might also have acquiesced in the use of instruments and manual force the more readily because many sixpennys were like the

self-described 'Chemist, druggist, surgeon, apothecary, accoucheur' who
kept a shop in the Camberwell New Road in the 1830s, and charged,
according to his handbills, sixpence 'Every morning before eleven
o'clock; After that hour, The usual charge will be made.'[103] By the mid-
1860s the usual night fee, even in country districts, was 'one guinea —
cash'.[104] There were also a few sixpennys at least, like Mr Edwards of
Chelsea, who practised in poor districts partly, it seems, out of altru-
ism.[105] Others, especially young men without capital, began as sixpennys in order to accumulate the funds to enable them to buy into a
practice in a more salubrious suburb. 'S' of London, for example,
argued that a quick turnover of lots of patients, at 6d. or 1s. a treatment
and 5s. a delivery in immediate cash, paid as well as a backlog of half-
paid or irrecoverable normal fees.[106] In the 1830s doctors in poor districts in Manchester and London expected to get only about one-third
of their possible fees. It was still at this level in the 1890s.[107]

Midwives

Midwives ranged from the able, clean and fashionable to the ignorant,
slovenly and very cheap. The ablest were undoubtedly very skilled
indeed. In Bristol, the daughter of Dr Spence studied with her father
during the 1820s and 1830s and practised on her own account very
successfully for several years, until she was stopped by a doctors'
boycott and ridicule fomented by them. She was succeeded by Mrs
Hockley, who built a splendid reputation for skill and gentleness and
had a large practice through the middle years of the century. Dr
Elizabeth Blackwell remembered in 1860 that many middle-class
women had confided to her that they felt 'ashamed and angry' at their
'rough handling' by male *accoucheurs*.[108] Emma Martin, midwife and
secularist lecturer on gynaecology and family limitation, also began her
career in Bristol. But ridicule came easily. As the career of Emma
Martin showed, the movement for skilled *accoucheuses* could be
labelled Owenite, socialist and atheistic.[109] The links undoubtedly exist.
Dr Spence and Elizabeth Blackwell's father were both unconventional
radicals. The subject needs exploration. Bristol would make an excellent
starting-point, but radical networks in other provincial towns such as
Birkenhead in the mid-1840s, where the Ladies' Charity, run completely
by females, made great inroads on the practice of local male *accoucheurs*, would be worth investigating.[110] Political objections apart, the
movement was suspect among Protestant heads of families because it
savoured of superstitious practices in Romish countries, where only
females were permitted to manage confinements and healthy male

rationality was excluded.[111]

As the mortality rates for lying-in charities suggested, midwives probably had a lower case-mortality rate than doctors because they delivered their patients at home, away from hospital streptococci and meddlesome students. They rarely used their own materials, but relied upon the patient to provide clothes, utensils and drugs.[112] But once a midwife became a carrier she was hard to stop. Until 1902 there was no legal bar to her continuing practice and no legal way of ensuring that she washed herself and her clothes. Mrs Tompsett of Maidstone had 'several puerperal deaths' traced to her in 1881, but she refused a coroner's request to stop practising for a month because she 'had her family to keep'. She compromised by having her clothes disinfected but refused to wash her hands in carbolic solution. Mrs Tompsett had conventional medical opinion on her side. The *Lancet* sympathised that 'in the urgency of practice . . . the difficulty is . . . to take these extreme and even exaggerated precautions'.[113] Medical opinion changed during the decade and by 1895 a midwife called Mrs Rake, of Packwater Street, Kentish Town, was charged with manslaughter on the death of a woman from puerperal fever, after she had been connected with eight previous cases, including five deaths, and had refused a request from the local Medical Officer of Health to interrupt her work.[114]

Some of the skilled women may have used instruments, especially catheters, but most did not. They were proud of their manual skills and the reach and strength of their fingers. It was not customary for midwives to introduce their hands into the womb, partly because they did not usually make ante-natal investigations, but mainly because midwives were not expected to turn a child when a breech or shoulder or other awkward presentation appeared.[115] These conventions meant less tearing of the womb and less infection. Probably, too, it meant that women who feared complications went to doctors. But these conventions, reinforced by ignorance, also meant that a woman attended by a midwife whose delivery became difficult was in for a very bad time indeed. The custom by which the mother supplied such drugs as might be used meant that only laudanum and alcohol were commonly available. Most midwives were afraid to administer chloroform.[116] But with an uncomplicated 'normal' delivery, and most births were uncomplicated and normal, there is no evidence that a competent midwife proceeded in any substantially different way than did an experienced medical man.

William Kibbey was a Bridgwater man whose family prospects shrank as his children multiplied. He told the Select Committee on

Medical Poor Relief in 1844 that his wife had had their first four children delivered privately by a surgeon, and the next two by the local midwife, Mrs Webber, when she had had 'a very bad time'. Kibbey had asked the Poor Law guardians to pay the surgeon for the seventh delivery but they had refused. His wife was 40, she haemorrhaged copiously under Mrs Webber's ministrations and died three weeks later, leaving a weakly child. Actually Mrs Webber had not been able to get the child out of the womb and it had been pulled out by the neighbourhood surgeon, gratis. He had been summoned by Kibbey in the midst of the emergency.[117]

In 1859 a woman was delivered of a healthy infant at Halling, in Kent. Her midwife was a neighbouring labourer's wife who had 'recently set up as a midwife'. The woman died 3 days later: the umbilical cord had never been removed from the womb.[118] At Northolt, near Uxbridge, Henrietta B—, a proprietress of a beer-shop and 'professedly a midwife', a woman without any education 'in any department of life, excepting the domestic', was engaged to deliver a farmer's wife, Mrs G—. Mrs G— was 44 and already had borne fifteen children. She haemorrhaged during an exhausting labour. Henrietta B— applied napkins soaked in vinegar and water, but could not stop the bleeding. She wanted to send for a surgeon, but Mrs G— refused. Her strength was kept up with gin and water. The haemorrhage continued for 14 hours. At last a child was born; but the placenta came away in pieces. Mrs G— was now unconscious and a surgeon was sent for, but apparently he never arrived. Mrs G— died 3 hours after the birth. At the post-mortem, most of the placenta was found in the womb. The coroner, Thomas Wakley, made Henrietta B— promise never to act as midwife again.[119] As with Mrs Kibbey, poverty shortened the odds for survival. The older the woman, the more children she had, the poorer she was, the more vulnerable she became and, short of charity, the more likely she was to be attended by a cheap midwife. At this level the ignorant destroyed the indigent.

At St Marylebone, Mary H—, aged 38, married to a man 'in very humble circumstances' was confined of her ninth child in 1840. She was in labour for 17 hours but her midwife, Mrs Moss, a lady with an extensive practice, refused to allow a surgeon to be called: 'she was quite confident of her business, and would not be laughed at by a parcel of doctors.' Mary H— was moaning and pleading that something be done. But Mrs Moss insisted that she was 'going on very well'. A baby was delivered alive after a labour of 26 hours, and then Mary H— died of exhaustion. Mrs Moss failed to get the placenta out because she broke it while dragging at it. A post-mortem revealed the 'whole body bloodless and flaccid'.[120]

Mr Moore, a surgeon, was urgently called to a woman at Dalston. She had been in labour for 24 hours, with 'no results'. He found the woman being 'forcibly held on her bed by several persons'. She was drunk and very violent. Two doctors had earlier arrived to attend her but had fled. The midwife, who had been dosing her patient and herself with brandy and opium, was 'half drunken and supercilious' and protested against Moore's intrusion; 'for if the people would hold the patient, she could and would deliver her without any doctor, and much the better than any of them'. The woman had 4 other children, each delivered by a surgeon, but the family had met financial reverses and this time had engaged the midwife. Moore, to quench the violence, 'determined to abstract blood . . . to 30 ounces'. The midwife denounced this proceeding. He also applied an 'evaporating lotion' to the head and eventually he produced 'a state of partial tranquility'. Next he examined the patient, something the midwife had omitted to do. He found the rectum full of faeces, and also drew off 2 pints of urine. Moore then decided he needed his enema apparatus and moved to return to his house to get it. But he found the door locked. The patients' friends were resolved not to lose their third doctor. So he sent for the enema and released an 'enormous quantity of faeces'. Moore then administered 40 drops of chloroform by means of a sponge fixed into a cone contrived from the cover of a copybook in the room. Fearful of the woman, he added 20 more drops 'from time to time' and kept his patient insensible for 40 minutes, after which he delivered a male child. It was dead, with one arm blackened by the midwife's pulling. He left soon afterwards, the midwife's abuse following him, 'medical men know nothing of midwifery'. The patient survived, so far as Moore knew when he wrote his report.[121]

The midwife's usual fee in the 1830s and 1840s attending a poor woman was an all-inclusive 2s. 6d. By the 1870s the common charge, even for poor patients, had risen to 4s. for the delivery and around 3s. weekly for 'subsequent attendance'. In 1908 midwives qualified under the Midwives Act of 1902 charged between 7s. 6d. and one guinea, leaving most poor women with the untrained (who were permitted to continue practice until 1910) at 3s. 6d. to 5s., and thereby largely defeating the purpose of the Act.[122] Midwives had no capital outlay. Their exclusion from legal medical practice meant that they did not have to spend money on education or instruments. The pregnant woman had to supply the bandages for the confinement and the rags to sop up the blood and urine. Moreover, their unqualified state kept them effectively beyond the law of negligence.

Midwives were cheaper and less fashionable partly because they were vulgar and slipshod, and partly because until 1902 they were not recognised by the state. Throughout the century the royal colleges thwarted plans to educate and qualify them, fearing them as a group which might trade among the middle classes. Between 1890 and 1902 the medical profession blocked five separate Bills. The pattern was established in 1813, during the period when men were moving extensively into midwifery. A draft Bill for the registration of apothecaries also provided for the examination and licensing of midwives by local committees of the Society of Apothecaries. This proposal in particular and the main proposal to legitimise apothecaries as GPs met the full hostility of the London colleges of physicians and surgeons. They forced the withdrawal of the Bill. When the Apothecaries got their Act in 1815, the midwives were excluded. They were similarly ignored when the Medical Act enabling the registration of 'medically qualified' practitioners was finally passed in 1858. The London Obstetric Society, founded in 1858, followed its Edinburgh and Berlin examplars in closing its membership and meetings to females. At least five later Bills, such as Foster's Midwives Bill of 1890, were also blocked by the Royal Colleges and the BMA. The Act of 1902 only survived after extensive concessions were made to the BMA.[123]

At various times through the century private schools, such as that run by Dr Dewhurst in London, sold diplomas to midwives; the standards seem to have been bad. During the 1860s some earnest surgeons in the provinces offered lecture courses for midwives on elementary cleanliness and antisepsis. But they appear to have won few pupils. The skilled midwives thought the instruction superfluous and begrudged the time and the unskilled could not afford the one guinea fee. In 1872 the Obstetrical Society instituted a course of instruction requiring attendance at 25 confinements, and offered a certificate permitting the midwife to attend 'natural' labour. But only 5,529 had been awarded the certificate by 1900. Good teaching in midwifery was still hard to find in the early twentieth century. I have found no evidence that midwives formally, beyond the very few trained at the lying-in charities, or indeed informally, taught each other.[124] Even more than their male competitors, midwives learned by trial and error.

A midwife with a good reputation could do 160 to 200 deliveries a year. (The National Health Service working party on midwives recommended an absolute maximum per midwife of 55 a year in 1949.[125]) Others, like Ernest Bevin's mother, a barmaid and part-time domestic servant in the 1870s and 1880s, attended confinements as occasion offered and as a neighbourly act.[126] After certificated midwives became available in 1903, many mothers continued with the old untrained women, not only because they were cheaper, but because they lent utensils, helped with the washing, fed the husband and cared for the other children. The starchy new midwives were above this sort of charring. Allowing that the pregnant women got virtually no ante-natal attention from skilled full-time, or unskilled part-time midwives, provided that it was a straightforward birth, she may have done better for post-natal help with the neighbour from the same street or village than the brisk professional from the next parish or nearby town. As the wife of an engine-driver in Upton-upon-Severn in Worcestershire explained in 1892, she

> always had the 'woman who goes about nursing' [as midwives were called in the West Country and elsewhere] [because] she did not see the good of paying a doctor a guinea just for the time, and looking after her and the baby for a few days afterwards, when she could get a woman who would do all that was needful at the time, and wash the child when it was born, and then attend her and the child for nine or ten days, all for 5/-.

Even when the poor in Worcestershire had to call in the doctor, they bargained for minimal attendance at a minimum fee and brought in a woman afterwards for 1s. per week.[127]

Midwives probably also helped the patient's morale by adhering to local childbirth customs. In Cumberland, until the 1870s at least, it was usual to seat a woman in labour over the gap between two chairs tied front to front. Her friends sat on either side of her and she put her arms around their necks. The midwife sat on a low stool behind to catch the baby when it appeared. It was a chancy method: the child's head was smashed if it was expelled suddenly and the midwife was slow. It was also agonisingly painful: the woman often was 'on the chair', screaming, for hours. Yet the power of custom was such that surgeons, however much they valued their training in delivery with the patient on her back or side, were 'not required' unless they agreed to conduct the delivery in this fashion.[128]

'Almost universally' in Yorkshire and in London even among 'better class people', against all medical protests, patients were confined, again at least until the 1870s, with all their clothes on: boots, stockings, drawers, chemise, stays, petticoats, dress, shawl, bonnet, some of the items borrowed or saved for specially for the occasion. If the first show began unexpectedly the neighbours rushed to dress the patient and place her on a bed, on the under-mattress, where she was delivered. A complaisant doctor reported:

> When the placenta comes away, the woman, without any further delay is 'got into bed' . . . This process consists in her standing up . . . while her clothes are taken off, and a clean night-dress is put on, and the bed made, when she mounts into it, as if nothing particular had occurred.

The ritual was messy and dangerous if the patient haemorrhaged. In 1875 a Bradford medical man sought 'a little firmness . . . on the part of the Yorkshire Accoucheurs [to] . . . end . . . a custom so unpleasant . . . to themselves and so dangerous to the women', but Dr 'XYZ' of London, while agreeing that it was 'inconvenient', added that 'a medical man . . . has his living to get by his practice [and] must not protest too much . . . [lest he] find himself voted fidgety'.[129]

Pauper Confinements

The remaining category of women could not afford to express their views. Paupers seeking their confinement at the public expense had no say in whether they were delivered in the workhouse or at home, by the parish midwife, or the parish surgeon or his assistant. These were decisions for the local Poor Law relieving officers. I shall write about Poor Law medical officers later in this book, but childbirth under Poor Law auspices raises four immediate points. First, the woman and her infant were charges upon public funds rather than objects of charity. Second, like the rest of the 'pauper sick' they were items in contracts made by principals whom they could not influence, and whose interests were not theirs. Third, their ambiguous situation as manifestors of a natural process rather than instances of 'impotence' often placed them among the 'able-bodied' and therefore subject to inhumanity enjoined by the less eligibility principle. Lastly, there can be no doubt that many thousands of women were confined as paupers through the century, although even near-precise figures are not recoverable. Poor Law doctors kept their books badly, Poor Law midwives usually kept no books at all, clerks to guardians reported erratically, and Poor Law Commissioners and Local Government Board officials had little interest in demanding better local records because they wanted total numbers rather than detailed analysis. The *Lancet* estimated in 1872 that 10 per cent of the total number of persons relieved inside and outside work-houses in England and Wales were childbirth cases.[130] This proportion tallies with my calculation that, after deducting 'widows' and females over 60 from the number of 'acute surgical' cases among 'able-bodied' females, the remainder runs at about 10 per cent of the whole. Assuming that this proportion is roughly constant, we have the enormous numbers of 140,000 pauper maternity cases in 1844, 79,000 in 1854, 100,000 in 1864, 79,000 in 1874, 73,000 in 1884 and 74,000 in 1894.[131] The great majority of these would have been delivered as out-door paupers, by midwives.

Pregnant paupers, who so often became contract charges on the public because of impurity, drunkenness or improvidence, had small claim on the doctor's or midwife's professional concern. Their self-esteem as practitioners was nourished by their charity and private practices, not their sideline Poor Law duties. Indeed, Poor Law attend-ance often harmed a doctor's standing as a private practitioner: middle-class women feared the contagion lodged on the hands and clothes that had touched workhouse women. Moreover, it was believed that Poor Law doctoring brutalised a man.[132]

The custom of handing over the medical management of the local poor to the lowest tenderer and the abuses that accompanied it existed before the Poor Law Amendment Act of 1834. In 1833, for example, the poor of Woodbridge in Suffolk were 'farmed' to a local dubiously qualified surgeon at £4 a year, or less than half the traditional going rate for the county. In the workhouse, Rebecca Bonner was simul-taneously dying of typhus and in the first stages of childbirth. Without waiting for the membranes to break, the parish surgeon ordered her to be held by the hands and feet while he performed a Caesarian opera-tion. The operation lasted seven minutes. Although she had been given opium (six grains of solid opium, in fact), Bonner was conscious throughout and attempted to follow the surgeon's orders, adding 'Sir' to each reply. The child was born alive, but died with its mother soon afterwards. The coroner's jury found 'death by misadventure'.[133] In the north of England, in rural north-west Yorkshire and Northumberland, for example, and in Scotland, there was no Poor Law medical service before 1834, indeed until into the 1840s. Some towns paid a local medical officer a retainer of about £12-£20 a year, on the understanding that he treated the poor gratis and delivered babies for what he could get the women to pay, but other towns throughout the countryside simply depended on private subscriptions to doctors to tend the poor. The Alnwick collection amounted to about £38 each year.[134] In other

places, and in Scotland, the poor went untreated, submitted themselves
to travelling charlatans or simply tended each other.

Most of the Amendment Act's other callous features existed before
1834 too, the illegitimacy and sickness provisions, for example, which
Dickens attached to the New Poor Law in *Oliver Twist*. Indeed an
incident which possibly inspired the opening chapters occurred in 1831.
In Rochester, Caroline Gilbert was 'over her time, and did not know
one hour from the other'. Her husband applied for her delivery by the
parish surgeon, who agreed and wrote a certificate to prevent her
being returned under the settlement laws to Cranbrook, her husband's
parish, twenty or so miles away. The mayor, apparently a local attorney, on hearing of the certificate, came and 'inspected' Mrs Gilbert.
He ordered her removal to Cranbrook. She had lived all her life in
Rochester and knew nobody in her husband's parish. The membranes
had now ruptured but she was placed on a cart, and the journey began.
Labour then commenced and the driver returned Gilbert to Rochester,
to be delivered by her husband's mother. She died twelve hours later,
after muttering several times that she 'felt jolted to death'. The coroner's
jury, composed of 20s. rate-paying vestrymen, returned a verdict of
'natural death' with a rider mildly censuring the mayor. He explained that
parish surgeons made money illicitly from 'suspended orders', that is,
orders for relief granted in the parish in which the sufferer currently
dwelt, but payable in his parish of settlement. The *Lancet* wasted little
sympathy on Caroline Gilbert or on the shortcomings of poor relief.
The Gilbert inquest was a battle won in the war against the supercilious,
interfering legal profession. 'The medical men have done themselves
real honour by their conduct . . . They have made the attorneys feel
their importance and have shown the public how to appreciate their
knowledge and ability.'[135]

None the less, the Act of 1834 probably made life harder for the
pauper sick. It weakened the doctor's motivation to do good by formal-
ising the loose mixture of casual goodwill, rough charity and greedy
callousness that prevailed before. Temptation to greed and callousness
was heightened by the curb on doctors' incomes, the increase in the
number of persons he was contracted to treat and the distances he was
supposed to travel, and by formally subjecting the doctor to the relieving
officer, to the guardians and to the Poor Law Commissioners, who were
keen to save money. The average payment for a confinement, formerly
a valued 'extra' on the contract, at 10s. 6d., was cut back in many places
in the south and west to 1s. The fee was edged up to 10s. 6d. again
during the 1840s and generally remained at that level until the end of

the century, but throughout it lagged behind standard private charges.[136]

In town parishes the guardians made special efforts, commendable in the view of the Commissioners, to reduce medical relief. The Limehouse guardians retrenched expenditure between 1833 and 1844 from about £36-£44 per week to £16-£17. Midwifery orders were thinned from an average of 112 orders a year to 32 in 1843, a 'year of distress' among a population that had more than doubled to 20,000. The relieving officer was ordered to attend his office only for two hours on Thursday afternoons and to refuse orders to paupers who called at his home. On Thursdays the officer was instructed to issue a 'provisional order' requiring the pauper to return for a 'midwifery order', but, as the relieving officer explained, 'in nine cases out of ten you will not find a poor man attend for a midwife's order'.[137] As the chairman of the Brentford Union guardians explained, paupers without a settlement hesitated to apply for a suspended relief order for fear of having a removal order issued, especially to husbands. At Brentford such orders were issued as a matter of course, even to families with 30 years' residence. Meanwhile the pregnant woman became anxious and turned to local charity for help.[138] At Stepney the guardians required both the man and woman to attend when seeking a midwifery order; the woman to prove her pregnancy, the man to prove his destitution. They rarely could attend simultaneously, and the rule eliminated nearly all single women. Even so, the clerk to the Stepney guardians, receiving about £275 a year, and himself the son of the vestry-clerk, confessed that he believed 'there could be more discrimination'.[139] The patient's countertactic throughout the country was to wait until labour was imminent and then to send for a 'one day midwifery order' and thereby secure a midwife or surgeon for the delivery. The central authorities condemned the practice but it seems to have continued at least until the mid-1860s.[140]

Single women were discouraged and forced back on their families by the rule compelling them to enter the workhouse for their confinement. The policy seems to have succeeded: by 1836 'the Commissioners claimed that the number of bastards born in workhouses and chargeable to the public had decreased by 10,000'.[141] Elizabeth Joyce, a single woman, was in labour when she walked to the St Giles Workhouse in 1855. She sought admission from the porter at the gate who, according to standard procedure to test for imposters, 'pushed her hard on the stomach'. He was unconvinced and sent Joyce inside to the midwife and an old pauper woman, who pronounced her not pregnant but diseased. Therefore Joyce had no grounds for admission and was

hustled out of the workhouse. In the street Joyce encountered a
friend, who took her to a common lodging-house and paid 1s. 6d. for
her to be confined there. The baby was born dead. This exhausted the
1s. 6d. worth of accommodation: the landlady hauled Joyce off the
mattress and put her out in the street again, where she died.[142] It seems
that only the isolated, rejected and desperate ended up in the workhouse wards; which might help to explain the death rates I shall illustrate below. Their status as 'able-bodied casuals' in many workhouses
also hurt their chances, because they were under the 'deterrent gruel
diet' rule for the 9 days of their confinement period and then on the
low standard diet for their remaining 14 days in the nursery. Because
the 'extra' fee was payable only on the 9 days of the confinement,
many guardians instructed the midwife never to call for a doctor's
help until the tenth day. In some cases, as at the Strand Workhouse
until the late 1850s, the medical officer was forbidden to enter the
labour ward.[143] At Worcester in the late 1860s, the midwife broke the
guardians' rule five times when the situation had become critical; on
the last occasion, after a severe warning from the guardians, a midwife
left a woman in labour from Monday till Saturday before finally
calling in the surgeon. But the guardians finally effectively stopped this
flouting of instructions by refusing the surgeons their 'extras' fee.[144]
The guardians of Halstead also taught Mr Budget a lesson when he
obliged a call from a Union midwife caring for a pauper's wife. Mrs T—
was 34, it was her first birth and she had been in labour for two days
and three nights with the foetus impacted on her pelvis. The midwife
had been told not to call for medical help. Mr Budget delivered the
child, alive, with instruments. He sent the husband for an order, which
was refused. Budget sent the husband back to the overseer. Again the
order was refused. Budget was left to seek his payment from James T—,
the husband, who was on wages of 10s. per week.[145]

Intransigent medical officers could be dismissed and thereby become
a warning to others. Francis Bonney was parish medical officer at
Brentford from before 1834 to 1843. Under the New Poor Law the
population of the Union was increased from 5,000 to 37,000. Before
1834 about 80 paupers received medical orders each year; in 1835 the
total rose to 535. Simultaneously Bonney's salary was reduced from
£84 to £45 a year. Yet he tendered for the job because he wanted to
keep strangers away from 'a [private] practice he had built over many
years', and he 'felt a sort of compulsion' to continue as local GP. Of
course he had an interest in raising his income by maximising the number of 'extras' among patients from whom he would otherwise receive

nothing. But the guardians disliked compassion at the public expense. Their letter of dismissal informed Bonney that they were 'dissatisfied with the manner in which you [have] discharged your duties, in giving orders for relief when not required, and in sending pregnant women to the Board for orders in their confinement, who otherwise would not have applied'. These allegations were founded on two cases. The first was a woman whose five children Bonney was healing 'for disease'. Her husband, after a long period of sickness, had lately found work at 15s. a week. She had offered to pay as a private patient, by instalments, for her approaching sixth confinement, but the family had no furniture, having previously sold it for food, they were ill housed, and Bonney had advised her to 'use . . . her newly acquired income to provide herself with necessaries, rather than to pay the medical man'. It happened that her husband lost his job even before the woman was confined, and the family was forced to re-enter the workhouse. There the woman developed 'epilepsy' and was found to have a prolapsed womb after a difficult birth. The guardian refused an order for Bonney's fee. The second case involved a woman who was delivered by her mother while the relieving officer 'deliberated' upon her case. No order was issued. Bonney concluded his explanation by noting that he believed that he had been finally dismissed after repeating complaints about the drainage of the Union, on lands owned by the guardians. The chairman of the guardians, Mr Pownall, disagreed: Bonney had not been dismissed; he had simply not been re-elected.[146] (Legally until 1847, and widely until the late 1860s at least, parish medical officers were usually re-elected annually or for strict contracted periods, at the discretion of the guardians.[147]) There must have been many Bonneys in the towns and parishes of Britain, but as elsewhere in this history, the evidence of the good that men do is sparse, while the evidence of their inhumanity is abundant. In Whitechapel in 1894 a 'poor woman' aged 19 was dying of blood poisoning a month after delivering herself of a stillborn child. A doctor was summoned, but when he found he was not to be paid he 'refused to do anything' and left. The Poor Law medical officer's locum was then called, but he refused to help without a fee or a relief order. During this month and for twenty days afterwards, the woman's only attention came from a 'handy woman' at a nearby newsvendor's shop. The woman was finally removed to the workhouse infirmary and died a week later.[148] In 1862 at Wapping a blacksmith's wife began labour, her husband obtained a Poor Law order and went to the Tower Hamlets parish midwife, at night. The midwife called from an upper window, telling the blacksmith to put the paper under the door and she would

come in ten minutes. The midwife never arrived and the wife haemorrhaged to death. The midwife claimed in court that she found no order
'among the papers put under her door', so she did not attend.[149]

The miserly nature of the Poor Law medical system almost enjoined neglect. Dr Defriez, the medical officer for Bethnal Green, was
charged with manslaughter after the death of a patient in 1871. He
founded his defence on the facts that in return for a salary of £150 a
year, he was expected to attend the parochial dispensary daily for two
hours; he had an average of 60 'special' (acute surgical etc.) cases a year;
100 midwifery cases; he paid 40-80 home visits each day and as fresh
orders were issued twice each day he often had to double back on his
route. He was overworked and overtired. The outcome of the case is unclear, but probably Defriez was released. The coroner told the jury that
'there was no possibility of a conviction'.[150] Parish midwives, who
sometimes got as little as 3*d*. per case, also overworked themselves in
order to make a profit. Throughout the century, midwives in populous
Unions were claiming for up to 600 cases every year.[151] Inevitably,
doctors appointed assistants, and hurried over cases. 'Scalpel' argued in
1846 that his low Poor Law salary compelled him to employ an assistant because he 'could not afford to neglect the private patients'. He
paid the assistant only £30 a year, the maximum going rate for an untrained man. Like other assistants, 'he attends midwifery cases, although he may never have seen a human uterus'. But then, 'Scalpel'
admitted, 'the poor people have no alternative'.[152] Jane Reeves died at
Powick in Worcestershire in 1842. After several hours of agony with an
incompetent parish midwife, her husband, after waiting several more
hours for the relieving officer to come home, secured an order for the
Poor Law surgeon. He was away in London. His assistant, Davis, arrived
some time later, did nothing, remarked that 'all would be well', and
left twenty hours later. At 3 p.m. next day, when Reeves was sinking,
Davis was summoned again. But Davis 'had a cold' and went to bed. The
husband went to him again at 7 p.m. and received a verbal direction to
go to another surgeon, Mr Herbert. Mr Herbert sent him to Mr Turley,
who refused to see the husband, but sent a note to the door saying that he
'was not in the habit of attending Mr Mear's [the parish surgeon's]
patients'. The husband went back to Mr Herbert. He had gone to bed.
Then the husband returned to the relieving officer, who issued, as was
necessary to guarantee him his fee, a separate order for Mr Turley.
Turley then sent his assistant, who helped the midwife deliver a baby
weighing 9 lb 3 oz. Jane Reeves died 30 minutes later. The post-mortem
showed a ruptured uterus. The *Lancet* remarked that this finding
showed that Reeves 'would have died anyway'. The coroner's jury

found Davis 'guilty of inattention'. The Poor Law rules never provided for alternative medical care.[153]

Dr Wood was charged with manslaughter in Boston in 1875 after he had been called to a woman in labour who was 'exhausted', 'haemorrhaging and very low'. He rapidly delivered the baby with instruments and while doing so he perforated the uterus. The woman was now 'in a state of collapse'. Wood stayed ten minutes after the delivery and then left. The woman lingered for three hours before she died. The *Lancet*'s comment indicates some norms of practice: 'it is a new idea that a doctor is to be . . . tried for manslaughter because he did not stay a certain number of minutes, or administer a certain amount of brandy. This is a doctrine at once absurd and intolerable.'[154]

Paradoxically, the payment for 'extras' sometimes produced unnecessary attention. From 1847 there was a differential for 'instrument cases' above the usual confinement fee; by 1905 it had reached £2, compared with the usual 10s.[155] At East Hetton, Durham, in 1859 a parish surgeon was called to a woman in a difficult labour. He arrived tipsy and immediately started a needless craniotomy. The untrained assistant of another doctor abetted him. Even after the craniotomy he could not extract the foetus, but went on pulling and probing with the crotchet until he perforated the uterus. Finally he penetrated an artery and the woman died in a rush of blood. He was imprisoned for one year for manslaughter.[156]

The labour wards in workhouses were wretched places until the workhouses and workhouse infirmaries were cleaned up during the late 1860s and early 1870s. At Sevenoaks, for example, there were, in January 1842, five women in two beds in a room 10 feet 9 inches long by 7 feet wide. The ward, according to the investigator, was 'beastly beyond description'.[157] In the 1860s the *Lancet* commission of inquiry into London workhouse infirmaries found that every lying-in ward was 'crammed' and noisome with old well-used 'bed-sacking, etc. stained with fetid discharges'.[158] The Poor Law Royal Commission reported in 1909 that affairs were much the same.[159]

The death rate was high, but was possibly less than we might expect. There are no official figures before the mid-1860s and thereafter the kinds of under-reporting that I have described earlier particularly apply. In 1865, 39 London workhouses reported 2,728 cases of childbirth, with 16 deaths, concentrated in nine of the workhouses. Over all the rate equals 6 per 1,000, or about equal to the reported rate of the British Lying-in Hospital for 1849-61, at 7 per 1,000, but much below the 40 per 1,000 rate for 1857 to 1863 at Queen Charlotte's, the hospital which admitted single women.[160] But the workhouse rate is almost twice the death rate for the outdoor midwifery department of St George's Hospital for 1853-63, at 3.5 per 1,000.[161] The Liverpool Workhouse Hospital had a notably good record from the 1860s. Two-thirds of its intake were single women, and about half were primiparae. In the late 1860s the maternal death rate was about 4 per 1,000, that is below the national average, almost the same as in the 1890s. But Liverpool led the country in having trainee obstetric nurses, fully trained midwives and monthly nurses for post-natal care. The Liverpool figures were probably exceptionally good also because the guardians were unusually generous with orders for outdoor deliveries managed by closely supervised midwives.[162] The workhouse at Brighton, newly built in the 1860s, with similar proportions of single primiparae mothers, and similar generous administration, also claimed exceptionally good results: only one death among 223 confinements between 1862 and 1868.[163]

Stability and Change in the Maternal Death Rate

This survey of the evidence about maternity practices and maternal death rates suggests three general conclusions. First a woman and her infant did best if the birth was managed outside a hospital. Second, mother and child were safest, if the birth was a normal one, with a midwife; and if not, they were in grave danger. Midwives carried less infection with them, doctors brought instruments that in the last resort could save life. Third, there was no overwhelming displacement of midwives by *accoucheurs*, despite assertions to the contrary in recent historical-polemical writing. *Accoucheurs* probably extended their practice among the comfortable classes, while the increase in disposable income and the spread of the Poor Law system after 1834 probably enabled a growing number of poor women to dispense with neighbours and relatives and to have attention from experienced midwives. By the mid-1870s Dr Farr estimated that about 70 per cent of all births in England and Wales were managed by midwives.[164] In 1892 one informed observer guessed that midwives were handling about half the 870,000 labours a year in England and Wales.[165] The variations through Great Britain are enormous, and inexplicable except in local contexts which we have not yet explored. In 1869 the Obstetrical Society asked its Fellows to report on the proportion of attendance by midwives in their neighbourhoods over the past few years. The results run: for three villages — Fleggburgh, Norfolk, population 554, reported 30 per cent; Gringley-on-the-Hill, Nottinghamshire, population 874, 46 per cent;

Bromyard, Herefordshire, population 1,300, 90 per cent. The average for the reports from 'small manufacturing towns' at 6,000-10,000 populations ran at about 5-10 per cent; Lewes was 'nil'; Long Sutton in Lincolnshire was 26 per cent; Altringham in Cheshire, 53 per cent. 'Large manufacturing towns', Glasgow, for example, ran at about 75 per cent, and Edinburgh almost none; Coventry 90 per cent. In Wakefield, all the Irish were delivered by midwives, all the English by doctors. The parishes of the East End of London varied between 30 and 50 per cent; the West End was 'very slight' at under 2 per cent. The availability of students from medical schools made a difference, because women preferred them, at least in Edinburgh and the East End. There was always a crisis and a rush for midwives during the hospital vacations.[166] The ratio of confinements managed by midwives was still varied through the country in 1909. Over all, it was said to be about 50 per cent, but in Newcastle it was only 11.2 per cent, in the London County Council area 25 per cent, in the West Riding 35 per cent, Liverpool 52 per cent, Manchester 60.9 per cent, Gloucester 83.6 per cent, and 93 per cent in St Helens. The availability of local charity funds must also have shaped the pattern of attendances, especially in richly endowed towns with a low birth rate, such as Exeter, or towns under local Acts outside the Poor Law, such as Coventry and Brighton.[167] This might explain the 100 per cent doctor attendance in Lewes. But as the Wakefield figures show, there are no simple answers. Were the Irish boycotting Protestant doctors? Were the doctors boycotting the Irish? At first sight it could be a case of Catholic women preferring to be delivered by women, but Irish women at home and elsewhere in Britain happily went to doctors for their confinements. Perhaps the Irish came within the rubric of a local Irish midwives' charity? But these speculations only illustrate how little we really know, and why sweeping assertions about the midwives/doctors question are ill founded. What is clear is that, whether delivered by a doctor or a midwife, the mother had to be strong, and lucky, to survive.

The stability of the maternal death rate throughout the century suggests that antisepsis and improvements in obstetrics made little difference. Indeed, as I have suggested, the increased resort to instruments might have maintained the rate during the last third of the century and into the 1930s. The death rate for 'accidents' held up until 1941-2. The servant-employing classes who retained expensive *accoucheurs* bought greater peace of mind, but no real lessening of their vulnerability. Fifty years of expensive education in midwifery ought to have made doctors

B. C.

less rough and more resourceful in a crisis, but measured against the death rate it does not appear to have done so. The spread of trained midwives must have helped lower the rate in the twentieth century, but again one would have expected their impact to have been greater than it appears to have been. This was partly because the trained midwives were not getting to the women who needed them most.

In Rotherham, for instance, where midwives were hand-picked by the health authorities and especially encouraged, 25 per cent of births in 1907 and 1908 were still 'unattended' and 25 per cent were attended by 'old un-qualified women'. 'Some women', Dr Robinson, the MOH, alleged, 'go un-attended or employ "unqualified women" because they have a reputation for having a large amount of what we call in Yorkshire "churchyard luck" [i.e. a high proportion of the infants they delivered were 'stillborn'].'[168]

The death rate from toxaemia also remained almost unchanged until it was halved between 1941 and 1945. Clearly the spread of the new penicillin drugs and the improved nutrition of expectant mothers during the war made the great breakthrough.[169]

The clue to the first transition in 1903-7 might lie in the decreased number of pregnancies past the eighth (and a consequent reduction in the number of women bearing children at the more dangerous end over 30) of the child-bearing age range. Maternal deaths at the eighth confine-ment, following Australian experience during the period 1892-1900, probably became statistically more likely that at primiparae.[170] There are no comparable data available for Britain, but there is no reason why the Australian situation should not apply. This reduction ultimately depends on greater recourse to contraception and its greater effective-ness.[171] We have no detailed information about the effectiveness of contraceptive practices and the sale of devices in this period,[172] but it is worth recalling that the decline in the English birth rate begins in 1877, in the same year as the rumpus in the daily press, the Church and the judiciary about the spread of information about family limitation. If family limitation is the key to the breakthrough, it is also worth recal-ling, in the light of the implicit medical cost-benefit sum, that medical doctors, with a few notable exceptions, determinedly fought the spread of contraception (at least in their public utterances) to mothers who practised or at least approved family limitation, and were themselves in the midst of their child-bearing years. And from what we know of present custom, it is a likely hypothesis that mothers encouraged daughters in family limitation and passed on contraceptive knowledge. Over all, it is worth emphasising that the maternal mortality is lower than we might have expected, given the poor nutrition and fatigue of overworked pregnant women, the risks of infection, the want of skill in the attendants and other hazards. But, as in modern Indonesia or Mexico, human reproductive processes outmatch poverty, ignorance and anaemia.[173] While 3,200 died in childbirth in England and Wales in 1847, over 450,000 lived (i.e. 1 death in 140); 3,000 died in 1861 and over 700,000 lived (1 death in 233); 4,400 died in 1891, and 860,000 lived (1 death in 198).[174] Here, the bias to mortality in our evidence is vividly exposed. One is left with an impression, both awesome and tantalisingly untraceable, of prodigious private stoicisms and strengths.

Notes

1. Dr William Farr, *Lancet* (hereafter *L*), 11 Aug. 1860, p. 138; *Parliamentary Papers* (hereafter *PP*), 1884-5, vol. XVII, p. lxxiii; Dr Thursfield, *L*, 7 Jan. 1893, p. 21; Janet M. Campbell, *Maternal Mortality* (London, 1924), p. 3; J.W.B. Douglas and G. Rowntree, *Maternity in Great Britain* (Oxford, 1948), p. 36.
2. *L*, 30 June 1866, p. 721.
3. Dr Farr, *L*, 26 Oct. 1872, p. 606; *PP*, 1895, vol. XXIII, part I, p. xxii; *PP*, 1904, vol. XIV, p. lxvi.
4. *L*, 13 Jan. 1872, p. 55.
5. *PP*, 1895, vol. XXIII, part I, p. xxii.
6. *L*, 3 June 1882, p. 919.
7. *PP*, 1895, vol. XXIII, part I, p. xxii; Dr W. Williams, *L*, 2 Jan. 1897, p. 50.
8. *PP*, 1895, vol. XXIII, part I, p. 685.
9. Anon., *The Ladies Friend* (new ed.) London, n.d. [c. 1800], pp. 147-8; Thomas Andrew, *A Cyclopedia of Domestic Medicine And Surgery* (London, 1842), pp. 429-30; Mrs Isabella Beeton, *Manual of Household Management* (first published London, 1860, reprinted 1968), p. 1034.
10. Robert Ferguson, *Gooch on some of the Most Important Diseases peculiar to Women* . . . (London, 1859), esp. pp. xliii-xliv, 98-123; Alexander Milne, *L*, 2 Nov. 1872, p. 659; Alexander Miller, 'Twenty Years' Obstetric Practice', *GMJ*, vol. LI (1899), p. 255.
11. James Blundell, 'Lectures on Midwifery', *L*, 24 Nov. 1827, p. 287; James Liston, *L*, 13 May 1871, p. 673; T.B. Grensdale, 'On the Use of Gloves . . .', *GMJ*, vol. LXV (1906), pp. 75-6; Curt Proskauer, 'Development and Use of the Rubber Glove in Surgery and Gynecology', *Journal of the History of Medicine*, vol. XIII (1958) pp. 374-80.
12. 'Censor', *L*, 25 Jan. 1845, p. 105, 22 Feb. 1845, p. 223.
13. W.N. Ryland, 'On the Stethoscope . . .', *Anderson's Quarterly Journal of Medicine and Surgery*, vol. III (1826), pp. 159-60.
14. Beeton, *Household Management*, p. 1023.
15. Dr Waller, *L*, 12 May 1828, p. 219; *British and Foreign Medical Review*, vol. II (1836), p. 79, 89; T.H. Jackson, 'Cannabis Indica – Its Uncertain Action', *Edinburgh Medical Journal*, vol. II (1856-7), p. 667; Alexander Milne, *L*, 2 Nov. 1872, p. 659; Alexander Miller, 'Twenty Years' Obstetric Practice', *GMJ*, vol. L1 (1899), p. 225; A.J. Pepper, 'Some Aspects of Forty Years' Hospital Experience', *L*, 11 Sept. 1909, p. 767.
16. Milne, *L*, 2 Nov. 1872, p. 659.

17. *L*, 10 Nov. 1877, p. 702; *GMJ*, vol. LXII (1904), p. 259.

18. *London Journal of Medicine,* vol. II (1849), pp. 971-2.

19. *L*, 14 Aug. 1847, p. 177, 18 Sept. 1847, p. 305.

20. *L*, 20 Nov. 1847, pp. 549-50, 11 Dec. 1847, pp. 626-31, 1 Jan. 1848, p. 17, 20 May 1848, pp. 554-68; Dr Samuel Ashwell, 'Late Obstetric Physician and Lecturer at Guy's Hospital', *L*, 11 Mar. 1848, p. 291; *London Journal of Medicine,* vol. I (1849), pp. 50-1; *Edinburgh Medical and Surgical Journal*, vol. LXXII (1849), p. 79. One prominent supporter of Simpson, Dr John Gardner, of Cavendish Square, drew much criticism for saying that his patients had expressed the 'liveliest satisfaction' under ether in childbirth. As Robert Barnes, Lecturer on Midwifery at the Hunterian School of Medicine, remarked, 'the question is not to be decided by the . . . female sex [or] by wanton abuse of medical practitioners' (*L*, 10 Jan. 1847, p. 55, 25 Dec. 1847, p. 678. W.E. Gladstone's entry in his diary on the birth of his first child in 1840 provides a vivid, sophisticated insight into the deeply held theodicy upon which childbirth anaesthesia was soon to intrude:

3 June 1840
At 6 P.M. [sc. a.m.] C. awakened me & sent me for Dr Locock, who was here before 7. The whole day was consumed in a slow but favourable labour. Till 11 the pains were slight — till 3 quite ineffectual, about 7½ they began to assume the expulsory character. Praise & thanks be to God for his mercies to her & for the fortitude he gives her. This is to me a new scene & lesson in human life. I have seen her endure today — less than the average for first children, says Dr L, yet six times as much bodily pain as I have undergone in my whole life. 'In sorrow shalt thou bring forth children' is the woman's peculiar curse, & the note of Divine Judgment upon her in Adam: so 'she shall be saved in childbearing' is her peculiar promise in Christ. — How many thoughts does this agony excite: the comparison of the termination with the commencement: the undergoings of another for our sakes: the humbling & sobering view of human relations here presented: the mixed & intricate considerations of religion which may be brought to bear upon the question of the continuation of our wayward race. Certainly the woman has this blessing that she may as a member of Christ behold in these pains certain especially appointed means of her purification with a willing mind, & so the more cheerfully hallow them by willing endurance into a thank offering. 'I offer these my sufferings O Lord unto thee as being precious gifts of thine, most calling for my gratitude, because most fruitful in promoting the work of my renewal'; whereunto also they were appointed.

Saw Farquhar & wrote confusedly on the U.C.C. case. Even there difficulties have been found! notes &c. about C. & spent most of the day in her room, read Buxton's Remedy (when all was over).

At 11¼ all was happily ended by the birth of a vigorous little boy [William Henry G.]. Catherine's relief & delight were beyond anything. She has been most firm & gallant, altho not only Lady W[enlock] & Lady B[raybrooke] (the only friends who have been in the house) but Dr L[ecock], encouraged her to scream. Weariness & a disposition to sleep protracted the latter stages. It seemed for a time as if there was not 'strength to bring forth'. — Her first wish after it was that I should offer a prayer. The child gave a faint chirp immediately on issuing into the world & then a longer cry when they were bringing him from under the bedclothes. He was declared to be extremely like me: with Catherine's mouth: he opened his eyes & looked deliberately at the nurse while she was enlarging his cap to put it on, as much as to say 'What are you about'? (M.R.D. Foot and H.C.G. Matthew, *The Gladstone Diaries* (Oxford, 1974), vol. III, pp. 32-3.

21. *London Journal of Medicine,* vol. II (1849), p. 1107.

22. *L*, 24 Dec. 1853, p. 611.

23. *L*, 11 Mar. 1848, p. 291.

24. *L*, 27 Jan. 1849, p. 100; *London Journal of Medicine,* vol. II (1849), p. 1107; *L*, 27 Mar. 1847, p. 321.

25. *L*, 24 Dec. 1853, p. 610. Compare the Paleyian cast of the argument as presented by Robert Barnes:

Nature has secured the safety and the end of parturition through so many admirable provisions, that she may be truly said to disdain assistance . . . No arguments . . . have hitherto proved that any one of the phenomena manifested in ordinary labour is hurtful or superfluous. Even pain . . . has its use . . . It is an outrage upon the fundamental law of adaptation to assume that a beneficient 'Creator' has associated pain with the parturient process for other than a wise and necessary purpose (*L*, 13 July 1850, p. 39).

26. I.B. Brown, *L*, 29 Apr. 1848, p. 476; Dr Neil Arnott, *L*, 14 May 1859; A.R. Simpson, 'The Jubilee of Anaesthetic Midwifery', *GMJ*, vol. XCVII (1897), pp. 178-9.

27. *L*, 18 Apr. 1857, p. 410, 6 Mar. 1858, p. 254, 22 Dec. 1860, p. 614.

28. Tyler Smith, *L*, 20 Nov. 1847, p. 544.

29. *L*, 9 Oct. 1841, p. 64, 2 Oct. 1847, pp. 345-65, 21 Dec. 1850, p. 697; T.W. Moody and J.C. Beckett, *Queen's, Belfast 1845-1949* (London, 1959), vol. I, pp. 257-9.

30. *L*, 5 Feb. 1842, p. 664.

31. Lyon Playfair, Select Committee on the Medical Act (1858) Amendment Bill, *PP*, 1878-9, vol. XII, Qs. 187, 192.

32. *L*, 30 July 1853, p. 111; Charles Newman, *The Evolution of Medical Education in the Nineteenth Century* (London, 1957), pp. 95, 163, 218.

33. John Simon, 'Address at Medical Teachers Association' (1861), *L*, 25 Jan. 1868, p. 117; Select Committee on the Medical Act (1858) Amendment Bill, *PP*, 1878-9, vol. XII, Sir James Paget, Qs. 2497-8, Lyon Playfair, Q. 2672, Appendix, pp. 404-8; R.R. Rentoul, *L*, 18 Apr. 1891, p. 875; F. de Havilland Hall, *Westminster Hospital Reports*, vol. XI (1899), pp. 29-33 (describing his 'education' in obstetrics in the late 1860s).

34. *L*, 27 Nov. 1847, p. 580; Select Committee on the Medical Act (1858) Amendment Bill, Sir Dominic Corrigan, Qs. 2979-83, Rev. S. Haughton, Qs. 3470-1; 'Metropolitan Hospital Enquiry', *L*, 20 June 1891, pp. 1411-12.

35. *L*, 27 Nov. 1830, pp. 301-3, 19 June 1841, p. 461.

36. *L*, 27 Nov. 1830, pp. 302-3; de Havilland Hall, *Westminster Hospital Reports,* vol. XI (1899), p. 29.

37. *L*, 13 Mar. 1897, p. 770.

38. *BMJ*, 5 Mar. 1892, p. 524.

39. *BMJ*, 16 Nov. 1907, p. 1435.

40. G.T. Hayden, Surgeon to the Anglesey Dispensary, 'A Case of Collapse, after Parturition . . .', *Dublin Journal of Medical and Chemical Science*, vol. I (1832), pp. 180-2. On 'binders', see *Medical Gazette,* 10 Sept. 1836, p. 915.

41. *L*, 22 Mar. 1845, pp. 341-2, 19 Apr. 1845, p. 452-75.

42. *L*, 4 Apr. 1846, p. 393.

43. John Clarke, *Observations on the Puerperal Fever* . . . [1790], reprinted, with introduction, by Fleetwood Churchill (ed.), *Essays on the Puerperal Fever* (London, 1849), pp. 376-7.

44. *L*, 5 Apr. 1828, p. 2.

45. *L*, 2 Nov. 1872; Dr Edgar, 'Is there Room for Improvement . . .?', *GMJ*, vol. L (1898), pp. 177-9.

46. Dr H.C. Rowe, *L*, 27 May 1876, p. 777; W.S. Playfair, Professor of Obstetric Medicine. King's College Hospital, *BMJ*, 27 Sept. 1890, pp. 715-16. In 1860 Dr Robert Dunn, in private practice, claimed 'amongst [his] . . . greatest achievements in midwifery practice . . . the personal attendance on seven labours in 30 hours' (*L*, 21 July 1860, p. 64).

47. *L*, 30 May 1835, p. 299, 19 Mar. 1864, p. 345.

48. *L*, 29 July 1865, p. 126, 19 Jan. 1867, p. 99, 7 Jan. 1870; *BMJ*, 21 Sept. 1912, p. 748.

49. F.B. Smith, *The Making of the Second Reform Bill* (Melbourne and Cambridge, 1966), pp. 9, 64-5.

50. *L*, 12 Feb. 1878, 4 Apr. 1885, p. 633, 28 Jan. 1888, p. 216, 9 Aug. 1890, p. 365.

51. Robert Dunn, 'Statistics of Midwifery in Private Practice', *L*, 12 Nov. 1859, p. 484; E.F. Funell, 'The New Workhouse at Brighton', *L*, 23 May 1868, p. 673; Dr Williams, *L*, 2 Jan. 1897, p. 50; cf: Douglas and Rowntree, *Maternity in Great Britain*, p. 60.

52. Mr E. Evans and William Pendle, Poor Law Surgeons, St George's Southwark, Select Committee on Medical Poor Relief, *PP*, 1844, vol. IX, Qs. 2265, 2406-7.

53. *PP*, 1909, vol. XXXXII, pp. 124-5.

54. *L*, 1 Apr. 1871, p. 454.

55. *L*, 30 Jan. 1897, p. 330.

56. *L*, 8 Mar. 1834, p. 899, 11 July 1868, p. 58; *BMJ*, 20 Mar. 1869, p. 266; Rev. S. Hansard, *Charity Organization Reporter*, 20 May 1874, p. 261; 'Inquiry into London Special Hospital', *L*, 10 Apr. 1897, p. 1041.

57. 'A Constant Reader', *L*, 19 June 1858, p. 618; the 'Constant Reader' was protesting against medical students being denied access to clinical material, not the delay experienced by patients; *L*, 11 Aug. 1883, p. 266.

58. John Langdon-Davies, *Westminster Hospital: two centuries of voluntary service, 1719-1941* (London, 1952), p. 61.

59. J.C. Steele, 'Numerical Analysis of the Patients treated in Guy's Hospital . . . 1854-61', *JSS*, vol. XXIV (1861), pp. 388-99.

60. *L*, 4 June 1864, p. 640.

61. *L*, 7 July 1877, p. 22.

62. Robert Jardine, 'Notes of 1028 Cases . . .', *GMJ*, vol. XXXIX (1893), pp. 32-5.

63. J.C. Steele, 'The Charitable Aspects of Medical Relief', *JRSS*, vol. LIV (1891), p. 278.

64. *L*, 31 July 1869, p. 190.

65. *L*, 4 Aug. 1849, p. 132.

66. *L*, 19 Jan. 1850, p. 89.

67. *L*, 3 May 1873, pp. 640-1.

68. Rev. George Weight, 'Statistics of the Parish of St George The Martyr, Southwark', *JSS*, vol. III (1840), p. 71.

69. Thomas Archer, *The Terrible Sights of London and Labours of Love in the midst of them* (London, n.d. [1870?]), p. 62.

70. 'Junius', *L*, 10 July 1830, p. 577.

71. J. Weatherill, *L*, 14 May 1831, p. 208; see also *L*, 18 Jan. 1834, pp. 635-6 for further evidence of the proprietary nature of this institution.

72. 'Mass meeting of Glasgow Southern Medical Society on "Medical Charities, Particularly Dispensaries   Their Abuse" ', *GMJ*, vol. XXVI (1886), p. 392.

73. Helen Bosanquet, *Social Work in London 1869-1912* (London, 1914, new ed., Brighton, 1973), pp. 406-7.

74. J. Robertson, *L*, 2 Dec. 1843, p. 310.

75. *L*, 4 Aug. 1849, p. 132.
76. *L*, 18 Oct. 1862, p. 423.
77. Dr Graily Hewitt, *L*, 29 Nov. 1862, p. 596; Dr George B. Brodie, 'Statistics of Queen Charlotte's Lying-In Hospital', *L*, 4 June 1864, pp. 639-40.
78. *L*, 7 Mar. 1914, p. 721.
79. *L*, 16 Jan. 1897, p. 155.
80. *L*, 7 Jan. 1899, p. 43.
81. *L*, 16 Jan. 1897, p. 155.
82. *L*, 2 Jan. 1841, p. 504.
83. *L*, 21 Nov. 1840, pp. 315-16.
84. *L*, 19 Dec. 1840, pp. 438-41.
85. *L*, 2 Dec. 1843, p. 310, 9 Dec. 1843, p. 325.
86. *L*, 7 July 1877, p. 22, 23 Mar. 1895, p. 776, 16 Jan. 1897, p. 155.
87. *L*, 16 Jan. 1897, p. 155.
88. M.C. Buer, *Health, Wealth, and Population In the Early Days Of The Industrial Revolution* (London, 1926), pp. 146-7; G. Talbot Griffith, *Population Problems in the Age of Malthus* (Cambridge, 1926), p. 24.
89. *L*, 18 Oct. 1862, p. 423.
90. *L*, 18 Oct. 1862, p. 427, 7 July 1877, p. 22, 23 Jan. 1897, p. 221.
91. *L*, 8 Nov. 1862, pp. 518-19.
92. Buer, *Health, Wealth, And Population*, p. 145; 'Harvey Graham' [I.H. Flack], *Eternal Eve* (London, 1950), p. 369, cf. *Edinburgh Medical and Surgical Journal*, vol. III (1807), p. 323, and *JSS*, vol. XXI (1867), p. 172, quoting *Pall Mall Gazette*, 25 Jan. 1867.
93. J.E. Burton, *L*, 3 June 1882, p. 937; cf. *Guy's Hospital Reports*, second series, vol. VI (1849), p. 136, third series, vol. II (1856), pp. 8, 31, for similar differences in mortality between in- and out-patients.
94. *L*, 29 Apr. 1882, p. 704.
95. *L*, 5 Dec. 1868, p. 749.
96. *L*, 19 Jan. 1875, p. 98.
97. *L*, 22 Apr. 1882, p. 663, 29 Apr. 1882, p. 704, 21 Mar. 1885, p. 538.
98. *L*, 14 July 1877, p. 71.
99. *L*, Clement Godson, retiring presidential address to Gynaecological Association, 23 Jan. 1897, p. 221.
100. *L*, 10 Sept. 1831, p. 752, 27 Dec. 1845, p. 703, 2 Oct. 1875, p. 512; *BMJ*, 24 Aug. 1907, p. 480.
101. *L*, 8 June 1839, p. 396, 5 Aug. 1848, pp. 160-2, 29 Oct. 1853, p. 430, 17 Dec. 1859, p. 623.
102. *L*, 10 Apr. 1841, pp. 102-4.
103. *L*, 8 Oct. 1831, p. 72.
104. *L*, 19 Mar. 1864, p. 345 (Lincolnshire).
105. *L*, 25 Apr. 1840, pp. 160-1; see also 'S' (London), *L*, 2 Oct. 1875, p. 512.
106. *L*, 23 Oct. 1875, p. 615.
107. *Medical Gazette*, 30 June 1838, pp. 585-6; *BMJ*, 2 Apr. 1892, p. 750.
108. Ingleby Scott, 'Dr Elizabeth Blackwell', *Once A Week*, 16 June 1860, p. 577.
109. *Reasoner*, Feb. 1848, pp. 177-9; *National Secular Society Almanack* (1871), p. 31.
110. *L*, 11 July 1846, p. 56.
111. 'Mogostokos', 'On The Necessity of Accoucheurs', *London Medical and Physical Journal*, vol. XXXVI (1816), p. 198.
112. *L*, 23 Feb. 1895, p. 499.
113. *L*, 28 Jan. 1882, p. 154.

114. *Truth,* 7 Feb. 1895, p. 327; *L*, 9 Feb. 1895, p. 360.

115. *L*, 8 Oct. 1892, p. 860.

116. *L*, 29 Jan. 1848, p. 122, 10 Apr. 1852, p. 369.

117. Select Committee on Medical Poor Relief, *PP*, 1844, vol. IX, Qs. 4787-813.

118. *L*, 22 Oct. 1859, p. 419.

119. *L*, 12 Dec. 1840, p. 399.

120. *L*, 12 Dec. 1840, pp. 401-2.

121. *L*, 29 Jan. 1848, pp. 122-3.

122. Select Committee on Medical Poor Relief, *PP*, 1844, vol. IX, Qs. 1919, 2903; *L*, 2 Nov. 1872, p. 644, 2 Oct. 1909, p. 1033; Report on Midwives Act 1902, *PP*, 1909, vol. XXXIII, Q. 6956.

123. This struggle is recounted by Jean Donnison, *Midwives And Medical Men* (London, 1977).

124. *L*, 17 Sept. 1831, p. 800, 29 Jan. 1848, p. 123, 25 Mar. 1882, p. 498; *Once a Week*, 16 June 1860, p. 577.

125. *L*, 18 Feb. 1899, p. 463; A. Lindsey, *Socialized Medicine in England and Wales – The NHS 1948-1961* (Chapel Hill, North Carolina, 1962), pp. 294-5.

126. Alan Bullock, *The Life And Times Of Ernest Bevin* (London, 1960), vol. I, p. 2.

127. Mrs Maria Martin, Select Committee on Midwives Registration, *PP*, 1892, vol. XIV, Qs. 690-5.

128. *L*, 17 Apr. 1875, p. 563; E.P. Thompson, *The Making Of the English Working Class* (Penguin ed., 1968), p. 320, quotes a surgeon of Hebden Bridge in the early 1840s describing a similar practice. Howard, the surgeon, says that the use of the chairs was necessary because of the want of a change of bedclothing. My examples suggest that by the 1870s, at least, the practice was common among a wide range of classes and was not simply imposed by poverty.

129. *L*, 29 May 1875, p. 781, 5 June 1875, p. 813, 11 May 1872, p. 655.

130. *L*, 20 Apr. 1872, p. 564.

131. P.G. Craigie, 'The English Poor Rate . . .', *JRSS*, vol. LI (1888), pp. 465-6.

132. *L*, 4 July 1868, p. 27.

133. *L*, 19 Jan. 1833, pp. 537-41.

134. Sir John Walsham, Assistant Poor Law Commissioner, SC on Medical Poor Relief, 1844, vol. IX, Qs. 9692-98, G.C. Lewis, Q. 9834 (on Scotland); *Medical Gazette*, 30 Apr. 1841, p. 231.

135. *L*, 5 Feb. 1831, pp. 629-31.

136. Poor Law Commission, *PP*, 1834, vol. XXVIII, Appendix A, p. 741A; Thomas Watts, Wheatenhurst Union, Gloucestershire, *L*, 30 Jan. 1836, p. 709; Walker *v.* Guardians of the Thame Union, *L*, 20 Feb. 1864, p. 238; Royal Commission on the Poor Law, *PP*, 1909, vol. XLII, pp. 110-11.

137. William Ford, former overseer at Limehouse, SC on Medical Poor Relief 1844, *PP*, vol. IX, Qs. 9508-41.

138. Henry Pownall, chairman of Brentford Union, SC on Medical Poor Relief, 1844, *PP*, vol. IX, Qs. 3334-42.

139. William Baker junior, SC on Medical Poor Relief, 1844, *PP*, vol. IX, Qs. 9570-612.

140. *L*, 9 Jan. 1864, p. 54.

141. Norman Longmate, *The Workhouse* (London, 1974), p. 71.

142. *L*, 3 Nov. 1855, p. 419.

143. Joseph Rogers, *Reminiscences of a Workhouse Medical Officer* (London, 1889), pp. 8, 15-19.

144. *L*, 24 Oct. 1868, pp. 549-55.

145. *L*, 12 Apr. 1856, p. 412.

146. SC on Medical Poor Relief, 1844, *PP*, vol. IX, Qs. 3200-55.

147. Ruth G. Hodgkinson, *The Origins Of the National Health Service* (London, 1967), pp. 116-19. Dr Hodgkinson over-states the degree to which Poor Law medical officers knew security of tenure under the Orders of 1847; the Order had to be re-issued in 1855 and 1857 and doctors were still under threat in the late 1860s; see *L*, 24 Feb. 1855, pp. 219, 223, 6 June 1868, p. 725, 1 Aug. 1868, p. 156.

148. *L*, 28 Nov. 1894, p. 1230.

149. *L*, 27 Sept. 1862, p. 349.

150. *L*, 11 Mar. 1871, p. 357.

151. *L*, 24 Dec. 1870, p. 903.

152. *L*, 16 May 1846, p. 560.

153. *L*, 12 Feb. 1842, pp. 680-1.

154. *L*, 29 May 1875, p. 771.

155. Dr McVail, RC on Poor Laws, *PP*, 1909, vol. XLII, pp. 110-11.

156. *L*, 12 Mar. 1859, p. 272.

157. *L*, 22 Jan. 1842, p. 588.

158. *L*, 1 July 1865, p. 19.

159. See Dr McVail's Report on Workhouse Infirmaries, *RC on Poor Laws, PP*, 1909, vol. XLII, pp. 45-6.

160. *JSS*, vol. XXXI (1867), p. 172.

161. Ibid.

162. *Liverpool Medical and Surgical Reports*, vol. IV (1870), p. 155; *L*, 20 Feb. 1897, pp. 545-6.

163. E.F. Fussell, 'The New Workhouse at Brighton', *L*, 23 May 1868, p. 673.

164. Donnison, *Midwives*, p. 77.

165. Dr J.H. Aveling, Registration, *PP*, 1892, vol. XIV, Qs. 251-3.

166. Dr W. Graily Hewitt, SC on Midwives Registration, *PP*, 1892, vol. XIV, Qs. 1149-82.

167. 'Report on Midwives Act', *PP*, 1909, vol. XXXIII, p. 4.

168. Ibid., Qs. 2458-9, 2597.

169. Richard M. Titmuss, *Problems of Social Policy* (rev. ed., London, 1976), pp. 512-23, 535-7.

170. Campbell, *Maternal Mortality*, pp. 6-10; 'Maternal Mortality in Connection with Childbearing', *PP*, 1914-16, vol. XXVI.

171. See N.D. Hicks, *This Sin and Scandal. The Australian Population Debate 1891-1911* (Canberra, 1978).

172. J. Peel, 'The Manufacture and Retailing of Contraceptives in England', *Population Studies*, vol. XVII (1963-4).

173. Alan D. Berg, *The Nutrition Factor; its role in national development* (Washington D.C., 1973), pp. 15-16.

174. Calculated from *PP*, 1884-5, vol. XVII, p. lxxiii, *L*, 7 Jan. 1893, p. 21 and B.R. Mitchell and Phyllis Deane, *Abstract Of British Historical Statistics* (Cambridge, 1962), pp. 29-31.

2 INFANCY

Throughout the nineteenth century infants under one year comprised the single largest group at risk. From the 1840s onwards, the period for which we have reasonably firm evidence for the nation at large, about one-quarter of all deaths recorded in England and Wales were of infants under one year, and almost half of all deaths were of infants under five. The incidence of infant deaths was highest among the poor and lowest among the comfortable, and highest in all classes among illegitimates.

The average figures for the nation and for some of the great towns, which are usually the only figures quoted by historians, mask as much as they reveal, but they are given here as a datum from which to measure the significant variations. For England and Wales the averages run as shown in Table 2.1.

Table 2.1: Infant Death Rate, England and Wales, 1839-1912 (per 1,000 live births)

1839 – 40	153
1841 – 5	147
1846 – 50	161
1851 – 5	156
1856 – 60	150
1861 – 5	151
1866 – 70	157
1871 – 5	153
1876 – 80	144
1881 – 5	139
1886 – 90	145
1891 – 5	151
1896 – 1900	156
1901 – 5	138
1906 – 10	117
1911 – 12	113

Source: B.R. Mitchell and Phyllis Deane, *Abstract of British Historical Statistics* (Cambridge, 1962), pp. 36-7.

In 1899 the rate was 163 per 1,000, the worst ever recorded. The

Registrar-Generals' reports for Scotland are available only from 1855, and are given in Table 2.2.

Table 2.2: Infant Death Rate, Scotland, 1855-1912 (per 1,000 live births)

1855 – 60	120
1861 – 5	120
1866 – 70	122
1871 – 5	127
1876 – 80	118
1881 – 5	118
1886 – 90	121
1891 – 5	126
1896 – 1900	129
1901 – 5	120
1906 – 10	112
1911 – 12	109

Source: ibid.

The main point shown by these tables is that the infant death rate remained steady, even rose, until the turn of the century, a generation after the general death rate began to fall.[1]

Too low though these reported infant mortality figures certainly are, it is worth recalling that excepting Scandinavia, where Sweden, for example, had reported rates of around 111 per 1,000 during the 1860s, British rates were the lowest in Europe. France had reported rates of 216 per 1,000 for the 1850s and 1860s, Prussia 220 per 1,000, Spain 226 per 1,000 and Bavaria 372 per 1,000 for the same decades.[2] In 1975 the English rate was 15.7 per 1,000 and the Scottish 17 per 1,000. Many nineteenth-century critics and some contemporary British historians blame the Industrial Revolution for the appalling British rates and there are good grounds for this as I shall suggest later, but the Continental averages imply that we ought to look to other conditions as well. Before we proceed, it is worth reminding ourselves of what these death rates mean in terms of actual individual lives and bereavements. In 1841, in England and Wales, there were 75,507 recorded infant deaths; in 1861, 106,428; in 1881, 114,976; in 1901, 140,648.[3]

The ways in which the British figures are understated are relevant to our explanation of the enormous variations from the mean. Civil registration of births in England and Wales, which began in 1837, was not

1837

compulsory until 1874. In Scotland there was no civil registration of
births until 1855, when it became obligatory. Historical demographers
have calculated under-registration of live births, especially among
illegitimates and the very poor at about 10 per cent over England and
Wales, and 20 per cent for London until about 1845, improving to 6
per cent for the nation in 1855 and 5.4 per cent by 1865.[4] These
corrections are probably still too low. The demographers have under-
rated 'stillbirths'. Only after 1874 in England and Wales and 1855 in
Scotland was a certificate legally required for the burial of a 'stillborn'
child.[5] Yet there is widespread evidence that this stipulation was often
ignored until the twentieth century. Merciful *accoucheurs* and midwives seem often to have arranged for the disposal as 'stillborn' of
infants who died within hours or days of birth. At a Glasgow medical
society discussion in 1888 Mr T.F. Gilmore is reported as implying that
he did not attempt to save infants born badly deformed. His remarks
apparently passed as nothing extraordinary.[6] Even among 'well-to-do
people, well nourished and carefully nursed', in one large private practice in the West End during the 1870s, one in 30 of the births was
'stillborn'. Many of these infants must have been premature, and the
few figures I have found for deaths of premature babies suggest that
babies born under 5¾ lb weight had poor chances.[7] (At present babies
are defined as premature at 5½ lb.) Research in 1946 showed that
prematurity was almost twice as common among agricultural workers
as among professional and salaried ones, and about a third more common among manual workers.[8] Presumably the same or worse ratios
obtained in the nineteenth century. But this is a subject that can only
be settled by intensive scrutiny of hospital and private practice records.

Deaths are said to have been more comprehensively registered. Dr
William Farr, effectively the Registrar-General for England and Wales,
claimed in 1839 a 98 per cent coverage for his first report.[9] My scrappy
evidence about uncertificated burials of illegitimate and 'stillborn'
babies suggests that Farr was over-confident. Old midwives in the larger
towns had understandings with local cemetery officials to bury small
coffins with no questions asked beyond, in order to meet a requirement in the Registration Act of 1874, a pencilled note from the doctor
or midwife to the general effect that the deceased was believed to have
been 'stillborn', 'prematurely born', or to have suffered 'fatal convulsions' or 'nine day fits'.[10] Midwives, sixpenny doctors and the mothers
themselves were happy to keep their distance from officialdom and
possible inquests. Moreover, the attendant's fee was more certain if she
could save her patient the burial charges, which ranged from 1*s*. 6*d*. to

over 7*s*. 6*d*. for a normally certificated child. An old midwife in Hanley in 1896 had throughout her career arranged for the disposal of infants up to a week old. When the father of one 'stillborn' child spoke of registering the body for burial, she told him 'he had no business with the police' and to leave it to her. Her fees for such all-inclusive service were 4*s*. for babies which lived beyond a few hours, and 3*s*. for the 'stillborn' ones.[11] In the mid-1860s the *Lancet* alleged that 56 such interments had been made during 1862 from just one poor London parish, St Giles.[12] The *Lancet*, reporting a case involving several such burials in Portsmouth in 1888, remarked that the practice was 'common' throughout the country.[13] During 1903, when registration presumably was tighter than fifty years before, a scrutiny of the records of the main cemeteries of Manchester over the last decade revealed that up to 1,500 infants had been unofficially interred each year.[14] If we allow that half this number had been live births, that is, had breathed and had existences distinct from their mothers', (the evidence from Portsmouth and St Giles suggests that was higher), and allot similar numbers for the dozen great towns and London parishes, we have a minimum addition to the unrecorded numbers of infant deaths of 10,000 a year.

It follows that the variations from the national average death rates among the poor are even greater than such official figures as we have.

The poorer the parents, the more vulnerable were their offspring, whether in city, town or countryside. In 1835 Dr John Roberton examined the burial registers for the Collegiate Church at Manchester over the period 1816-23 and Rusholme cemetery for 1821-5. Burials of 'stillborn' children had not been entered in either register. The 'poorest class' buried their dead at the Collegiate Church and 'a class somewhat above the very lowest' at the general cemetery. Over 50 per cent of the burials from both groups were aged under five, as shown in Table 2.3.[15]

In York, Dr Laycock calculated from the reported deaths under one year old for 1839-43 that the 'highest' parishes, topographically and socially, had a percentage rate of all deaths of 17.6, 'middle' parishes 20, and 'lowest' 23. Children under five comprised 42 per cent of all deaths in the town during the period.[16] Alexander Finlaison, the vital statistician, concluded from returns for Bath in 1839 that one in two of the offspring of 'Agricultural and other Labourers, Artisans and Servants' died under five years, while the rate for the offspring of 'Gentry and Professional Persons' was one in eleven.[17] During the late 1850s and early 1860s in Preston the death rate under five years among the 'upper classes' was said to be 18 in 100 deaths, 36 in 100 among dass.

the 'middle classes' and 62-64 in 101 among the 'industrial or insuring
classes'.[18] Enormous disparities still existed at the end of the century:
in 1899 the upper-class wards of Liverpool had an infant death rate of
136 per 1,000, the poor wards 274 per 1,000. A few streets within
these poor wards had rates of 509 per 1,000.[19] By 1902 the Sefton
Park division of Liverpool had a rate of 120 per 1,000, and the Scotland
Division 222 per 1,000.[20] Throughout the period agricultural or grazing
counties were below or near the national average death rate, while
counties with industrial towns were above it. London had much the
worst rate, although this may partly be a result of better registration.
By 191·1 the differences between rural and urban rates had narrowed,
but country infants still had a slightly better chance of survival.[21]

Table 2.3: Roberton's Findings on Child Deaths

	Total Deaths in Register	Under 2 Years (per cent)	2–5 Years (per cent)	5–10 Years (per cent)	Total Under 10 Years (per cent)
Collegiate Church	8,656	50.40	14.78	4.47	59.63
Rusholme cemetery	3,559	40.06	12.36	3.82	56.31

Source: *Medical Gazette*, 21 Feb. 1835, p. 733.

The persistence of these high rates in the face of advances in medical
science prompted several fashions in explanation. Those explanations
which laid the blame on the mothers were attractive to doctors and
moralists because they were at once economical, exonerative of the
profession, and often fitted the facts. The clearest example was the
correlation between high infantile death rates and illegitimacy.

Illegitimacy

In Marylebone Vestry district between 1843 and 1858, 516 of 1,109,
that is 46 per cent, of infants born illegitimate died at under 12 months
old. In All Souls' district, of 145 born, 87 died, or 53 per cent; in
Christchurch, of 223 born, 209 died, or 93 per cent; in St John's, of 148
born, 129 died, or 87 per cent.[22] For 1874 in Glasgow Dr J.B. Russell,
the city's Medical Officer of Health, calculated that illegitimates formed
27.7 per cent of the total mortality compared with 14.9 per cent for

legitimates, yet illegitimates comprised only 8.5 per cent of the registered births.[23] In Sheffield during the mid-1870s illegitimates died at a
rate of 582 per 1,000 live births, while legitimates averaged 162 per
1,000.[24] At the end of the century illegitimates in the Rhondda were
still dying at more than twice the rate of legitimates.[25]

Moralists had two main interpretations of these figures. Feminist
purity campaigners, such as Miss Wolstenholme, argued that the law
placed an unfair burden on the mother. She was legally responsible for
the child. The father, if he could be found, summoned and brought to
court, was only liable for 5s. per week for the first six weeks and
2s. 6d. for the next thirteen. But this process rarely eventuated: and
the mother was responsible for all the legal expenses.[26] The other line
of argument, strongly held by the Rev. Henry Butter and Dr Curvengen
(a founder of the Infant Life Protection Association in the mid-1860s),
was that illegitimates, as offspring of peculiarly degraded parents, were
especially vulnerable to all the dangers that beset infants in Victorian
England, to constitutional weaknesses, violence and the diseases that
ensued from neglect.[27] Implicit in both sets of diagnosis, although
neither Miss Wolstenholme nor Mr Butter drew the moral, was that
illegitimates were peculiarly the victims of poverty.

The mothers of illegitimates lacked the will and the neighbourhood
support that enabled their more fortunate working-class sisters to marry
when they became pregnant or obtain an abortion. George Moore may
have gathered his information second-hand, but his delineation of
Esther Waters' travails is almost a textbook case of this situation. Girls
dishonoured by social superiors had no chance at all, as the mid-nine-
teenth-century venereologist, William Acton, noticed.[28] Girls isolated
from their families, domestic servants, dressmakers and fashion-trade
workers, were especially open to seduction and appear to have been the
least capable of remedying their plight. On the other hand, the highest
registered illegitimacy rates occurred in the most rural counties,
Cumberland, Hereford, Norfolk and Westmorland, and the lowest in
metropolitan Middlesex and Surrey. Monmouthshire, Cornwall, Staffordshire and Lancashire had low illegitimacy rates, but were said to have
high rates of 'early marriage'. In general, mining districts had low illegitimacy rates, agricultural districts high ones. In Scotland, illegitimates were often legitimated by the subsequent marriage of their
parents. Clearly, local marriage and abortion customs, inheritance
systems, masculinity ratios, local patterns of housing, household income and savings were important, but the elucidation of these variations must wait again for local studies. The results of such studies are

likely to be surprising. One contemporary observer remarked of Norfolk, which had a relatively high illegitimacy rate, that the males were below the national average in 'education' while the women were well above it, and that the proportion of women who married under the normal age of marriage was much below the national average, thereby implying among other possibilities that Norfolk women preferred to raise their children as illegitimate rather than yoke themselves to dolts.[29]

Wet-Nursing

One outcome of poverty and isolation peculiar to single mothers was wet-nursing. This was the negotiation by which a woman with milk suckled the child of another woman for money and keep. Wealthy mothers who feared to ruin their figures by prolonged lactation, or who, like Catherine Gladstone in 1842, found themselves unable to nurse their infant, or who tired of the broken hours and coarseness of suckling; like Jane Austen's sister-in-law, and Lady Arabella in *Doctor Thorne*, all engaged wet-nurses;[30] as did bereaved fathers left with infants and wanting the best rearing for them, like Mr Dombey. As Dr Haden explained in 1827: '*Wetnurses* are unfortunately a necessary evil. Without them the children of the better classes . . . would suffer very materially; . . . they form one of the conveniences which money can command.' Mr Gladstone worried about the rights and wrongs of obtaining a wet-nurse for his infant son. But he did not spend too long thinking about it. It was a question of survival.[31]

Occasionally married women undertook this job, like Mrs Toodles, but most doctors advised against married wet-nurses because they were likely to have taken the job only after family disturbances and might therefore prove greedy and hard. The ideal was a single woman, without encumbrances, possessing, as Mrs Beeton advised, a good 'ruddy tone of the skin' and 'full, round . . . elastic' breasts. 'Young and healthy, tidy and clean servants' were recommended by doctors as being safe and knowing their place.[32]

The recruiting system was described by Dr Rogers, a Poor Law doctor: a medical man came to his London workhouse in the 1850s and asked the matron whether he might 'look over the women near confinement,' so that he might select 'some healthy young woman' as a wet-nurse for 'a lady under his care'. He picked out a girl who turned out to be a German and safely friendless. The workhouse master brought the girl to him, whereupon he instructed the sister 'to send her next day to his consulting-room, where the lady's friends might see her'. There the doctor inspected her for signs of venereal disease, and the friends inspected her face and breasts for evidence of smallpox or other diseases, or signs of a malign temperament.[33]

The lying-in hospitals also served as employment agencies for wet-nurses. Most hospitals had a maximum time of fourteen days during which the mother had to use her baby to get her milk flowing, then wean the baby and leave the hospital for the wet-nursing position found for her by the matron or ladies' committee. Donations by grateful mothers to these hospitals for this service formed an important source of income.[34]

Once engaged, the wet-nurse was required to live in, so that she should be totally separated from her own offspring and any temptation to feed it, and isolated from her presumably lowering family and companions. Wet-nurses had necessarily to be fed well, but Dr Haden and Mrs Beeton warned against designing females of the lower orders who tried to gorge themselves and thereby spoilt their milk: such females, Haden explained, sought to wheedle from their mistresses 'two meals of meat in the day, with from two to three pints of porter, besides their breakfast and tea'. They were partial to coarse foods, too, like uncooked vegetables; these had to be forbidden because they 'gripe the children'. Wet-nurses were also, in Haden's experience, averse to washing their bodies. He advised their mistresses to ensure that they were put under a 'warm shower' every morning. But the women were well paid for their milk. The going rate among middle-class employers in the 1820s and 1830s was 10*s*. to 12*s*. and all found.[35] Esther Waters at the end of the century hoped to receive one pound, but had to settle for 15*s*.

Doctors who had links with moral rescue societies, Dr Acton for example, occasionally recommended as wet-nurses girls they knew to be part-time prostitutes. It was, Acton argued, 'the most harmless of all forms of reclamation'.[36] Apparently they had to hide the girl's previous history from her prospective employer, because mothers and fashionable *accoucheurs* strongly opposed such appointments. Recourse to such creatures, as 'Mater' pointed out, showed no regard for the infant to be suckled. 'Undoubted authority', she continued, had 'proved that the moral taint was transmitted through the milk', although the trend was so 'insidious' that it hitherto had escaped 'normal methods of chemical detection'.[37] 'Mater's' missing science was supplied by 'Pro Re Neta' [*sic*], a medical man, who produced four clinical proofs: first, quoting an authority on insanity, Dr Forbes Winslow, he noted that 'criminal children were often the offspring of mad parents', thereby proving that bad fallen women could transmit insanity with their

milk; second, he explained that 'where a nurse's milk has by emotion
. . . been altered in nature, it may give rise to diarrhoea'. Fallen women
proved by their very condition that they possessed uncontrollable,
ill-disposed emotions. Third, experiments with animals demonstrated
that their tempers could be altered and 'their instincts' degraded by
the 'quality of food supplied'. Fourth, fallen women were likely to
'convey cancer' with their milk.[38] A variety of substances are transmitted in milk, some favourable, some not. The materialist cast of
nineteenth-century British beliefs on the question could have encompassed modern findings that milk conveys antibodies against infection, but the argument that the physical security of familiar body contact is also favourable is absent from nineteenth-century ideas about
the matter.

Appointment as a wet-nurse for nine months or more must have
come as a life-saver to many mothers who found themselves alone,
penniless and unemployable otherwise. The appointment also commonly meant death for their own infants. As Dr Haden noted, 'the
majority of London wet-nurses, at least those who go out at an early
period after lying-in, lose their own infants.' Those infants who survived the separation, he added, 'lost their health'.[39] In 1848-9 Dr
Webster traced 347 deaths in Westminster among infants whose mothers
had gone wet-nursing. In the first quarter of 1850 he counted 39 more
infant deaths 'from want of breast milk, . . . sacrifice[s]', he added, 'to
lucre and fashion'.[40] Some women, like the unwed mother of Bessie
Pay, who died in 1869 aged nine months, surrendered each of their
babies in turn while they went wet-nursing. Among these women, as
with Bessie Pay's mother, there is a strong implication that successive
pregnancies were mere unavoidable preparations for a near full-time
trade as wet-nurse.[41] In the 1880s, infants of women who became wet-
nurses were still the most vulnerable group born in Lancashire 'benevolent institutions'.[42]

The fates of these children illustrate in a concentrated way the
dangers which beset their age group in all classes. As especially poor
children, they were especially subject to violence, neglect and sloppy
management born of ignorance.

Abortion and Infanticide

A great many infants were born unwanted: hundreds must have been
the survivors of unsuccessful attempts at their abortion. Ordinary
people clearly accepted abortion as a normal means of limiting their
offspring and avoiding family difficulties. To judge from the hundreds

of cases which ended up as the subject of inquests, attempted abortions conducted by women upon themselves, or by the 'midwives' of the village, must have been widespread throughout the country.[43] One common abortifacient, feverfew (*Pyrethrum Parthenium*), was universally known as 'kill-bastard'. In 1898 at King's Norton, a married woman aged 23 died after taking pills prepared from croton oil, a violent, poisonous purgative, to bring on an abortion. She was three months pregnant, and had aborted a child only six months before. The use of drachyton for abortion, a cheap ointment made at home usually for cuts and sores, was, the *Lancet* said, 'common practice in this [North Worcestershire] and adjoining districts'. It was also commonly used for this purpose in the Potteries.[44]

Midwives, chemists, herbalists and sixpenny doctors often served as neighbourhood abortionists as well as *accoucheurs*. Elizabeth Goddard, a midwife, was convicted of the wilful murder of Sarah Kellam in Leicester in 1861. Kellam had left her husband to live with another man. She became pregnant and went to Goddard, who operated with instruments. Kellam died a few days later from a punctured womb and sepsis. In 1869 a single girl travelled from Mansfield to Nottingham to get an abortion from a policeman's wife who practised as a midwife. When the girl died a local surgeon, who appears to have escaped charges, helped cover up by issuing a death certificate stating that the girl died of 'normal haemorrhage'. In the following year William John Wells, a chemist, was convicted at the Central Criminal Court of 'feloniously assaulting' a woman for the purpose of procuring an abortion. Wells was sentenced to eighteen months' hard labour. He had been tried and acquitted of another abortion charge only a few weeks earlier. Then he had been charged with using instruments, namely a syringe, to inject water into the uterus. The woman had paid him £3. She had died soon afterwards from, it was certified, 'disease of the lungs'. In 1853 the daughter of a keeper of a select lodging-house in Holborn became pregnant by a clergyman lodger. An old servant of her mother's advised her to go to George Thomas, a chemist, in Leather Lane. He confirmed the pregnancy and gave her 'powders', which failed. Then Thomas directed her to Charles Cunningham and James Currie, surgeons, who told her to move into lodgings. She was now four to five months gone. At the lodgings the two surgeons, assisted by midwives, aborted the daughter with a silk ligature 'placed around the uterus'. The charge was £10, paid by the clergyman. The daughter died. The surgeons were transported for seven years. The midwives and others were acquitted. In 1880, John Colmer and his wife, respectable herbal practitioners of

Yeovil, were convicted by a coroner's jury of wilfully murdering Mrs Bridge, who died after her womb was 'lacerated by the improper use of instruments'. But it appears that the Colmers were never sent for trial. Charles Tipple, a cheap surgeon of Baldock, was acquitted of similar charges at the Hertford Assizes in 1857. He had administered 'powders' and then resorted to instruments after the powders had not worked.[45] The records contain dozens of similar instances.

Their greedier, more shifty colleagues openly advertised in the newspapers, religious weeklies and ladies' magazines, *Leach's Family Dressmaker*, for instance, and had handbills distributed in towns, especially in the kitchen areas of houses.[46] Typical of advertising throughout the second half of the century is: 'Ottley's Strong Female Pills quickly and certainly remove all OBSTRUCTIONS . . . where Steel and PennyRoyal fail. Invaluable for married women. By post, under cover, for 14 and 33 stamps . . . Please mention the *Derbyshire Times*.' Professor Leslie's 'Infallible Safeguard for Preventing Irregularities', at 4s. 6d., 10s. 6d., 31s. 6d. were all alike, containing 98 per cent water and 2 senna, the last with a little peppermint added. These abortifacients worked but indifferently. Wrapped around the cheapest of Ottley's Pills was a leaflet advising that 'If these don't do all you wish send for the Extra Strong Pills at 5/3, or the Strongest at 10/- per box, and say how far over. If these don't do it the Strongest will shift anything.' The 'Strongest' contained 22 per cent iron and 61 per cent savin (dried tops of the shrub, *juniperas sabina*, a severe purgative and poison).[47] At the recommended dose of three or four pills a day, the savin could kill. The 'Strongest', like the aloes, pennyroyal, arsenic and other concoctions, the inserted boot-hooks and the rest, probably worked because they were the last drastic onslaught on constitutions already debilitated by hunger, anaemia, overwork and anxiety. None the less, as purchasers of Ottley's and Professor Leslie's products discovered, abortion was a difficult, expensive business with a high failure rate.

Even so, abortion was probably very common, not least because the law against it was ineffectual and, until the 1870s, relatively leniently applied. Abortion was made a statutory felony carrying the death penalty in England in 1803. Before this Act the prosecution had had to prove that the foetus had quickened and that it had been killed in the womb: this was practically impossible and so prosecutions were few and convictions fewer. These weaknesses in the law suited public opinion. Abortions were, after all, conducted by mutual arrangement to remove encumbrances and sources of distress. And amidst so much infant mortality and death it was unnecessarily harsh and intrusive of the state to prohibit the service and punish the benefactor. Foetal and infant existence was worth less than the mother's life. Jurors continued, after the law of 1803 and its strengthening in 1828 and in 1861, under the Offences Against the Person Act, to block moves to conduct post-mortems on likely cases and were reluctant to convict abortionists, at least until the 1870s. The Offences Against the Person Act of 1861 made attempted self-abortion a crime, effectively for the first time. Women who died after attempts at self-inflicted abortion were generally found to have died by 'Visitation of God'. At Beccles in 1839 a surgeon was called to an unmarried girl who had fainted and was dying, from 'poison', her friends hinted. She was seven or eight months pregnant. She died soon afterwards. Her family refused to admit to the surgeon that she had been pregnant. The coroner's jury tried to stop the surgeon conducting a post-mortem, and, after the post-mortem, refused to support his demand for a legal inquiry. He secured the inquiry, but the (non-medical) coroner happened not to arrive in the town until after the time for an inquiry had elapsed, and in the meantime the jury refused to inspect the body and therefore remained unable to report on it. Their verdict was: 'Died by Visitation of God'. When a woman called Barker died after an abortion performed by the fashionable French doctor, Dr Gaudin of Wardour Street, in 1863, the coroner's jury found she had died 'from peritonitis' and exonerated Gaudin. Barker had been five months pregnant and Gaudin had charged £4.[48] He seems never to have gone to trial.

The narrow construction of the Act of 1803 and subsequent judicial interpretation in the case of Pizzy and Codd (1808) (Pizzy was a farrier who had tried 'medicines' which had failed, used an instrument, and finally his hand, to try to abort Codd's unmarried servant, seven and a half months pregnant — the girl later delivered herself of a dead child — and lived) effectively precluded the prosecution from leading evidence about 'instruments' in attempted abortions, probably until the Act of 1861.[49] Legal dispute about the meaning of the word 'noxious' in the Acts also helped the defence.[50]

Those abortionists who did end up in court usually did so only after their client had died from the savin, croton or arsenic they had given them, or from sepsis. Alfred Thomas Heap, an unqualified surgeon in Manchester, appears to have been the only person to have been hanged for criminal abortion, in 1875. He procured the abortion with an instrument and was therefore technically convicted of the murder of his client. After the sentence was passed, the foreman of the jury declared that they would never have found him guilty had they known he would be hanged.[51] Seven more were sentenced to be hanged for murder as the outcome of criminal abortion up to 1882 and each was reprieved – and seemingly found guilty by the jury only on the understanding that they would be reprieved. They and other convicted abortionists until the end of the century usually received sentences of three to seven years' hard labour.[52] The authorities had to move carefully. When Andrew Carmichael was acquitted on an abortion charge in York in 1857 a 'huge crowd . . . consisting chiefly of females' cheered him through the streets. They carried flags and, preceded by a band, pulled his cart through the town.[53] In 1897, when a jury at his second trial found John Lloyd Whitmarsh guilty of murder as a result of criminal abortion, by direction of the judge, the jury added 'the strongest possible recommendation to mercy'. The judge none the less sentenced Whitmarsh to death. The trials – there were two, for the jury refused to convict at the first – aroused enormous public interest. It was the first murder case in England in which the accused was constituted a competent witness, and Whitmarsh made the most of his chance. The *Lancet* and spokesmen for the medical profession wanted Whitmarsh hanged, but the Home Secretary bowed to public protest and reprieved him amidst exuberant popular relief. He was struck off in the following months by the General Medical Council. (In 1881 Whitmarsh had lost a suit for fees he had levied on 'a poor aristocratic family' in Southgate. He had boldly argued then that 'doctors were entitled to charge according to the rental of the house in which *they* [the doctors] live'. The *Lancet* thought his argument right, but imprudent.)[54] The abortionist's service was worth the comparatively small risk involved. Doctors charged up to £10, sixpennys and midwives varied between 10s. and two guineas. In the 1890s Madame Graham, a proprietress of a typical clinic, was aborting 12 or 13 women every day at about two guineas each. When the Chrimes brothers, proprietors of a business selling abortifacients by post, were tried for blackmail in 1898, they were found to have 8,100 women on their current books.[55]

We have no way of knowing how many pregnancies were terminated or how many foetuses survived attempts at termination. But one set of figures is indicative of the numbers involved. In 1859 Dr Charles Clay, the Senior Medical Officer at St Mary's Hospital, Manchester, published the results of his 'Observations on the liability to Abortion', meaning in his context deliberate termination of pregnancy. Clay counted 790 females in his hospital and private practice who had completed their child-bearing age: 430 had had abortions and had living children, 350 had never been aborted and had living children, and 10 had had no abortions and no children. The entire number of pregnancies was 6,970; the number of abortions was 1,000. One woman had had 28 abortions.[56] Incidentally, the mean fertility of this group, around seven to eight children born per female, is close to the mean fertility for women in contemporary poor tropical countries who practise abortion, for example Papua-New Guinea. Edward Moore, a medical officer for part of Bethnal Green, reported handling 702 pregnancies between 1851 and 1861. Of these, 485 were normal deliveries, while 217, almost a third, were 'cases of abortion, mostly produced by herb pills'.[57] Abortion must have been a main means of family limitation.

The infants of wet-nurses and working women were lodged with other members of the family or with baby-farmers, to be reared by hand. Baby-farming was centuries old, but we only have firm evidence about its nature and extent from the 1860s onwards, when doctors and reformers became alarmed at the scandals which emerged. Baby-farming as a sort of paid fostering was undoubtedly necessary and beneficent in a society with a high maternal death rate. Helmsley in the North Riding, for example, had one of the highest illegitimacy rates in England. Traditionally, the mothers sent their babies quickly out of the district to villages 20 or 30 miles away where women who were not relatives reared the children, for a fee, and effectively adopted them. This kind of arrangement must have operated widely through Great Britain, although we know virtually nothing about it. The depositing of infants with relatives was probably even more common.

Revelations in Helmsley in 1880 show how easily the system was abused. One such child had died of starvation, on a diet of bread and water. The corpse was found to have sores on its scalp and burns on its arm and shoulder: it had 'fallen against the fender', the baby-farmer explained. A second farmer of Helmsley children remarked that she had not previously noticed that the leg of one of her charges stuck out at right angles to its body. She had known that the child had earlier broken its thigh, but had not bothered to call anyone to set the bone.[58]

Criminal baby-farmers contributed in probably a small, but steady, way to the infant death rate throughout the century. Some, like Charlotte Winsor in Exeter in the 1860s, simply smothered the infant while the mother waited in the next room. Winsor had a sliding scale of fees for her service, according to the means of the parent.[59] Joseph and Annie Roadhouse disposed of at least 35 children in London in the late 1880s.[60] Mrs Sach and Mrs Walters kept an 'adoption' home in South Kensington around the turn of the century. They accepted one-day-old infants and 'quietened' them with chlorodyne (tincture of chloroform, morphine and prussic acid) before dispatching them on the train as parcels to prospective custodians.[61] Apart from the initial fee of up to £5 and the usual 5s. to 7s. 6d. per week per infant, often paid up to a theoretical age of eight or ten, usually paid without the intermediary or mother seeing the child, there was money to be made by selling the children's clothes after death and by insuring their lives. George and Mary Heys had seven children in their charge in Swindon in 1888, four of whom were insured with friendly societies. The Heys were surrounded by unproven rumours about several earlier deaths. One of their insured charges in 1888 was a girl aged two, who weighed only ten pounds and could not walk.[62] Mrs Flannigan and Mrs Higgins in Liverpool in 1884 had collected insurance on at least eleven infants who had died in their charge. The going rate was between £3 to £10 per child.[63] In this company Mary Ann Cotton, the famous mass poisoner with about 20 victims, mostly insured children, during the 1870s in Durham, is not as unusual as historians have claimed.

Other baby-farmers operated on a pyramid-selling basis. Given the high opening fee and the weekly 7s. 6d., many women made a business of 'introducing' babies to other minders, who then farmed them to third and fourth parties. Mrs Dyer of Bath Road, Bristol, ran such a business in the 1870s. Each contractor had an incentive to take as many babies as possible and keep them as cheaply as possible. Mrs Dyer farmed out about a dozen infants within weeks in 1879. Two were already dead from 'atrophy and convulsions'; two others still with Mrs Dyer were found to be 'wasting away'. Twenty years later her more notorious namesake in Reading simply strangled the babies and threw them into the Thames.[64]

More desperate or more callous parents killed the infants themselves. The usual method was by drowning the new-born infant in a river or cesspool. Even the recorded numbers make a sizeable contribution to the total mortality. Between 1855 and 1860 in London coroners found verdicts of 'murder' on 1,120 infants. In the eighteen months ending in June 1862 there were 902 findings of 'murder' associated with infant deaths in England and Wales.[65] Mothers of children found abandoned were frequently placed on trial under the concealment of bastard births clause in the Act of 1803, but throughout the century juries consistently refused to find them guilty, or when they did, made strong recommendations to mercy. Because there was no legally conclusive method by which the deceased baby could be proved to have breathed and lived distinct of its mother, defending counsel and juries could nearly always thwart the prosecution.[66] The simple test of placing the lungs in water to see whether they would float, as a test of whether the child had breathed, was difficult to introduce as evidence.

By the mid-1860s reformers believed the numbers of children destroyed in these ways to be great enough to warrant a campaign for legislation. Led by doctors such as Curvengen and Ernest Hart, churchmen such as Oscar Thorpe and concerned MPs, the Society for the Protection of Infant Life sought to make everybody do his duty. Charities were to multiply foundling hospitals, poor law authorities were to establish crèches in workhouses to assist mothers to go to work, and some extremists even wanted a kind of motherhood allowance.[67] Parliament and the more hard-hearted ratepayers among the doctors took fright, while the Society itself alienated some important potential supporters by declaring itself, in Curvengen's words, 'determinedly anti-Malthusian'. The *Lancet*, speaking for rate-paying doctors, dismissed the programme as too expensive. The only solution was to make fathers pay, by altering the law to compel registration of the father's name on the birth certificate. In the event, Parliament carried a weak Infant Life Protection Act in 1872, which required baby-farmers to register and keep records of admissions or deaths, but it excluded day 'minders', did not make parents liable, and did not require contracts between parent and baby-farmer to be authenticated. The Act remained ineffectual. Infant burial clubs were suppressed in 1875 but the friendly societies blocked subsequent attempts to control the insurance of infant lives. Children were still dying, neglected but insured, in the 1890s.[68]

Neglect and starvation easily slipped into violence. Emma Rideout of Croydon was charged in 1895 with neglecting and ill-treating two infants 'for whose maintenance she was paid'. One baby was 'emaciated'; the other, aged two and a half years, had two black eyes, a broken nose, both cheeks and temple bruised, bruises all over its body, and was 'very thin and weak'. Rideout was fined £5 and went back to her charges. In the same week at Cambridge Petty Sessions, two lads were convicted of stealing a pair of boots from a shop door and were each gaoled for three months. In two other cases, typical of hundreds, Arthur Taylor and his wife were charged at Nottingham County Police Court with 'neglecting' an infant, aged six months, probably not their own, and allowing it to die. They had been previously 'cautioned' about an apparently similar happening. Each was fined 10*s*. 6*d*. On the same day at the same court, Joseph Boot was convicted of 'trespassing in search of game' and fined two guineas.[69]

Neglect

While violence was a steady and undoubtedly under-recorded cause of death, 'neglect, want, cold, exposure and natural diseases' were more widespread contributors. In 1861, for example, a fairly healthy year in London, coroners found verdicts of 'wilful murder or manslaughter' in inquiries upon 71 children under two years, and found 'neglect' etc. in 614 cases, of a total of 1,104 inquests on children.[70]

'Neglect' covered a vast amount of ignorant mismanagement, bad feeding and uncleanliness. The younger the baby, the less experienced or intelligent the mother, the greater the mismangement, the more the chances of death or damage. Over the period 1889-93, Dr Porter, the MOH for Stockport, made a pioneering investigation of each infant death. The general average was a high 225 per 1,000. He found that the number of deaths on the first day of life was three times greater than on any succeeding day; that the number of deaths in the first week was above half the total deaths in the first month; and that the infant mortality in the first month was nearly double that of any other month.[71] Modern studies show that these proportions persist to our own time.

The main sets of causes adduced for present perinatal (that is, in Great Britain, up to seven days) mortality are congenital malformation, intrapartum anoxia (haemorrhages of body organs and congestion of lungs) or trauma, respiratory distress and pulmonary infection.[72] These causes undoubtedly obtained during the nineteenth century and we may reasonably assume that they effected a major part of the mortality. Anoxia and cerebral trauma due to precipitate or prolonged labour might have been proportionately more common among working-class mothers than now, because these would have been more weak rachitic women. We can also reasonably assume that infection was more destructive than it is now amongst all classes, but especially those pauper mothers delivered in hospital. But I know of no data which would enable us to make precise statements about the incidence of these factors regionally, chronologically or by class. Dr Tatham, the sanitarian, calculated round figures for eight principally reported causes of death under one year for Salford in the 1880s; of the annual total of 1,200 or so, 'premature births' at 80-120 deaths, 'consumption' at 180-200, and 'lung diseases' at 100-300 occur among the leading causes, and very likely they relate to perinatal deaths.[73] But at this stage we cannot be sure. Possibly we could recalculate Tatham's figures from local records and do the same for other places: the project would be worth the effort, given the probable fundamental importance of the perinatal component in Victorian infant mortality rates.

The doctors' simplistic functional notion of childbirth and their narrow view of 'poison' and 'disease' blinded them to the processes happening before their eyes. Processes that lay beyond the reach of medical intervention provided no motive for minute investigation. Their explanations of the high infant mortality rate, as I shall illustrate later, are based on transactions and diseases which kill at lower rates at later periods of infant life. However, we now know that perinatal deaths from congenital malformations and the rest are most prevalent among the infants born to women of smaller stature, poorer health and low social class. We also know that perinatal death rates are highest in Wales, the north-west and Scotland, and lowest, at around one-third less, in the east, south-east and south of England.[74] The same pattern existed in the nineteenth century in an even more striking form: the north and west had twice the reported infant death rate of the south and east.[75] And, as I suggested earlier, such figures as we have show that the death rates were much higher among the poor than the rich.

Lay custom, and the medical opinions which echoed it, endangered new-born babies. Grandmothers in all classes, midwives and doctors agreed that the first aliment for new babies should be 'something of an opening nature'.[76] Professor Evanson recommended 'a little castor oil', but warned that it had to be 'perfectly fresh and free from rancidity'.[77] Midwives liked to 'stuff . . . an infant with sugar and butter' as the best means of 'evacuating the bowels'.[78] By the late 1820s some advanced mothers were turning against the practice, and giving nothing but cow's milk and water, but it remained general enough for successive writers of child management manuals to warn against it. Typically, the author of *Plain Observations on the Management of Children during the First Month* (1828) warned 'families of rank and respectability', and presumably other readers who wished to think themselves such, that it was now 'unnatural' and unfashionable to force into the infant's throat 'a solid mixture of nutmeg, butter and brown sugar within an hour of . . . birth . . . succeeded by a tea-spoon of castor-oil, and a boat of gruel'. There was also no need to apply blisters to the infant's back, to 'clear the complexion'.[79] Dr Buchan, who also counselled against feeding infants too early and too much, invoked Rousseau when he asserted that the powers of 'nature' had been undervalued and too much reliance placed in artificial strengthening.[80] However, the upper classes were still giving new-born babies wine, at least until the 1860s and 1870s, and probably the other customs lingered, too.[81] It was the standard medicine for 'scrofulous' (that is, probably tuberculous with glands enlarged and sometimes discharging, especially in the neck) children who, as Sir Astley Cooper had demonstrated, suffered that 'congenital debility' common among 'pthisical persons'.[82] Among the poor and ignorant it was usual to give the child a 'taste' of 'whatever was going', possibly, as happens in present-day South America and Africa, as a gesture of acceptance (and also because there was not much else). Deaths are recorded from projectile vomiting and 'convulsion' in all social classes throughout the period.[83]

It was usual, among the poor at least, to press the breasts of new-born infants 'to get out the milk', a process which often developed 'inflammation' (abscess) and fretfulness. The navel string was rubbed with tallow or candle grease to soften it and facilitate its removal; if, as sometimes happened, the string was cut before the part underneath was healed, a raisin or fig was pushed into the navel to seal it. This procedure, too, was often followed by 'inflammation' and 'peritonitis'.[84] The babies of wealthy mothers were washed in brandy. This irritated the skin, caused 'inflammation of either the bowels, lungs, or of . . . the nostrils, producing what nurses call the snuffles'.[85] Advanced medical opinion seems to have been against 'unnatural' cleansing, at least until the 1860s. But washing weak babies in beef tea and washing in alcohol babies born to syphilitic mothers persisted into the twentieth century. Infants whose deaths were ascribable to syphilitic lesions were registered as dying from 'constitutional debility', marasmus infantum, or some other inherited weakness. Some doctors, Dr Rigby of Preston, for example, believed the number of such deaths to be considerable.[86]

Wealthy women, in the early part of the century at least, customarily waited until the child was three days old before they began to suckle it. Doctors opposed this delay, pointing out that weak babies sometimes became unable to suck after their forced artificial feeding, and that the mothers developed sore breasts and 'fevers'. But the regularity of the doctors' warnings against the practice suggest that it persisted for much of the period.[87] Poor women, with less food to bestow and less chance of resorting to a wet-nurse if things went wrong, apparently began to suckle on the first day. And if they had adequate milk they probably continued to suckle longer, perhaps in the not completely unfounded belief that prolonged lactation was a form of contraception. East Lincolnshire women into the late 1820s at least were reported to suckle their children to seven or eight years of age.[88]

Recent findings in the United States suggest that only about 5 per cent of (presumably adequately fed) American mothers are totally incapable of lactation.[89] Throughout the nineteenth century British doctors' reports agree that the majority of upper- and middle-class women at least made a start at breast-feeding their children. But reports from Doctors Buchan, Cheyne and Haden in the first third of the century, and from Doctors McMillan, Wills and Barclay Ness in the last third coincide in noting that 'excitable and delicate' upper-class women had too little milk and too little patience, and that they quickly dried up, and that lower-class women also had too little, or only sour, milk.[90] Among the poorer classes the 'habitual intemperance and violent passions of the mother', according to Cheyne, converted 'the naturally salubrious food . . . into a noxious aliment'; with the result that many children of the poor were 'reared artificially'.[91] As elsewhere, we can discover more about the cases which went badly than the enormous amount of breast-feeding which presumably went well. I have been unable to find figures for the proportions of infants who were breast-fed among the comfortable classes and my only set of figures for the poor are suspect. However, Dr Hugh Jones surveyed 500 out-patients at the Liverpool Infirmary for children in 1893. These infants would have come almost exclusively from working-class and poor, casual labourers' families. Jones' findings are given in Table 2.4.

Table 2.4: Extent of Breast-Feeding by Liverpool Out-Patients, 1893 (per cent)

	'Totally' Breast Fed		'Partially' Breast Fed	
At 0 – 3 months	50	[*sic*]	70	[*sic*]
At 3 – 6 months	40		60	
At 6–12 months	35	[*sic*]	60	[*sic*]

Source: Dr Hugh Jones, 'Infant Life', *JRSS*, vol. LXII (1894), p. 32.

Even allowing for answers meant to please the doctor and a probable high Irish component which would increase the breast-feeding proportion, the figures are impressively high for a city population.[92] In Mexico in 1968, for example, the comparable figure for totally breast-fed babies at six months was 45 per cent, and in Chile in 1970, at thirteen months, only 6 per cent.[93] In England present-day advocates of natural feeding say that 'the great majority of babies . . . were breast fed' until the 1930s. In 1894 Dr Brown, MOH of Bacup, claimed that the great defection from breast-feeding had occurred in the 1850s and 1860s. In 1892, Dr Webster of London traced the onset of artificial feeding to the 1820s. The figures for 1965 show that almost 33 per cent were never breast-fed and another 25 per cent went over to cow's milk during the first month, while in Scotland 49 per cent were never breast-fed.[94] One wonders about such global claims and the class, regional and ethnic continuities or discontinuities involved. Enthusiasts for breast-feeding seem always to posit a golden age a generation before their own bleak age of bottle-feeders. One possible continuity, reflecting the better nutrition, greater leisure and a closeness to doctors of women in class I is that 79 per cent of them in the 1960s initially tried to breast-feed their first babies, compared with 65 per cent in class V. This differential increased with second and subsequent babies.[95]

Feeding and Diarrhoea

One leading malady of infants who were partially or wholly artificially fed was diarrhoea. It matched prematurity and the other principal destroyers on Dr Tatham's Salford list by causing between 100 and over 200 deaths every year. Diarrhoea was a seasonal disease which reached its peak in late summer and was worst in years with mild winters and long sultry summers. Attacks in infants were always acute with a probable high case-fatality rate. The illness lasted about a week in a strong child and death was often preceded by distressing convulsions, while young babies and weaklings could be carried off in less than 48 hours. Other members of the family, especially the children, were generally also affected, indicating, amongst other causes, poor food handling and much personal dirtiness.[96]

Doctors had long recognised diarrhoea as a major killer, but until the late 1850s they regarded its visitations as a natural hazard, no more to be evaded than teething.[97] Suddenly, from 1856 onwards, doctors became curious about the environmental and social etiology of the disease and thereby began to suggest ways of preventing it. Clearly, diarrhoea was a scourge which accompanied maternal improvidence and insanitary surroundings. Mothers and nurses, Dr Herbert Barker lamented in 1856, consistently did the wrong thing. Those who did breast-feed were not content until they also stuffed their infants with bouillie (flour mixed with cow's milk and water). At night, in attempts to evade their duty to give the child the breast every three or four hours, they filled the child with 'tea, coffee, spirits, anything', toast in water, oatmeal mash, opium, in order to make it sleep. Wine, especially, was administered too freely. It was the substitute for opium among the comfortable classes. Wine had a 'tenfold pernicious effect' by inducing a premature 'appetite for alcoholic stimulants'.[98]

Dr Barker's objections to over-reliance on bouillie or pap were justified, and not only for the reasons he adduced. The recipe in *The
Female Instructor* of 1841 is typical:

> To two-thirds of new milk, after it has stood five or six hours from
> the time of milking, add one-third of river or spring water, and set it
> on a quick clear fire. Temper some good wheaten flour into a batter,
> with either milk or water; and when the milk and water is near
> boiling, but before it actually does boil, add a little salt, and let
> it stand to cool.
>
> A good spoonful of flour is sufficient to thicken a pint of milk
> and water. This will make it about the thickness of common milk
> porridge, which is what will eat the sweetest and be the easiest kind
> of digestion.

Bread pap was made by pouring scalding water over thin slices of white
bread, letting it cool, pouring off the water, mashing the bread and
adding milk and usually sugar.[99]

In cases where artificial feeding was unavoidable Dr Barker recommended cow's milk and water and then, as the teeth grew, milk, sugar
and yolks of lightly boiled eggs, toast in water and wheatmeal in milk.
All 'vegetable matter' was forbidden. After seven months the baby
could be given bread crusts and milk. At two years, the child could
begin the day with 'a little bread and milk'; at nine a.m. he could
have a breakfast of 'bread softened in hot water, with milk and sugar
added'; at one o'clock dinner was to consist of meat broth and a slice
of bread, and if the child had fully formed teeth, boiled meat with
thoroughly cooked potatoes, turnips and cauliflowers. No drinking was
to be permitted during the meal, but afterwards, 'toast-water, freshly
made' was permissible. At 6 p.m. the child could have more bread and
milk and then be put to bed. 'This course of food . . .', Dr Barker
warned, would 'not suit all stomachs. Meat or broth every day would
perhaps lead to fulness of the system in some.' When this occurred a
lightly boiled egg was to be substituted for the meat. Cocoa was to be
preferred to tea. 'Ripe fruits . . . the orange, strawberries, currants, a
few grapes, the skins being rejected, and roasted apples, may be allowed;
but stone fruits and nuts must be avoided, also dried fruits, with the
exception of figs.' 'Avoid pastry, pork, veal, salt beef, new or heavy
bread, tea-cakes, strong tea, sweetmeats, and especially . . . all alcoholic
beverages.'[100]

Dr Appleton in 1858 strongly commended a new baby food daily recipe which required two pints of white flour, one pint of oatmeal, four ounces of milk, sweetened with white sugar. This he pronounced to be 'a most strengthening and fattening diet'. The first baby show in Britain was held in Manchester in 1905. The object was to 'find the heaviest and fattest babies', and to encourage breast-feeding. The champion weighed 23 pounds at four months (the average weight at this age is about 12 pounds). The runners-up were twins, each 17¾ pounds, at eight months (average weight at this age is around 15-16 pounds).[101] This fashion for 'bonny babies' was to last into the 1950s.

As they had to do with pregnant women, doctors called in to manage babies perforce had to dogmatise about the daily regimen in order to mask their clinical incapacity. 'It may seem', Dr Barker remarked, 'to an undisciplined mind, something beneath the dignity of the profession to give advice on the preparation of food for a babe', but he went on to point out that medical students rarely encountered infants during their course, unless they were surgical cases, and that medical teachers passed over the treatment of infants 'lightly and briefly'.[102] This situation remained much the same until the turn of the century.[103]

Doctors had no sure resource when diarrhoea struck. Dr Ashby was repeating in 1898 what Dr Haden had recommended in 1827. Despite the advance of germ theory, in desperate situations doctors could only assert their relevance by exhibiting heroic doses to 'drive out the poison'. Dr Ashby's standard procedure was to order calomel as an 'evacuant drug' in one-grain doses during the worst of the attack, succeeded by doses of one-sixth of a grain every half-hour; opium, in the form of enemas of starch and opium, every one or two hours; bismuth nitrate as a 'throat disinfectant', five to fifteen grains every 'two or three hours'; no milk, but only white of egg in sugar water, chicken tea and diluted brandy. Dr Haden had in addition administered castor oil and rhubarb.[104] This treatment might have been effective in reducing the discomfort of straining painfully. Equally, it would cause even more dehydration and increase the danger to infants.

The death rate from diarrhoea, Haden noted, as did Dr Hugh Jones in 1894, was considerably underestimated because it did not include the subsequent deaths reported as resulting from 'atrophy and debility'. After the purging ceased, Haden explained, 'the infant often developed a loathing of food, emaciation, restlessness, thirst and fever follow[ed] . . . by swelling of the extremities and drowsiness'. The 'most effectual treatment' was a fresh course of calomel, castor oil and beef tea. Dr Jones calculated that in 1873-5 in England 17.1 per 1,000 were reported as dying from diarrhoea, but 39.5 per 1,000 were reported to have died of 'atrophy and premature birth'. In Scotland, with, Jones thought, more breast-feeding and better infant care, diarrhoea carried off only 7.1 and 30.7 per 1,000 from 'atrophy and premature birth'.[105]

The doctors' new concern about diarrhoea in the mid-1850s was linked with the increase of information about adulteration of milk and other foods, and the slovenly cooking and housekeeping of lower-class mothers.[106] The cheap milk they bought was skimmed, watered and old.[107] The doctors came across innumerable cases of bad management. In 1869 at Carlton Worksop Dr Rogers was summoned to attend an eight-month-old child. It had choked on a piece of raw ham the mother had put in its mouth to quiet it while she prepared her husband's dinner. The practice of giving infants solid substances, he remarked, seemed universal among the poor.[108] In St Helens in 1902 an eleven-week-old child had died during convulsions. It had been fed since birth on 'boiled bread'. Pieces of meal and cinder were found in its stomach. The final bout of convulsions had begun after the father had given the child a feed of ham and the mother had given it a drink of 'cinder tea' (brandy tea). At West Gorton in the same year a fourteen-month-old child died of 'pneumonia and diarrhoea'. It had been fed since three weeks old on bread and milk, with the addition of potatoes at six months. Both parents were 'hopeless drunkards', living in 'hopeless squalor'. The family's clothes were all in pawn. This child was their fifth to have died in infancy.[109]

The new concern of the 1850s also coincided with what contemporaries believed to be a dramatic spread of feeding by bottle. There probably was some increase, because the introduction of the indiarubber nipple in place of the old stitched parchment, or leather, teat or tube, or ivory teat, must have made the operation easier and quicker. New shaped bottles were also being marketed in the 1850s and 1860s. The new 'Edwards Feeding Bottle', for instance, was commended by the *Lancet* in 1858, because it was horn-shaped, with an indiarubber nipple at the pointed base and a finger-sized hole in a removable rubber cap at the top, so that the flow could be regulated. Unlike the older bottles with narrow necks it 'could be cleansed with the greater facility by merely rinsing it out with water'.[110] The 'Mamma' bottle of 1869 was shaped like a horizontal gourd, with the cap and finger stop at the narrow stalk end and a removable rubber full breast and nipple at the round end. Like the others, it could be purchased in either glass or steel. The *Lancet* writer declared the 'Mamma' to be the best he had seen, particularly because of its ease of cleansing.[111] 'Marshall's Patent Sectional Feeding Bottle', which came on the market in 1881, was one of several which permitted the top to be screwed off to allow the 'fingers to be introduced to clean the interior'.[112] But even the best invention could falter under female usage. Mrs Beeton in 1861 advised her readers to ensure that the servant washed the bottle in warm water, but added that there was no need to remove the teat because that upset the twine which normally bound it on.[113] Dr Chavasse in 1869 recommended keeping two bottles, in case one was broken. He remarked that they ought to be kept clean but did not mention boiling them.[114] In 1894 the standard bottle in workhouse nurseries, and doubtless in many poor homes, was still the old, any old, bottle with a narrow neck and feeding tube of pig's skin or rubber.[115]

There was no clear guidance as to the contents of the bottle. The author of *Plain Observations* in 1828 recommended for the first week or two 'one pint of fresh cream, to four, five or six pints of water, according to the richness of the cream', and thereafter a gradual transition to plain milk. This was to be boiled each morning, with the 'scum that rises, carefully removed when it is cold'. Thereafter the milk was not to be heated again, but warmed if need be by standing in a basin of hot water.[116] Esther Copley in her *Catechism of Domestic Economy* of 1851 suggested 'fresh, pure cow's milk, with boiling water just enough to warm it, and a very few grains of salt and sugar'.[117] Dr Chavasse's recommendations were very similar, although he objected to boiling the milk or water unless the baby had 'difficulty with its bowels', and he was more liberal with the sugar, proposing that it be added in lumps. He also repeated (without explaining why) the very sound old wives' advice of ensuring that the milk came only from one cow.[118] This made for milk of greater daily consistency and diminished the chances of catching tuberculosis. Catherine Buckton in *Food and Home Cooking* in 1883 was more scientific. She advised three pints of cow's milk daily until teething began. Other goods were not to be given until nine months. Flour and bread, she admitted, were nourishing, but they caused 'agonies' in young children 'because the saliva in the mouth cannot digest the starch . . . and turn it into sugar'.[119]

The reader will appreciate that young mothers in the nineteenth century received little help from the manuals. They were left, the poor and illiterate especially, like their mothers before them, at the mercy of their mothers and the neighbours in discovering how, what, how much and when to feed their babies. In general, the pattern seems to have been feeding on demand; that is giving 'sugar and water, castor oil, rusks, porridge, or arrowroot without rule, save that when an infant cries it must be fed'.[120] By the 1880s, however, some careful middle-class mothers were obeying their doctors' injunctions to feed their

children more 'regularly'. So far as I have discovered, the first tentative
plea for measuring a baby's feed, and adjusting the feed to particular
babies, was made by Dr A.H. Carter, at a meeting of the Midland
Medical Society in 1897. Carter wanted the baby's intake controlled by
regular weighing. His plea seems to have had no immediate response.[121]
The control of feeding was a development of the late nineteenth century, a development which under the aegis of Dr Truby King and
similar medical systematisers was to become Procrustean in the 1920s
and 1930s.

Doctors disliked artificial feeding because it offended their conception of the natural. The inhabitants of nineteenth-century Britain, Dr
Buchan, invoking Rousseau, remarked, no longer lived 'as nature directs'
and therefore many mothers were in no condition to give suck. Dr
Haden regretted that so many people lived 'close and unhealthy' in
larger cities; nature's retribution came in the form of high infantile
death rates. Village children, by contrast, 'live almost hanging at the
breast of the mother'; she kept them near her as she went about her
daily tasks and they grew up robust and rarely ill. City mothers had to
forsake their infants as they left the home each day to work.[122]

Haden had outlined a situation which undoubtedly existed, although
there were then no detailed data to prove it, and which seemed insoluble.
Doctors continued to advise their patients to breast-feed their infants,
but it was not until the advent of the improved feeding-bottles that
prospects opened up for improving infant feeding and management.
The Registrar-General began to collect data about the distribution of
deaths from summer diarrhoea from the early 1870s. The information
confirmed the existing assumptions. Over all, 80 per cent of summer
diarrhoea fatalities in England and Wales were reported among children
under two years. In the 18 largest cities and towns the rate was 4.4 per
1,000 deaths; 3.5 per 1,000 in the 50 next largest towns; and 1.5 per
1,000 in the whole of England and Wales exclusive of these 68 cities.
Farr concluded by speculating that diarrhoea deaths were peculiarly
linked with female labour in textile towns.[123]

Farr's calculations initiated a series of investigations into the links
between diarrhoea, artificial feeding, urban living and mothers in factory work. Dr Yeld in Sunderland reported that the 102 deaths ascribed
to diarrhoea and convulsions in 1874 included 71 fed only by the
bottle.[124] Dr William Johnston, the Assistant Medical Officer of Health
for Leicester, the textile town with the worst infantile diarrhoea death
rate at 6.2 per 1,000, set about refuting the slur on factory work by
producing more general explanations. In 1878 he investigated 238

deaths from diarrhoea, selected apparently because they were ones about which full details could be obtained. Without telling the proportion which the 238 represented of the whole diarrhoea or atrophy group or anything else about his sample, he asserted that 165, or 69 per cent, were 'breast fed'. Diarrhoea, he argued, was an effect of summer conditions, not neglect resulting from factory employment.[125] Mr Pilkington, the MOH for Preston, the factory town with the second-worst diarrhoea death rate at 5.5 per 1,000, also argued for more general causes. Diarrhoea occurred

> among the operative and labouring classes, those of the Irish being comparatively exempt . . . due to the fact that the latter are almost always fed at the breast. Bronchitis added largely to the deaths of infants, . . . attribut[able] to their removal in the cold in the early morning from warm and ill-ventilated rooms . . . to houses in which they are nursed while their mothers are at work.

The 'discovery' about the Irish, later corroborated from many towns, must have surprised sanitarians. Indeed, the comparative fewness of Irish in a town could raise the infant death rate, as in Preston. Hitherto doctors and health visitors had regarded them as more careless and dirty and even greater contributors to the death rate than their English compeers.[126]

The national averages confounded Farr and the sanitary statisticians and reinforced the arguments of the textile town doctors. The mortality varied with the hotness of the summer. The average for 27 provincial towns during the mild summer of 1886 was 4 per 1,000 and ranged up to 4.3 per 1,000 for the sweltering one of 1884. Some textile towns, like Leicester at 6.2 per 1,000 and Preston at 4 per 1,000 for the 1880s, were decidedly bad. But others, Blackburn, for instance, with a rate during the 1880s of 2.8 per 1,000, and Huddersfield, at 1.4 per 1,000, were not. The worst town of all was Norwich, with around 8.2 per 1,000 during the 1880s.[127] When set in a European context it is even more likely that factors other than breast- or bottle-feeding were involved. Even the Norwich rate looks almost benign when compared with the reported 26.9 per 1,000 for Berlin in the 1880s, the 14.4 per 1,000 for Munich, the 13.3 per 1,000 for Budapest, or the 6 per 1,000 for Vienna and 5.8 per 1,000 for Stockholm.[128]

Among the more general causes of diarrhoea was sheer callous mismanagement and starvation. Dr Partridge of Stroud reported in 1882 that in his (cloth-making and small manufacturing) town among the working classes, where the mother leaves home early and returns late in the evening, the children are placed out to nurse. The sopped, heavy bread and sugar, or milk kept in unclean bottles, or until it is sour, soon cause irritability of the mucous membrane leading to . . . [diarrhoea, debility, convulsions] . I have often seen infants, of a few months and upwards, standing crying, spoon in hand, before their sour mess of fermenting stuff, loathing and rejecting it, until the grandam had added more sugar to tempt the unpalatable stuff down.[129]

In 1884 Dr Taylor, the MOH for Scarborough, reported that over the period 1876-84 there had been 163 deaths attributed to diarrhoea. Of these 131 had occurred among children under one year, concentrated in the two poorest parts of the town. In 1873 a weekly crèche had been established to cater for the children of women who lived in these districts and went out to casual work during the summer season. The children brought to the crèche often had diarrhoea when they arrived. During their full-time stay the children generally rapidly recovered. The mothers collected them on Saturday and when the children were returned on Monday they had diarrhoea again; the result, Dr Taylor concluded, of 'improper feeding on the Sunday'. At his instigation, 10,000 circulars on 'right feeding' had been distributed in the town.[130] The circulars can have done little to counter the emotional disturbances now recognised, together with infective agents, as major causes of the increased peristalsis, and secretion of mucus in the colon that leads to rapid evacuation.

Doctors welcomed condensed milk when it came on the British market about 1871. The industry had boomed during the Franco-Prussian War and condensed milk had become the main food in Paris after the lifting of the siege. Unlike cow's milk, it arrived in a clean container, it did not sour quickly, it was not adulterated with water or anatto (an orange dye from the fruit of the South American *Bixa Orellana* used to colour foods), it was filling, and relatively cheap. Dried milk had been available since the mid-1860s, but it was generally more expensive, and troublesome to make up. Children did not fatten on it as they clearly did on condensed milk. None the less, Dr Daly noticed among his patients in Dalston in 1872 that infants raised on condensed milk seemed to sink rapidly under very mild, generally non-lethal, attacks of diarrhoea. Even children drinking the ordinary 'bad London milk' did better. He also noticed that condensed milk babies would not take easily to other foods. They rejected meat and potatoes, and would only eat 'farinaceous food saturated with sugar'.[131] Condensed milk contains the di-saccharide sucrose (sugar) which has to be split by an enzyme before it is absorbed. Small children, especially when malnourished or with diarrhoea, are deficient in the enzyme, so condensed milk causes more diarrhoea simultaneously with producing a dependence upon the sweet taste of the sucrose.

Repeated doctors' warnings suggest that condensed milk became a major stand-by for instant baby food among working-class families until into the twentieth century. The patent dried milk foods, Bengers, Glaxo and the others, seem to have been restricted to the comfortable classes. One of the difficulties with condensed milk was that individual tins varied. Nestlé's in the 1880s contained solid pieces of starch 'of different sizes and different forms'. The company apparently attempted to reduce the free starch in the early 1880s, while enlarging the proportion of sugar. Dr Borchardt of Liverpool was convinced that the new recipe increased 'chronic indigestion and in consequence . . . the disposition to rickets'. Possibly it did. In 1904 this 'perfect food for infants', according to the label, was still 77.4 per cent carbohydrate, one-third of which was starch.[132] Condensed milk could hardly have supplied adequate vitamin D. An analysis in 1889 of 'Standard' brand condensed milk 'for infants' revealed that 90 per cent of the original cream had been abstracted. The label said: 'especially prepared from richest cow's milk with nothing but cane sugar added' and directed that it be made up with five parts water to one of 'Standard' milk.[133] The cheaper the tin, the greater the hazard. In 1898 the label of one brand offered 'Advice to Mothers: If condensed milk on opening the tin has any smell, such as a sour or fishy smell, the milk is not fit for use.'[134] Some cheap brands came in big tins: once opened they could stand on the shelf for days. In the following year the medical profession sent a deputation to the President of the Board of Agriculture, Walter Long, to ask him to have skimmed, concentrated and condensed milks compulsorily labelled 'not fit food for children or invalids'. Public analysts told him of the 'poverty' of most brands; Dr Stocker of Willesden claimed that diarrhoea was 'rampant' as a result of feeding on the stuff. Long was unmoved: inconsequentially he answered that 'if the public liked to buy a thing they must be allowed to buy it'.[135]

Meanwhile the sanitarians kept up their campaign against bottle-feeding and slovenly child-raising. Some doctors blamed factory work, others, especially in factory towns, blamed the new-found 'desire for freedom from maternal ties'.[136] Others pointed to female fecklessness and stupidity. In Bradford one doctor said that he had found that 80

per cent of the infants who died of diarrhoea in 1880 had been unwashed, fed from bottles fitted with dirty drinking-tubes, with milk
that was 'days old', followed with arrowroot, cornflour and bread
sops. One-quarter of the total infant deaths comprised illegitimates.[137]

Doctors and health visitors moved in the 1890s to inculcate regular
feeding timetables because they found infants often left hungry or
dosed with sedatives while their parents worked or slept. Dr Wills of
the Westminster Hospital devised one of the first routines after tracing
the irregular feeding habits among his poor out-patients and their
'miserably pale and thin' babies. Feckless mothers who breast-fed did so
on demand during the day and filled the child with opium at night; this
had to stop because it spoilt babies. Feckless mothers or minders who
raised infants by hand fed them too little and too intermittently. Wills
proposed the schedule given in Table 2.5.

Table 2.5: Dr Wills' Feeding Routine

	Numbers of Feedings in 24 Hours	Interval in Hours During Day 7 a.m. to 9 p.m.	Numbers of Feedings During Night from 9 p.m. to 7 a.m.
Third day to end of first month	10	2	2
Second month	9	2½	2
Third to sixth month	7	3	1
Seventh to twelfth month	6	3	0

Source: *Westminster Hospital Reports*, vol. XI (1899), p. 59.

The feedings in this routine are about twice as frequent as the 'four-
hourly plus demand' system which has become general since the 1940s.
Wills' apparently more strict scheme partly represented an attempt to
incorporate existing feeding on demand customs. It also represents the
opening of the brave new age of strict infant routines.[138]

The medical advocates of breast-feeding regarded the employment of
women in factories as 'unnatural' and sought to link female out-work
with neglect of babies, artificial feeding and high infant mortality rates.
Dr McMillan remarked in 1885 that women in 'modern society' sought
employment and resorted to the feeding-bottle 'to free them[selves]
from what ought to be their "first duty" '.[139] Dr James Mackenzie
reported as MOH for Burnley in 1886 that 'the strong desire in the
feminine mind to earn high wages cause[s] married women to work

longer in the mill than is good for their offspring'.[140]

These assumptions apparently were not tested until the early 1890s when Dr George Reid, the MOH for Staffordshire, produced figures to substantiate them. Reid divided the populous districts of his county into two: the northern part in which many women were engaged in the pottery manufactures, and the southern iron- and coal-producing areas, where few women were employed outside the home. Over the ten years 1871-80 the infant death rate for the northern part was 182 per 1,000; for the southern, 152 per 1,000. Reid then took all the English towns with over 50,000 inhabitants and calculated the proportion of women reported in the census as employed. He claimed that the infant death rate ran parallel to the proportion employed. His finding strengthened the doctor's existing knowledge that infant mortality had fallen, despite great deprivation, both during the Lancashire Cotton Famine in the 1860s and the Siege of Paris, when women were unemployed and at home. Reid concluded with a call for legislation forbidding women to work within three months after childbirth.[141] Hitherto women in textile factories worked, if they could, until their actual confinement and returned within five days. The Factory Act of 1891, effective from 1893, forbade resumption of work within a month of confinement, but did not prohibit work during pregnancy. The women themselves, as one reformer admitted, would have fiercely opposed any such constraint. The Act of 1891 placed the onus on the employers to report breaches of its maternity provisions and hence made prosecutions most unlikely. In the event, new mothers and their employers connived to evade the Act and women commonly returned to work within ten days.[142]

Many reformers linked factory work and maternal neglect with deaths from overdoses of sedatives. The practice of giving infants 'quieteners' was much older than the nineteenth century but it probably became more widespread among all classes as supplies of Eastern Mediterranean opium increased through the growth of the French drug industry, and distribution in Britain became more effective. Opium-taking among adults, as I shall explain later, was as common as alcohol-drinking (indeed the tincture *was* alcohol), especially in the manufacturing towns of Lancashire, Yorkshire, Nottinghamshire, the Fen Country and London, and among some sections of the intelligentsia.[143] Opium was a household cure-all. Thus it was nothing extraordinary to give opiates to infants. George Crabbe, the country surgeon turned poet, described the custom in the *Borough*, published in 1810:

The boy was healthy, and at first expressed
His feelings loudly, when he failed to rest;
When cramm'd with food, and tightened every limb,
To cry aloud, was what pertain'd to him;
Then the good nurse (who, had she borne a brain,
Had sought the cause that made her babe complain)
Has all her efforts, loving soul! applied
To set the cry, and not the cause, aside:
She gave the powerful sweet without remorse,
The sleeping cordial – she had tried its force,
Repenting oft: the infant freed from pain,
Rejected food, but took the dose again.
Sinking to sleep; while she her joy express'd,
That her dear charge could sweetly take its rest.
Soon may she spare her cordial; not a doubt
Remains, but quickly he will rest without.

This moves our grief and pity, and we sigh
To think what numbers from these causes die.

The 'powerful sweet' came in several guises. In 1823 the recipe for
'Dalby's Carminative' was: tincture (alcohol) of opium, four and a half
drachms; tincture of assafoetida, two and a half drachms; oil of cara-
ways, three scruples (one scruple = 1/24 ounce); oil of peppermint, six
scruples; tincture of castor oil, six drachms and a half; rectified spirits
of wine, six drachms; put two drachms into each bottle (size unspecified), with magnesia, one drachm, and fill up with simple syrup (usually
sugar and water) and a little rectified spirits of wine. The specifications
for 'Daffy's Elixir', another good seller, were senna leaves, four ounces;
santile (presumably sandalwood) shavings; dried elecampane root (a
stimulant with a bitter taste, from the yellow flowering *Inula
Helenium*); aniseeds; caraway seeds; coriander seeds; liquorice root; of
each two ounces; raisins (stoned), eight ounces; proof spirit, six pounds.
And the famous 'Godfrey's Cordial': Venice treacle (a kind of universal
mixture – believed to possess anti-poisonous qualities; ginger; of each
two ounces; rectified spirits of wine, three pints; oil of sassafras, six
drachms (this improved the appetite); water, three gallons; treacle,
fourteen pounds; tincture of opium, four pints.[144]

The want of information about the quality and amounts of opium
re-exported make it impossible to determine how much was imported
and consumed in Great Britain. The leap in import figures occurred

Opium.

between 1820 and 1838, when the Customs reported an increase from
16,000 lb to 131,000 lb. The total apparently stayed at a little over
100,000 lb until into the 1850s. The figures for 1852 suggest that
slightly under half the total imported was eaten at home.[145] Applying
this ratio to the other figures, we have roughly 40,000 to 50,000 lb
consumed each year. Some of this was used in veterinary medicines,
but the bulk of it was said to have gone for human consumption. The
sale of opium was completely unrestricted until the Poisons Act of
1868, when straight opium-taking is said to have begun to diminish.
But my impression is that opium-taking in the form of patent medicines,
which burgeon in the late 1870s (partly as a result of the Poisons Act
and Sale of Food and Drugs Act of 1875) continued to be widespread
until the First World War.[146]

In 1808, a local surgeon asserted that 'upwards of 200 pounds of
opium' were sold each year by grocers, corner shopkeepers and chemists
in Nottingham, together with 'above 600 pints of Godfrey's Cordial',
retailed to the 'poorer classes'. *The Times* in 1844 reported that almost
every druggist and village shopkeeper sold large amounts of opium and
'quieteners' every week.[147] Mr Calvert, a Manchester chemist, told a
Committee of the House of Lords in 1857 that chemists in the town
sold between twelve and fifteen gallons of laudanum (alcoholic tincture
of opium) each week and that between 100 and 150 customers called
every day to buy opium.[148] In Clitheroe about 1850, 6,725 people,
predominantly calico printers and factory workers, bought four pints
of Godfrey's Cordial every week, and 4,000 poppy heads to make their
own 'sleepy stuff'.[149] In 1862 a chemist who was also a member of the
Nottingham Town Council remarked during a discussion on the indiscriminate sale of drugs that he sold about 400 gallons of laudanum a
year, half of which he believed was administered to infants.[150] A
chemist from Goole, giving evidence at an inquest on the death of an
infant from laudanum poisoning in 1886, admitted that he sold 'plenty
of it' every week. In Lowestoft in 1875, which had a population of
about 10,000, a chemist sold 100 pennyworths (half a cup-full, sometimes claimed to contain ten grains of opium) of Godfrey's Cordial each
week. In the 1890s it was usual for mothers in north Wales mining
villages to brew a 'punch' for their infants before they went out to
work. The 'punch' recipe was one lump of sugar in a teacup, one to five
drops of laudanum on it, according to the infant's age, with a teaspoonful of hot water added. The child was then dosed and with luck slept
until the mother returned. (Incidentally, our perspective might be
opened a little wider if we recall that over 200,000 children under 11

Adulteration of opium

were being doped with doctor-prescribed tranquillisers in Britain in 1974.)[151]

The population was saved from mass poisoning because the opium mixtures were adulterated. Wholesalers sold all drugs until 1875 on a sliding scale, with up to nine levels of decreasing quality and increased adulteration. Not until 1887 was it established that tincture of opium had to conform to the standards of the *British Pharmacopoeia*.[152] Most dealers bought the cheap Malwa or Turkey opium. The dearer Patna or Smyrna opium at over thirteen shillings per pound in the early part of the century was likely to be even more adulterated than its cheaper counterparts.[153] In 1838 the opium from a 'first-rate' shop in Edinburgh, sold as high-quality stuff containing 130 grains of opium to the ounce of fluid, was found to be only 17 grains to the ounce. In that same year five samples purchased from London druggists contained added water varying from 35 to 63 per cent of the mixture.[154] The situation improved after the Sale of Food and Drugs Act of 1875, but adulteration remained common. In 1897 a druggist in Nottingham was fined for selling laudanum with water comprising 63 per cent of the alcohol tincture and 90 per cent of the claimed *BP* standard opium missing.[155] The drug was adulterated before it left Turkey, adulterated by French middlemen (although the French laws about the purity of drugs for home consumption were strict), adulterated by British wholesalers (who were not included in the adulteration acts) and adulterated by retailers. Between them they extracted the valuable morphine from the drug, and added any or all of water, pea-meal, honey, gum, poppy capsules, wheat flour, powdered wood, sugar and sand. Nineteen of 23 samples examined in London in 1854 were adulterated.[156] The standard mix for 'best quality' pharmaceutical opium on sale in England in 1847 was one half pound of pea-meal and honey, beaten into a mass, to every pound of Turkey opium, which generally already was thick with crushed poppy capsules.[157]

When parents found that the usual dose did not induce sleep in their infants or stop their diarrhoea, they enlarged and multiplied the dose. Tired, ignorant, bewildered parents, worried and exasperated by their inability to succour babies made restless by infection, stomach upsets, hunger and drugs, readily administered extra drugs and medicines as the only means of survival, as they saw it, for their baby and themselves. Babies under a month old were started on a teaspoonful of 'Godfrey's Cordial' at evening but soon built up to three teaspoonfuls. In a typical case at Langport in Somerset in 1841 a mother gave her twelve-day-old baby 'a pennyworth' (about ten grains in tincture) of

M iasma.

Godfrey's Cordial because it 'was disordered in its bowels'. The coroner's jury attributed its death to a 'visitation of God'. In 1876 at Basford in Nottinghamshire a child of four months old had been 'continually' dosed with Godfrey's Cordial, 'ten drops every evening', according to the father, 'to send it to sleep'. This proved ineffectual on the night of the baby's death. The father got up and 'gave it four or five drops of laudanum and some castor oil'.[158] Inquests on such deaths are reported at the rate of about one per week until the first decade, at least, of the twentieth century.

The doctors' faith in miasmic infection theory, intrinsically wrong though it was, none the less led them rightly to concentrate on proving the aetiological links between dirt, dampness and neglect and the disease; these were conceivably remediable sources, unlike the poverty that underlay much, but by no means all, of the diarrhoea mortality. In 1875 Doctors Buck and Franklin investigated an outbreak in Leicester which had killed 238 infants in three months, three-quarters of them under twelve months. Only 22 had been totally breast-fed; 133 had been 'partially' breast-fed; and 61 had been fed wholly by hand. The dwellings were not notably insanitary, the doctors decided, nor did they uncover any more 'narcotics or maternal neglect' than was general in textile towns. With an almost unconscious reversion to simple miasmic theory, they concluded that 'the fatality was concentrated in low-lying ground', where — although Buck and Franklin did not say so — the poorest people dwelt.[159]

Yet the sanitarians were justified by common sense in associating diarrhoea with dirty living, the dirty living and low expectations that accompanied poverty. In 1878 Dr Butterfield, the MOH for Bradford, studied 101 diarrhoea deaths remarkably concentrated in back-to-back houses. He found that the deaths were twice as numerous in the front dwellings as in the even darker rear ones, which were also adjacent to the privy or ashpit for the block. Butterfield then learnt that the front dwellers kept their excreta in a corner of their room under the food shelf, until their single trip each evening to the ashpit. The back dwellers (some of whom jointly owned the contents of the ashpit which was sold as manure), simply threw their excreta on to the heap through the front door or window. Habits such as these, reinforced by the absence of good piped water and ready heating devices for cooking purposes, commonly meant, as Professor Jardine complained in 1904, that 'the poor simply will not take care about cleanly feeding of babies, utensils, storage of milk etc.' As a local doctor remarked of the infant mortality of Northwich, Manchester, in 1900: 30 per cent of all deaths were aged under one year at a rate of 214 per 1,000 live births: 'ignorance, apathy, neglect with in far too many cases no great wish that the child should live'.[160]

The first report, apparently, which directly associated an infant's death from diarrhoea with inadequate family income and the malnutrition and inadequate care which resulted from it, comes from a doctor in Salford in 1888. The father of this family, the size of which was not specified, was earning only 16s. per week. The mother had to go out to work in a mill, the investigator reported, to help maintain the household. The deceased infant, four weeks old, was left each day with a relative, and fed on cornflour and milk.[161]

This case did not initiate similar studies. Elaborate investigations in the 1890s were still based on assumptions about miasmic poisoning. In 1893 Dr Cameron of Leeds inquired into the mode of feeding of 153 infants who died of diarrhoea or convulsions during the six weeks ending 30 September. He reported that among infants under three months three times as many 'bottle fed' babies died as those wholly breast-fed, at three to six months almost five times as many, and at six to nine months thirty times as many.[162]

Cameron's finding inculpating artificial feeding was reinforced by two large surveys conducted in Liverpool by Dr Hope. The second survey, published in the early 1890s, covered 1,000 cases of death from diarrhoea at under five years (see Table 2.6).

Table 2.6: Baby Deaths and Type of Feeding

Mode of Feeding	Age at Death					
	Under 3 Months	3-6 Months	6-12 Months	1-2 Years	2-5 Years	Total
Breast alone	16	7	7	—	—	30
Breast and food	70	50	55	34	—	209
Breast, bottle and food	40	35	30	4	—	109
Bottle alone	33	19	13	—	—	65
Bottle and food	69	115	115	16	—	315
Cow's milk and food	5	3	5	—	—	13
Breast and any kind of food	—	1	16	20	—	37
Any kind of food	—	—	14	156	52	222
	233	230	255	230	52	1,000

Source: *BMJ*, 3 Aug. 1899, p. 255, quoted in Dr Hugh Jones, 'Infant Life', *JRSS*, vol. LVII (1894).

I give this table in full because it provides an insight into the assumptions of the investigators and the ablest medical statisticians of the day. In their view, the results vindicated the prevailing beliefs about the worth of breast-feeding and the culpability of mothers who hand-reared their children. Doctors Hope and Jones and their medical audience were satisfied that artificial feeding, and especially the careless artificial feeding indicated by 'bottle and food', was revealed as sixteen times more dangerous than straight breast-feeding. If the numbers of deaths from 'subsequent chronic wasting' and 'atrophy' were included, the indictment of artificial feeding was even grimmer. This conclusion is very likely true. But Hope's figures do not prove it. He apparently did not collect the totals in each feeding category who survived. And his single-cause categories exclude consideration of other characteristics possibly associated with each: 'poverty' and 'poor management', for example, with 'Bottle alone and food'.[163]

Some of the other components of the infant feeding problem are indicated in Dr Hope's earlier investigation in 1899, although Hope did not follow them up. He looked into 1,096 deaths among 1,082 families. These particular families had already collectively lost in infancy 51 per cent of the children born to them; nearly two-thirds of them from diarrhoea. The rate of deaths among breast-fed babies was 20 per 1,000, compared with 300 per 1,000, or 15 times as many, among those artificially fed. The average age at death was 7.4 months. Somewhat puzzled, Dr Waldo, who reported Hope's findings, noted that the

> people among whom the deaths occurred were by no means of the lowest class; in many it would appear that the families were in fairly comfortable circumstances, the husbands being men in steady work, and there were numerous instances of care and attention having been paid to the children.

Only 180 of the mothers went out to work, and only 124 of the families were 'dirty'; although 254 of the parents were 'intemperate'. Forced reluctantly on to the germ theory, Dr Waldo compromised with his environmental assumptions by concluding that diarrhoea was contained in horse dung which entered the atmosphere, and thence got into milk, but added that the disease was probably transferred only by personal contact.[164] This last finding is consonant with recent theories, which postulate a reserve of infection among adults in families. Henry Tonkin, the MOH for Leicester, had noticed in 1888 that the mortality from diarrhoea was 'principally infantile, but by far the largest proportion of *sufferers* [were] much older'. But his insight, with its implications about family hygiene and overcrowding, was never developed.[165]

Younger doctors and advanced middle-class mothers began boiling milk, in order to kill germs and make the milk more 'refined', in the late 1880s. As one enthusiast remarked, 'We would no more think of using raw milk than of using raw meat.'[166] But older doctors suspected the germ theory and thought boiling needlessly fussy, while mothers often abandoned the practice when their babies refused boiled milk. Moreover, boiled milk seemed to lose its keeping qualities: milk was not regarded as needing special cooling or protection during the summer; and there was still no simple, effective apparatus for keeping it cool.[167]

Apparatus for 'pasteurising' milk at home became available in 1898. Milk in glass-stoppered bottles was boiled in water at 90°C for ten minutes, and then the bottle was plunged into cold water.[168] The corporation of St Helens, at the instigation of Dr Drew Harris, the MOH, established the first depot for 'sterilized' milk in 1899. Harris modelled his depot on the infant clinics which had recently developed in France. The milk was boiled in closed bottles at 102°C for 45 minutes and then cooled. Each bottle contained sufficient for one meal and was sold cheaply to working mothers. Similar depots were opened at Battersea, in 1901, Ashton-under-Lyne and Liverpool.[169] The proponents of the Battersea experiment claimed instant success: their infant mortality rate in 1902 was 33 per cent less than the average for England and Wales. The St Helens depot was similarly successful (see Table 2.7).

Table 2.7: Death Rates for St Helens, Depot and District, 1899-1901

	Number of Children on Books	Death Rate per 1,000 among Children at Depot	Infantile Death Rate, St Helens Urban District
1899	232	103	157
1900	332	102	188
1901	282	106	175

Source: *Lancet*, 16 Aug. 1902, p. 478.

But the idea did not catch on. The St Helens depot managers complained that 'the people' were 'apathetic' about using the depot. Presumably more middle-class mothers than working-class mothers took advantage of it. By 1901 it was losing money at the rate of £157 a year.[170]

Less than a dozen other depots were opened in Great Britain and they can have made little impact on feeding patterns.

Doctors resisted boiling, too, on the grounds that it reduced the nutritive quality of the milk. Given the fierce heat to which the milk, which was inherently of poor quality, was exposed (60°C for 30 minutes is the normal present standard) they were undoubtedly right. If the pathogenic bacteria were reduced, so was the vitamin C content. The conservatives were still opposing the boiling of milk in 1914. The process destroyed the 'vital property' of milk and made it easy for mothers to avoid breast-feeding and careful motherhood.[171]

The average age at death from diarrhoea which Dr Hope found in Liverpool, 7.4 months, confirmed older practitioners in the belief that the malady was the inevitable concomitant of 'dentition', which was regarded as a disease in its own right until the 1880s. (At about this age the influence of maternal antibodies has diminished, the child is beginning to crawl about and is weaning on to adult foods, often difficult to digest.) Until the late 1850s, the standard procedure was to give a strong emetic 'as long as the case required'.[172] Calomel [usually mercurous chloride] with resin of jalap [another fierce purgative derived from the root of the Mexican climbing plant, *Exogonium (Impomaea) Purga*, a variety of convolvulus], scammony [yet another strong purgative from the root of a variety of convolvulus native to Asia Minor, *Convolvulus Scammonia*] or Rhubarb' was the mixture generally recommended to get 'rid of undigested sordes [impure matter collected about teeth and gums] and accumulation of slime'.[173] In addition to the emetics, the milk teeth had to be let through by lancing the gums. This last procedure had the extra advantage attaching to normal bleeding, of reducing the pressure of blood in the skull which led to convulsions and hydrocephalus. Desperate situations required resolute interventions. The usual method, as Dr Marshall Hall, MD, FRS, instructed his students, was to lance the gums either along the base or on the line of teeth, before, during and after the teeth appeared, for as often as the infant's continued irritation or convulsions rendered necessary. A child's irritability subsided with lancing. Throughout, the bowels had to be 'kept moving with the blue pill [mercuric compounds] and a little calomel'.[174]

Some independent-minded doctors began to question the medical approach to teething and diarrhoea in the early 1880s. One of the first to do so was Francis Bonney, the Poor Law doctor dismissed by the Bradford guardians for his over-zealous humanity. In 1852 he had asked whether the haemorrhage that ensued upon lancing gums did not cause at least as many deaths as the upsets lancing and dosing were supposed to cure. It was in the doctors' interest to consider the question, he added, sardonically. Most of the cases were private. Yet most of the deaths were among pauper children. The death of an occasional pauper child did not harm a surgeon's reputation; but a bad haemorrhage death in a socially superior private case might cost the surgeon his career.[175]

The transition through the 1850s and 1860s, among advanced thinkers at least, from the internal inflammatory to an external environmental explanation of dentition is summed up in the *Glasgow Medical Journal* in 1869, in an anonymous approving review of Eustace Smith's exposition of the new theories in *The Wasting Disease of Infants and Children*. Smith was Physician to the North-West London Free Dispensary for Sick Children. No doubt dentition did irritate the bowels and cause diarrhoea, he argued, but the link was not uniform. Diarrhoea during dentition was much more common, Smith asserted, during summer and autumn than winter, 'that is, at a season when the changes of temperature are so rapid and unexpected, and when . . . the child is particularly exposed to sudden chills'. Moreover, dentition often coincided with the introduction of new foods into the child's diet and these were often 'articles . . . unsuited to his age'.[176] Routine lancing fell into disuse among younger doctors during the 1860s and 1870s, and they set about the environmental investigations I have described earlier. By 1884 Dr Joll was telling Liverpool medical students that dentition was 'normal'. The shock of lancing the tense nerves in the gums only exacerbated the diarrhoea: certainly there was no evidence that it stopped it. He advised them to leave their 'lancet in their waistcoat-pocket'. His published advice evoked wrathful denials. Mr Hope of Shrewsbury declared that he always lanced and dosed, and so did 'dozens of others'. It ended convulsions 'instantly'. Mr Walford of Finchley said it 'instantly' stopped fretting, especially if the baby was also given potassium bromide. Mothers expected it from the doctor. Presumably the procedure died with this last generation of doctors; and thereby the infant mortality rate was diminished. None the less, between 1881 and 1890, over 25,000 infants were registered in England and Wales as dying from 'dentition'.[177] 'Dentition' itself gradually gave way in domestic medical manuals and journals to 'teething', a descriptive term without the connotation of disease.

Whooping Cough

The remaining major set of reported causes of death among infants under two were the 'zymotic' diseases (a general term covering infec-

whooping cough (handwritten)

tion in various ways from various forms of putrefying matter — see
below, p. 106) — whooping cough, croup, measles and smallpox.
Measles and smallpox have wider bearings and I shall discuss them in
later chapters.

Whooping cough is still one of the most deadly infectious fevers. It is
infectious and at work before it can be certainly diagnosed. The causative organism, _Bordetella Pertussis_, is spread by the victim's coughing
and sneezing and by objects he has touched. Dr Edward Smith, a
founder of the science of nutrition and already a brilliant investigator,
estimated in 1854 that among infants under twelve months, where it
was most prevalent, whooping cough and its complications had a case-
fatality rate of 1:2. Two-fifths of all deaths were under one year; two-
thirds were under two years; 19/20 were under five. These estimates
remain no more than well-informed guesses, because whooping cough
was not a notifiable disease.[178] The total numbers of deaths from
whooping cough in England and Wales were reported as shown in Table
2.8. The reader will notice that whooping cough killed more females
than males, making it unusual among nineteenth-century infections.

Table 2.8: Whooping Cough Death Rate, 1841-1910

	Male	Female	Total
1841	NA	NA	8,099
1855	4,658	5,617	10,275
1861	5,510	6,799	12,309
1871	4,546	5,814	10,360
1881	4,798	6,032	10,830
1891	6,051	7,561	13,612
1901	4,573	5,632	10,205
1905	3,954	4,755	8,709
1910	3,862	4,935	8,797

Source: *PP*, 1916, vol. V, p. 60; *PP*, 1914-16, vol. IX, pp. cvii-cix.

Dr Creighton, the epidemiologist, noticed this excess of female deaths
in the 1890s. He speculated that the female glottis was weaker, while
adding that females always showed more convulsions when attacked by
a paroxysm of coughing. This could imply that initially stronger female
infants were able to prolong their agonies and, ultimately, more completely exhaust themselves. The figures for 1968-72 show no preponderance of female deaths.[179]

Dr Edward Smith calculated in 1854 that between 1844 and 1853 whooping cough ranked only after consumption and pneumonia (to which it was — and is — often the forerunner) as a recorded cause of death among the general London population, at about one in every 30 deaths; it caused almost the same number of deaths as measles and smallpox combined, although the latter was much more feared and written about, and still preoccupies historians. Whooping cough apparently had its highest incidence in East Anglia, the south-east and Yorkshire and its lowest in the south-west, Wales and the north. In 1847 this reported incidence ranged as shown in Table 2.9.

Table 2.9: Whooping Cough Death Rate, 1847

East Anglia	1:28.1 deaths
South-east	1:32.8 "
Yorkshire	1:35.5 "
London	1:37.0 "
England and Wales	1:45.7 "
North	1:53.8 "
Wales	1:72.0 "
South-west	1:94.8 "

Source: *Medico-Chirurgical Transactions,* n.s., vol. XXXVII (1854), p. 233.

The same pattern obtained in England and Wales in 1972, with East Anglia even further above the national average, at 0.85 per 1,000,000 deaths, against the average for England of 0.42 per 1,000,000 and Wales 0.29 per 1,000,000, in a total death toll of 2,069.[180] As this general table shows, whooping cough was not a zymotic disease peculiar to great cities and, before 1870, was not regarded as such. By the 1870s, when deaths from scarlatina (an acute streptococcal infection of the throat, skin and middle ear) declined, whooping cough joined measles as a leading killer in Great Britain. The death rates are shown in Table 2.10.

Table 2.10: Whooping Cough Death Rate, 1851-90 (Scotland, 1871-90)

England and Wales	1851-60	5.7/10,000
	1861-70	6.0/10,000
	1871-80	6.1/10,000
	1881-90	6.0/10,000
Scotland	1871-80	6.1/10,000
	1881-90	6.0/10,000

Source: Charles Creighton, *A History of Epidemics in Britain* (London, 1891-4), pp. vol. II, pp. 673-5.

It had also become apparently more virulent in towns and less so in the countryside. In Scotland in 1889, the death rate was 0.91 per 1,000 in the eight principal towns against 0.25 per 1,000 in mainland rural districts.[181] Its real impact was probably even greater, for it was often the accompaniment to cholera and measles and the precursor of pneumonia and severe respiratory affections. In 1849 and 1853, for example, both cholera years in London, the average number of weekly 'hooping cough' deaths rose from the usual 36 to 45 and 50 respectively. The number of 'whooping cough' deaths also jumped in the cholera year of 1866.

It is relevant here to remind ourselves that the English reported rates, and even the higher Scottish ones, were still among the lowest reported in Europe (see Table 2.11).

Table 2.11: Whooping Cough Deaths per 1,000 Living at All Ages

	1881-5	1886-90	1891-5	1896-1900	1901-5	1906
England and Wales	0.46	0.44	0.40	0.36	0.30	0.24
Scotland	0.60	0.61	0.52	0.51	0.49	0.29
Austria	1.10	0.97	0.71	0.53	0.44	0.48
Prussia	0.52	0.51	0.45	0.42	0.36	0.31
Sweden	0.19	0.17	0.17	0.20	0.18	0.17

Source: *Medico-Chirurgical Transactions*, n.s., vol. XXXVII (1854), p. 234; Royal Commission on Smallpox and Fever Hospitals, *PP*, 1882, vol. XXIX, pp. 320-1; Jones, 'Infant Life', *JRSS*, vol. LVII (1894), p. 17; *PP*, 1909, vol. XI, p. lxx.

Then, as now, doctors had no sure remedy. Lancing the throat near the glottis was standard procedure until the 1850s, together with the usual doses of calomel and antimonial wines (normally tartrate of antimony in white wine or Spanish sherry — an emetic — often given in water, barley water or sarsaparilla). In 1823, Dr Webster, Physician to the Royal Infirmary for Sick Children, claimed great success with cases of severe whooping cough and what probably was middle ear infection with leeches on the forehead and calomel, together with rosewater and magnesium sulphide. One typical case, Charles Forrest, aged 16 months, apparently received the whole battery simultaneously and recovered! Dr Armstrong, lecturing on physic in London in 1825, said that he believed that whooping cough was 'far more fatal in London than in the country'. This resulted primarily, he thought, because the children were delicate and the 'mucous irritations' were 'more urgent'. But he could not help suspecting, too, that the higher death rate derived from the 'more active treatment' generally followed in the metropolis. 'A very common plan' was 'to sicken children two, three, or more times in the day by ipecacuanha or antimony'. Armstrong had often traced, he said, the origin of the irritation of the mucous membranes and the bowels to these medicines, or to doses of prussic acid 'and generally the affection of the brain has succeeded'. He, in advance of his time, recommended a warm room, bland diet, fresh air and mild aperients.[182] Mrs Beeton's surgeon contributor in 1861 recommended (and was still recommending in the 1880 edition) ½ to 1½ teaspoonsful a day of equal parts of antimonial wine and ipecacuanha (prepared from the root of the South American *Ceptaelis Ipecuanha*, a fierce emetic), together with a mixture, given by dessertspoon every four hours: of syrup of squills, ½oz (prepared from the sea-onion plant – it excites vomiting and 'clears the chest'); antimonial wine 1oz; laudanum 15 drops; syrup of tolu (prepared from bark of the tolu tree, *Myrospermum toluiferum*, of tropical South America – used in flavouring) water 1½oz; and leeches were to be applied to the breastbone and a 'small blister' to the throat. By 1880 the prominent physician Dr Sigismund Sutro was reported as administering quinine and, rather drastically, fuming, corrosive hydrobromic acid. Two country GPs with allopathic leanings, Dr Evans at Beaumaris and Dr Garraway at Faversham, used belladonna, 1/200th of a grain (they claimed) late each morning after the patient had been made to fast through the night and morning. They remarked that the paroxysms were much weakened by the treatment. By 1886 Dr Barlow of Manchester was using the new resorcine (a compound of potash and South American resin) in a solution of 1 or 2 per cent, swabbed on the glottis every two hours night and day. The whooping stage can last a month. These drastic, elaborate treatments could only have been given to private patients. The doctors' attentions may well have made the incidence of death a little less uneven between the unprofessionally treated, or hastily dosed, infants of the poor and the medically harassed infants of the rich.[183]

The first controlled experiment with the disease came two years later at the City of Glasgow Fever Hospital. Dr R.S. Thomson treated one group of 60 children over two years old with dilute nitric acid in 20 minim doses every four hours; a second group of 49 cases was given 10 minims in liquid extract of ergot every four hours; a third group of 95 was given five grams of chloral hydrate. The nitric acid gave 'poor results', the ergot had 'no effect' and the chloral hydrate, administered as an anaesthetic and hypnotic drug since 1869, 'mitigated' the severity of the paroxysms. Chloral hydrate was still commonly given during whooping cough attacks in the 1920s. Thomson's work seems not to have excited interest. Nineteenth-century doctors and sanitarians did not spend time on problems which appeared insoluble.[184]

Parents seem to have agreed with the doctors. Patent medicine preparations for whooping cough were few compared with the dozens of remedies advertised for coughs and colds. Two typical late-nineteenth-century lines were *Dr Assmann's Whooping Cough Remedy*, which came in both powder and pill forms, but contained only lactose. *Tussothym* was sold as especially good for whooping cough: it contained a weak distillate of thyme in alcohol.[185]

The failure of orthodox medicine left folk practice in possession of the field. The full range of sympathetic, symbolic rituals survived to comfort parents faced with a horrifying, intractable, unpredictable disease. One standard procedure was to seek out a donkey and then perform actions usually associated with the old magical number of seven. The donkey was used in several curing rituals because of its association with Christ. In 1818, at Wath in the North Riding, Benjamin Newton observed a woman, carrying a child with whooping cough, asking permission of the owner of a donkey to set her son on the beast and lead him seven times around a pear tree. At Croydon in 1858 Sir Francis Bond Head saw an Irish reaper stop a gypsy boy riding a donkey, take his child about two years old and pass it three times over the back and three times under the belly [so Head reports, but he probably miscounted] of the donkey, each time making the boy, who was 'sqalling', kiss the donkey's withers. The boy did not have whooping cough, but the Irish reaper was taking advantage of meeting the donkey to prevent an attack.[186] Usually the owner of the donkey charged for the use of his beast: in Dundee in the 1870s the going rate was sixpence for a child in arms and fourpence for the less endangered toddler. Proprietors of donkeys who worked the fairs and beaches during the summer, travelled the whooping cough circuits through the winter.[187] In northern Shropshire in the 1880s parents watched for a particular canal boat and then brought their children with whooping cough to meet the boatman who was the seventh son of a seventh son. Once met, the parents sought the boatman's advice about the illness. What happened next is not reported, but if other incidents are representative, the boatman would have attempted cures by touching, giving or recommending herbs, and would have made predictions, usually comforting, about the outcome. Riders of piebald horses were also frequently summoned to cure infants with whooping cough.[188]

The menacing power of whooping cough is also illustrated by the other rituals which coexisted in Shropshire with visits to the seventh-seventh boatman. Parents and relatives would pass the child over and under a briar bush seven times. Then they would draw three yards of black ribbon through the body of a frog and hang it around the neck of the child, or make a live frog breathe into the child's mouth, presumably on the old transference principle that the frog would incorporate the cough in his croak. Thrush, which was called 'frog' in the north-west, was also treated in this way. The frog had to hang in the mouth until it died. One man remarked in 1898 that his son had worn out four frogs before he died of convulsions. The frog was sometimes replaced by a mouse. The procedure in Hampshire in the 1890s was to roast a mouse over a candle and then make the child eat it whole. In Scotland the larvae of the tiger moth, 'hairy oubits', were used in season.[189] A wise woman of Ilkeston in Derbyshire in 1892 advised a mother of a child with the disease to shave the child's hair completely off and to put it with a piece of butcher's meat in the ashpit. The business had to be performed in absolute secrecy, or it would not work. (This is a rare revelation of the difficulty of finding evidence about these presumably widespread practices.) Probably, by analogy with other folk-medicine beliefs, the whooping cough was to diminish as the meat decayed, on a kind of diminishing life-force principle. But the near impossibility of keeping the child's bald head a secret provided an irreproachable escape clause when the ritual failed.[190]

Some folk techniques possibly did help the infant to breathe and to destroy some of the organisms associated with the *Bordetella putussis*, which primarily caused the disease. Cecil Torr, recounting oral traditions around Lustleigh in Devon, reports that in 1856 a child was treated (but apparently not cured for whooping cough by being laid in a sheep's 'forme'. The child was taken out into a meadow in the early morning and placed face downwards in the warm imprint left in the grass where a sheep had lain through the night. He was told to breathe the rising vapours in through the nostrils and mouth, until the ground grew cold (after about five minutes) and there was no more vapour. Then he was taken home to bed. When Lady Muriel Paget got whooping cough at the age of 20 in 1896 a friend begged her 'to go to a gasometer and smell the gas'. It had cured her friend's whoop 'instantly'. The coal-tar derivatives possibly did some good. In 1950 parents in Hertfordshire still took their children to the gasworks during an outbreak of whooping cough. Scots preferred the air about distilleries. The two leading herbal remedies were preparations of dropwort (chiefly *Spiraea filipendula*) and comfrey (*Symphytum officinale*). The latter has antiseptic qualities and might have had occasional good results.[191]

Croup

Croup was not a major killer but it was common and was regarded seriously by parents or doctors. The disease, as described in the 1820s by Mr John North, a London surgeon, was often seen as the prelude to consumption and other respiratory diseases, and began between the third and seventh month. It disappeared as the teeth appeared, but returned later at intervals until the child was about four years old. North recommended that 'the gums should be freely lanced ... purgatives must be freely given: calomel, in combination with powder of jalap (a purgative drug chiefly derived from the root of a Mexican climbing plant, *Exogonium (Ipomoea) Purga*), is perhaps the best remedy.' North casually added that the child should be put in a warm bath, the vapour of which probably did help.[192] North was more advanced than the country surgeon of Blegborough on the Yorkshire coast 'where croup frequently occurs'. He found that the 'copious extraction of blood from the jugular vein, during the first stage of the disease, has proved very successful'. He also administered an 'active dose of scammony with calomel' and ordered blisters on the legs.[193] Mr Jewell, of London, remarked that he and other town practitioners preferred cupping the neck as a more efficacious means of extracting blood (cupping consisted of making numerous scarifications of the flesh, heating glass cups about 2 inches deep and 1¼ inches in diameter, usually with narrow necks, with a spirit lamp to exhaust the air and then quickly setting them over the scarifications; the blood flowed strongly into the vacuum). But, he added, parents usually preferred leeches as being more direct.[194] By the 1840s these heroic measures had softened. John Savory, for example, recommended a mixture of ipecacuanha wine, ½oz; tartar emetic, 1 gram; distilled water, ½oz; one teaspoonful to be given every ten minutes during the attack until the child began to vomit. After the mixture produced this effect the child was to be put into a warm bath and given calomel and James's Powder (an antimonial medicine intended to promote perspiration). If the child was still coughing, the 'entire throat' was to be covered with leeches and the bowels emptied with a mixture of turpentine, yoke of egg, decoction of camomile flowers and an ounce of Glauber's salts. If these did not succeed within twelve hours the routine was to be repeated.[195] Mrs Beeton in 1861 proffered much the same advice, adding mustard plasters to the feet and mercurial ointment to be rubbed into the armpits and angles of the jaws. As Dr North admitted, elaborate treatments were only for the children of wealthy parents. Occasionally such a patient died after lancing and dosing 'after painful dentition, and from paroxysms of convulsive breathing'.[196]

The poor seem not to have sought medical help for their cases of croup. Possibly their more huddled humid family existence reduced the incidence of croup among them and made its attacks less oppressive. Their standby for attacks was a decoction of hyssop (usually *Hyssopus officinalis*) gathered from local gardens or bought from herb-sellers.[197] The child might have benefited from its volatile oils and at least would not have suffered from them. The parents and neighbours were probably helped by the bustle involved with gathering, preparing and administering the herb.

Syphilis

Syphilis is not reported as a leading cause of infant deaths in the nineteenth century but three informed observers claimed that it was very important. Dr Reid, writing about Preston in the 1880s, remarked that the high infant death rate of the town was 'partly due to the high syphilis rate . . . yet this was never mentioned as a cause of death'. Another doctor remarked that the use of 'marasmus infantum' on death certificates was 'as good as any other . . . indifferent term. . . when congenital syphilis [was] suspected'. Dr Lapage of Manchester noted in 1910 that the Registrar-General's report for 1905 listed 'congenital syphilis' as causing only 1.30 per cent of the infant deaths; yet a survey at the Manchester Evelina Children's Hospital revealed that 5.2 per cent of the deaths resulted from congenital syphilis and Lapage's own dispensary had a death rate of 7.2 per cent, 2/3 of which occurred at under six months of age.[198]

Congenital syphilis is a leading cause of miscarriage and the high rates reported by Lapage help to make sense of the puzzlingly high incidence of some of the conditions, the damaged facial skin and mucous membranes and disturbed development of facial bones, for example, apparently subsumed in 'hydrocephalus' through the century. The liver, eyes and ears are also often affected and undoubtedly congenital syphilis contributed to the morbidity rates at all ages of jaundice, and to blindness and deafness. This disease must have caused enormous personal suffering, family dislocation and public expense, yet it is virtually unnoticed by historians. Research could begin on the records of asylums for imbeciles.

Stability and Change in the Infant Death Rate

It is easy enough to see why the infant mortality rate held up throughout the nineteenth century. It is much harder to explain why the mortality rate turned downwards during the period 1903-8. This abatement occurred nearly thirty years after the decline began in adult mortality rates, and explanations of the transition of the total population between 1840 and 1900 from about 27 per 1,000 to 17 per 1,000 are regularly generalised by medical and social historians to imply a similar pattern for infants, with the same chronology for the turning-points. But the causes invoked by historians, declines in incidence and case fatality of scarlet fever, smallpox, cholera, tuberculosis and typhoid fever do not primarily relate to infants, for none of these was a consistent leading destroyer of life under 12 months, where the bulk of the mortality obtained.

The other causes implicit in the cost-benefit equation, sanitary improvements and advance in medical science and surgical skills seem also to be inapplicable. I know of no advance in public sanitation which could explain the sudden change after 1902, nor of any major innovation in medicine which affected infant lives in these years, although, in the long run, we can partly explain the gradual decrease in the infant death rate from the 1860s by the slow abandonment by the profession of gum-lancing, bleeding and massive dosing. In this respect the poor were more realistic than the comfortable classes. When members of a parliamentary committee in 1909 asked why the poor did not summon doctors to sick infants, Alderman Broadhurst of Huddersfield remarked that, apart from the difficulty of the expense, the poor believed that 'doctors [were] very little use for babies'.[199]

Possibly the gradual improvements in nutrition, especially through the period of increasing real wages from 1891, attained a point where the generation of mothers born after 1880 were both freer of tuberculosis and better able to bear stronger infants with a higher birth weight, and to breast-feed them. But even this development must have been very slow. Rates of death from 'immaturity' and 'congenital defect' remained constant through the first decade. And there were still great numbers of mothers, especially those bearing feeble infants, who had impaired health: 76 per cent of those mothers in Finsbury whose infants died of 'immaturity' had previously had at least one miscarriage.

Dr George Newman, who investigated this situation in 1906, found that 10 per cent of the mothers were 'under-fed'; 22 per cent 'did hard work during pregnancy'; and 50 per cent 'suffered from ill-health and poor physique'. Over the period 1902-8 the fall in the death rate for the first three months of life was only 4 per cent. This decline was due to a diminution in the numbers dying from 'atrophy and debility', suggesting that their feeding had improved.[200]

The practice of boiling milk spread among working-class families after 1900 and the Board of Agriculture instituted minimum legal standards for the quality of milk in 1901.[201] But still the very poor consumed very little milk. Urban working-class families bought less than two pints a week in 1905, that is they bought a pennyworth — 1/3 of a pint — per day; 48 per cent of working-class families in Finsbury depended entirely on condensed milk. Rural working-class families in 1908 consumed under one pint per day. Families did not buy milk in worthwhile quantities unless the breadwinner brought home at least 30s. per week.[202]

The years of transition coincide with the real take-off of the health visiting movement, and it is reasonable to conclude that the movement did have a sizeable impact on the infant death rate. Contemporaries thought they 'did good' but admitted that they had 'no clear evidence'. Health visiting grew out of the old cottage-visiting custom during the 1870s. Before then, like Jane Austen's Emma or the aristocratic sisters at Manor Cross in Trollope's *Is He Popinjoy?* the ladies brought clothes, food and wine to the ill and elderly and exercised a certain charitable terror by ordering the cleansing of the 'habitations of the vicious and most unfortunate' and systematically returning to check that their orders were obeyed. As J. Cordy Jeaffreson, a surgeon turned novelist, remarked in *Sir Evarard's Daughter* (1863), 'a call from them soon becomes to those on whom it is made little better than an insult'. In 1868 the pioneering Manchester Ladies' Sanitary Association developed the system of employing a 'sanitary mission woman', rather than themselves visiting. Or rather they visited to check on the work of the missionary.[203] This arrangement left little scope for personal gratification to the ladies and the Association stagnated until the late 1880s. During the next decade of concern about infant mortality the movement spread throughout England. By 1891 the reanimated Manchester Ladies' Health Society was employing 13 'female visitors', who made 7,000 visits 'to poor people' and 650 'special enquiries'.[204]

These spreaders of the 'gospel of carbolic' did not, at this stage, wear uniform. They were selected as

> superior women belonging to the classes among whom they work
> . . . [with] a fellow feeling and more thorough understanding of the
> difficulties . . . the failings and the sorrows of the poorer classes than
> women brought up in greater refinement and luxury would have.

In Salford they were paid 16s. per week. Each had to reside in 'her'
district and spend six hours visiting six days per week. Each visitor was
paid and supervised by a lady who had selected the district. By the late
1890s municipal corporations had been induced to help pay for the
service: Manchester paid for nine of the sixteen visitors supervised by
the Health Society. Birmingham corporation advertised for four
'women' visitors in 1899. But they were to be full corporation employees at 25s. per week and in uniform.[205]

The entry of the corporations into the system encouraged the
growth of schools for health visitors, such as that founded by the
Liverpool Ladies' Sanitary Society about 1894. The schools equipped
their alumni with qualifications which formed the first step to promotion as 'health inspectors'. Professionalism had begun. By 1897 the
Liverpool school had trained eighteen visitors. Most medical doctors
and the BMA bitterly opposed this development. Untrained deferential
assistants were acceptable: qualified professionals were a threat.[206]

The visitors made house-to-house investigations, supervising the lime
washing of bedrooms, selling pieces of wood as chocks for windows to
induce the poor to ventilate their dwellings, and lending scrubbing
brushes and buckets from the corporation pool for cleansing operations.
They reported 'nuisances' and, as their numbers grew in the late 1890s,
they began to visit every house containing a mother and new infant.
The Battersea Health Visiting Committee, run under the auspices of the
Charity Organization Society which entered this field in 1904, undertook 'to visit all mothers of young babies, both before and after confinement, with a view to teaching them the precautions and care necessary for the successful rearing of young children. All the visitors . . . are
fully trained and qualified.' The Battersea visitors, like those employed
by the City of Westminster Health Society which also commenced this
work in 1904, obtained the names and addresses of expectant mothers
from the hospitals where they booked in for their confinements. In
1907 the Westminster visitors inspected over 2,000 infants during
10,000 visits. They were reported to have achieved great success 'in the

realm of what should be termed "personal hygiene" '.[207]

The transition years also saw the creation, in Huddersfield in 1905, and the extension to London and the other great towns, of 'mother-craft' centres. These 'schools for careful mother-craft' were linked with training courses for midwives and again were run by voluntary ladies' committees financed by municipal corporations. The centres at Fulham, Poplar, Shoreditch and Stepney were by 1914 supplying meals to deserving mothers for six months before and a year after the birth of their child, and giving instruction in washing, feeding and handling the child, and making clothes for it, at a fee of one penny per month. These services were an elaboration of the old child-minding crèches which had an insecure existence since the 1870s. The charitable organisers of such nurseries had faced continual financial difficulties and frequent resistance from parents. The charges had to be low enough to encourage the mother to leave her baby at the crèche rather than with a sibling or a neighbour, and so 2*d*. to 4*d*. a day until the 1890s and then up to 6*d*. were the maximums. This left the crèches dependent upon charitable donations. That at Patricroft needed £60 a year in the 1880s, to cover the nurses' salaries and 'the good milk diet' for the children. It seems that £60 was not always forthcoming. Mothers were also indifferent or suspicious of the nursery sisters and their methods. The crèches at Ordsal in Manchester failed in 1883 because the women considered it too far, some hundreds of yards, from their factories. At Patricroft, the nurses were ordered by the medical director 'not to be too fussy'. The children were 'very dirty when brought in' at 5.45 a.m., but the 'mothers [were] very touchy' and would take the child away again if a nurse complained or set out to instruct the mother. In the Potteries the crèche movement failed completely and there were still none in 1904. The working classes feared the nurses' alien routines and alleged that they were 'taking the bread out of the mouths of the elderly people'. Thus, blighted by working-class hostility and lack of middle-class financial support, the nursery movement languished until the corporations began to help them in the 1890s. By 1906, under the impetus of anxiety about national efficiency, the movement had founded sufficient nurseries and became confident enough to institute the National Society of Day Nurseries.[208]

The health-visiting and nursery movement deserves much more study than I provide here. It was wide in coverage, even in rural counties by the turn of the century (it was exceptionally strong in Buckinghamshire, where it was backed by Florence Nightingale), assiduous in its work and its sensible advice about infant management could only have helped preserve life. But there are indications that the movement was not uniformly successful. The visitors' insistence upon carbolic, soap, milk and whitewash was often beyond the means of the poor. Instructions about regular feeding times, sobriety and neatness upset the accommodating pace of existence that made survival possible amidst the hugger-mugger of family living in a single room or tiny back-to-back, and the debility induced by malnutrition. The Reverend W.H. Verity of Huddersfield confessed in 1909 that the 'very poorest . . . who need[ed] the advice most' resented the lady health visitors, whereas the 'upper working classes' welcomed them. He thought that between 1905 and 1909 the health visitors had made 'mothers more proud of their babies', but there were still outbreaks of the disorder that had been common when the mothercraft movement began its systematic visiting in 1905, with neighbours jeering the visitor as she approached the door of a house containing a new infant and shouting 'bribery' if the mother let the lady in. Dr McAllister-Hewlings of Leicester also remarked that 'people resent their intrusions' and added that doctors got 'angry' if they 'interfered with private patients'.[209] The late Dr George Kitson Clark told me that when, before 1914, his mother was associated with the Leeds Baby Welcome Committee, the local doctors remained uncooperative and ridiculed as both pettifogging and intrusive on the doctors' domain the Committee's procedure of weighing babies and keeping records of growth. Further study of mothercraft centres might well reveal that the movement educated the medical profession, as well as mothers.

If mothers were becoming more proud of their babies because of the lady visitor's interest and their private confidence in their increasing skills in mothercraft, they might also have valued their infants more because they had fewer of them. This change might be linked with the spread of compulsory attendance at elementary schools after 1880, on a hypothesis similar to that offered by some demographers who relate decreases in the birth rate in modern Africa to the spread of schooling, because attendance at school reduces the proximate economic value of children to parents and dramatically alters the transfer of intergenerational wealth within the family. There is no need here to enter the intricacies of this hypothesis. I simply wish to point out that while the birth rate fell compulsory schooling increased, and to add that the market for child labour, even in the countryside, shrank at the same time.

Between 1876, the peak year since registration of births began in

England and Wales, and 1909, the birth rate fell as shown in Table 2.12.

Table 2.12: Births in England and Wales, 1876-1909

	Per 1,000 Population	Per 1,000 Women Aged 15-44
1876	36.3	156.7
1881	33.9	147.6
1886	32.8	140.4
1891	31.4	132.6
1896	29.6	121.9
1901	28.5	114.5
1902	28.5	114.6
1903	28.5	114.3
1904	28.0	112.7
1905	27.3	109.7
1906	27.2	109.2
1907	26.5	106.2
1908	26.7	107.6
1909	25.8	103.6

Source: Mitchell and Deane, *Abstract*, pp. 29-31.

1876 was also the peak year for Scotland. The decline matched the English and Welsh rate through the 1880s, but lagged by about two to four years thereafter. The 'transition years' to the new low fertility rate come between 1910 and 1914.

Table 2.13: Births in Scotland, 1876-1914

	Per 1,000 Population	Per 1,000 Women Aged 15-44
1876	35.6	153.9
1881	33.7	146.4
1886	32.9	142.2
1891	31.2	134.4
1896	30.4	127.9
1901	29.5	122.1
1902	29.3	120.6
1903	29.4	120.6
1904	29.1	118.6
1905	28.6	116.4
1906	28.6	115.8
1907	27.7	111.9
1908	28.1	113.0
1909	27.3	112.7
1910	26.2	108.0
1914	26.1	108.5

Source: ibid.

fall in b·r.
etc.

If we posit 1876 and 100 as the peak of the birth rate among women of child-bearing age in England and Wales, the birth rate of illegitimates, the infant population at greatest risk, with a death rate twice that of legitimates, fell to 55.6 between 1876 and 1908, with the decline accelerating after 1900. The birth rate of legitimates fell from the same peak to the still remarkable figure of 73.4. The overall decline might partly be accounted for by a change from coitus interruptus to more effective mechanical contraception. Completed family size fell in every social class, fastest in class I (landowners and professionals) and slowest among class VII, the miners. The decline can be demonstrated after 1851 for class I and between 1871 and 1881 for miners. Over all, completed fertility fell from 701 per 100 wives in 1861 to 611 in 1871-81 to 554 in 1881-6 to 217.6 (legitimate births) in 1908. The numbers of females and males under 24 years married in Great Britain also dropped sharply between 1901 and 1911, while the total numbers of married rose, after falling continuously since 1861. This change in marriage patterns, which was possibly accompanied by an increase in the worth ascribed to premarital chastity in both sexes, helps to explain the fall in the illegitimacy rate.[210] But these are all basic social processes about which we presently know very little.

Some alarmists saw the fall in the birth rate as 'race suicide'. The dismayingly high rejection rates for volunteers for the Anglo-Boer War, which I shall discuss later, increased the anxiety about Britain's 'national efficiency' which had festered since the Prussian triumph of 1870. An Inter-Departmental Committee on National Deterioration was set up in 1904. But Sir John Gorst's speech in the House of Commons announcing the Committee also announced the findings he intended it to make: that mothers were lazy, drunken, shiftless and, in limiting their offspring, careless of their duty to the Empire. The race was being vitiated by overcrowding, want of air and light, juvenile smoking and consumption of stewed tea.[211] In fact, the Committee, led by Sir Almeric Fitzroy, clerk of the Council, proved resistant to the alarmists and reported that the people were gradually improving in physique and personal hygiene. But the alarmists had much to be alarmed about. They noted that towns with high proportions of lazy mothers had continuing high death rates: Bilston and Burslem, Barnsley, Merthyr Tydvil, Widnes, Liverpool, Abertillery all had infant death rates of above 160 per 1,000 live births, and showed small improvement from the bad rates of the mid-nineteenth century. By contrast, 'residential towns such as Croydon, Richmond (Surrey), Hendon, Swindon, Handsworth, Stretford, all reported infant death rates around 100 per 1,000.

Not Effic

But the towns with slipshod mothers also had the highest birth rates, at around 35-37 per 1,000, that is about 10 per 1,000 above the national average, while Croydon and other salubrious places had birth rates around 25 per 1,000. Gorst and his comrades concluded that the 'unfit' were outbreeding the fit: the Empire would be bereft of leaders.[212]

This conclusion gave a fillip to the eugenics movement. Medical sanitarians added to the anxiety. Doctors Heron, Newsholme and Stevenson all proved that the pauper class was overrunning the 'prosperous classes'. Newsholme and Stevenson ingeniously divided the London boroughs into six groups according to the average number of servants reported for 100 families in each. They then took the number of women married in each district (their conclusion would have been even more dramatic if they had included single women), corrected the figures for age and the average marital state at each age for England and Wales, and then they 'corrected' the reported birth rate of each district, presumably according to its deviation from the national average by age and marital state.

Table 2.14: Newsholme's and Stevenson's Study of London Birth Rates

Group I	with only 10 servants per 100 families	31.56
Group II	" 10-20 " " " "	25.82
Group III	" 20-30 " " " "	25.63
Group IV	" 30-40 " " " "	25.50
Group V	" 40-60 " " " "	25.36
Group VI	" over 60 " " " "	20.45

Source: Physical Deterioration Committee, *PP*, 1904, vol. XXXII, pp. 38-9, Qs. 11790-5.

Group I, the very poor, about one-quarter of the population of London, were producing at a rate 33 per cent greater than that of the very rich. Moreover, the reproducing masses were demonstrably of low 'mental capacity'.[213] Professor Karl Pearson in his Huxley Lecture of 1903 had warned that 'looking round impassionately from the calm atmosphere of anthropology', he had discerned that England was 'breeding less intelligence' than she had done fifty or a hundred years ago. Given the 'scientific fact' that intelligence was inherited, the 'only remedy ... [was] to alter the relative fertility of the good and bad stocks in the community'. Gorst in 1904 was more blunt: the state had to thwart marriages among the 'least fit' to enable the 'superior stocks' to catch

proto-fascism

up on reproducing themselves. The prohibition of early marriage seemed the most practicable starting-point.

Selective human breeding for patriotic reasons had appealed to some doctors since the period of national disquiet from 1855 following the disclosures about bad management in the Crimean War. As one doctor put it, 'we can breed good horses . . . now for good men . . . for the protection of the home land'. The phrase 'sterilization of the unfit' had entered the language in 1888-9, in the clinical context of preventing the 'incontestably established' hereditary transmission of syphilis, gout, phthisis and insanity. Here the end was not national power, but medical power: 'We are responsible', the editor of the *Lancet* proclaimed, 'for the employment of our peculiar authority in promotion of the purification and well-being of human society.' Dr Gordon Dill called for state support of medical certification of applicants for marriage, with the object of eliminating the reproduction of syphilitics and alcoholics. Dr Rentoul in 1904 also wanted a state board to protect doctors as they sterilised degenerates by sealing the vas deferens or the Fallopian tubes. Idiots, persons likely to transmit disease to offspring, children of prostitutes, 'sexual degenerates', confirmed tramps, criminals, weak-minded children, were all to come under the board's scrutiny. The British Medical Association remained non-committal until the battle against National Insurance in 1911. This Bill, as the doctors saw it, threatened private practice. It was promoted, the President of the BMA, Sir James Barr alleged, to cherish 'malingerers and the unfit', and to hasten the destitution of the higher physiological 'castes'. Thereafter Barr and other BMA leaders, such as E.B. Turner, became tireless advocates of doctor-state controlled eugenics as the 'new form of preventive medicine on behalf of the race as well as . . . the individual' and private practice.

The transition years were also the period of take-off for the psychological 'measurement' crusaders. They joined the eugenists (they were often the same people) in working for a virile, organic Empire comprising a selectively bred populace led by intellectually proven Platonic guardians. Consonant with Gorst's and Pearson's concern with overcrowding, want of fresh air and light, and juvenile smoking, the transition years were also the foundation years of garden cities such as Port Sunlight and Bournville, the Boy Scouts and school Cadets.[214] Socialists such as H.G. Wells, Bernard Shaw and Keir Hardie saw the solution in terms of uplifting the whole population by creating a system of family allowances. But this suggestion implied a massive reallocation of wealth and was never taken seriously by the Tory and Liberal leaderships. Moreover, Wells and Shaw had not excluded single or deserted mothers from their proposal and it was therefore deemed immoral as well. Government involvement extended only to legislative provision for municipal subsidising of school meals in 1907.[215] Eugenists and measurers of mental capacity found consolation in pressing for the sterilisation of the unfit and the objective vertical stratification of society as a means of preserving the class-divided nation.

In their perplexity the 'national deterioration' believers overlooked, as historians have continued to overlook, the crucial point which the socialists had glimpsed. The great question for the nation was not simple birth rates, but the fostering and increase of viable life.[216] Measured in this way, the increase in the number of human beings surviving infancy, about 8 per cent between 1901 and 1911, is probably the largest and quickest advance in modern British history. These calculations suggest a new hypothesis to explain the general decrease in infant mortality: more effective family limitation meant that mothers could care more effectively for the fewer children they had, that the family income went further, and that the earlier completion of the family meant fewer defective children born to older mothers. I have to confess that there is at present no way of verifying the application to the past of this contemporary demographic commonplace, but it could be approached through family reconstitution methods. Moreover, if we surmise that one primary motivation for producing offspring is the parents' desire for 'immortality', then the enhanced likelihood of the earlier-born children surviving to adulthood could weaken the disposition to have additional children. In this situation contraception, as in the present world, becomes more carefully applied and efficient.

We can explain the 1902-7 breakthrough in the decline of infant mortality more precisely by noting the percentages of decline in Great Britain at various ages (see Table 2.15).

Table 2.15: Decline in Infant Mortality, 1902-7

0–3 months	(about 50% of the mortality under 1 year)						4%
3–6 "	(" 18% " "	"	"	"	"	)	9%
6–12 "	(" 32% " "	"	"	"	"	)	14%

Source: Calculated from Stevenson, *PP*, 1909, vol. XI, p. lxxix, and Mitchell and Deane, *Abstract*, pp. 6, 12-13.

These dramatic improvements reflect a fall in mortality ascribed to whooping cough by one-third in England and Wales and one-seventh in Scotland. The other zymotic killer which diminished was 'diarrhoea and convulsions', which fell in England and Wales by 12 per cent, in urban counties by 13 per cent and in rural counties by 26 per cent, resulting in an annual saving of about 20,000 lives, in a normal total of about 76,000 deaths ascribed to this disease, in a total number of deaths averaging 120,000.[217] A succession of cool summers helped, but the basic cause must have been improved feeding and mothering. France, which had a much higher infant diarrhoea and twice the mortality rate of Britain, introduced mothercraft incentives and teaching in 1895 and reduced the rates to equal the British ones before 1900.[218]

The 4 per cent decline of mortality in the first three months of life is almost solely attributable to a fall in deaths ascribed to 'Debility, Atrophy and Inanity'. The rate of deaths registered as from prematurity and congenital defects even rose slightly between 1890 and 1908. Again this pattern suggests better feeding and handling, and no improvement in the ante-natal health of the mother. Moreover, by 1911, the mortality rate for infants under one month was only 8 per cent higher in towns than in the countryside. But thereafter the gap widened enormously — at 2-4 months, the town rate was 11.6 per cent higher; at 4-7 months 43 per cent higher; at 7-12 months 67 per cent higher. The class differential remained, too, as shown in Table 2.16.

Table 2.16: Infant Death Rate, 1911

Among	'families of the upper and middle classes'	77 per 1,000
Among	'textile operatives'	148 per 1,000
Among	'miners' (i.e. coal)	160 per 1,000
Among	'agricultural labourers'	97 per 1,000

Source: Dr. Newsholme, *Lancet*, 10 Jan. 1914, p. 129, 31 Jan., p. 339.

These groupings hide even greater extremes: as against the miners' 160 per 1,000, naval officers' and solicitors' families had a rate of 41 per 1,000 and medical practitioners' families 39 per 1,000.[219] Moreover, as the rate for the comparatively well paid miners shows, infant mortality was not a simple outcome of poverty, nor of whether mothers worked outside the home, because wives in mining communities were inhibited by custom from taking outside work. It would seem that middle-class mothers valued their babies more than wives of coal-miners and had much greater material and intellectual help in caring for them. Mining communities, moreover, then as now, might well have been relatively severely male-dominated, with a consequent devaluing of female and infant life. The normally static stock of poor housing and the rental or leasehold tenure of that stock must also have contributed to the poor sanitation and amenity normal in mining villages and the bad health that distinguished such communities. These complex factors were apparently still at work despite the social welfare revolution of the Second World War. By the 1960s neonatal mortality had declined at the same proportions for occupational groups as obtained in 1911.[220]

Yet the deprivation that imprisoned working-class life remains crucial to any understanding of high infant morbidity and mortality rates. A brilliant pioneering investigation by Mrs Barbara Drake in Westminster in 'the twelve months beginning June 1907 demonstrated relationships between infant morbidity and living conditions that had long been postulated but never, so far as I know, tested. Mrs Drake was the favourite niece and working companion of Beatrice and Sidney Webb, and the lucidity of her exposition may well owe something to her distinguished mentors. She was a member of the City of Westminster Health Society, founded in 1904. Using the visitors' records of the Society she analysed the 'health of infants under different conditions of housing, poverty, mother's work, mother's health, and mode of feeding', in 1,237 cases. In each classification her figures show a close link between low income, poor housing and high morbidity and mortality among both infants and mothers. In general, twice as many infants in low-income families in poor housing were sickly or dead. Her classifications are unexplained in her paper and are very likely impressionistic, but they are based on detailed knowledge of individual cases and they probably err on the side of severity. The definition of a 'comfortable' family income at 25*s*., for example, puts the topmost class in her ensemble below the level of a moderately regularly employed ordinarily skilled London cabinet-maker, engine-driver or carpenter at 30*s*. to 36*s*. per week.

Healthy children are distributed by housing type in about the same proportion as each type of housing is to the total number of cases. Children of delicate health, children who die under one year of age and, most markedly, children who die at under one month are disproportionately distributed towards tenement housing.

Housing with good sanitation contained proportionately more healthy children, fewer, though less pronouncedly so, infant deaths and, significantly, a proportional share of deaths at under one month.

Table 2.17: Health of Infants and Level of Income, Westminster, 1907/8

Cases No.	Per Cent	Income Levels	Healthy No.	Per Cent	Delicate No.	Per Cent	DEATHS Under 1 Year No.	Per Cent	Under 1 Month No.	Per Cent
546	45.0	Comfortable (25s. +)	427	78.2	86	15.7	33	6.0	23	4.2
402	33.1	Poor (21s. 25s.)	294	73.1	80	19.9	28	7.0	14	3.4
266	21.9	Very poor	136	51.1	93	35.0	37	13.9	14	5.2
21		Unstated								
1,214			857	70.59	259	21.33	98	8.07	51	4.2

Source: Mrs Drake, 'A Study of Infant Life in Westminster', *JRSS*, vol. LXXI (1908), pp. 680-6.

Table 2.18: Health of Infants and Mother's Health, Westminster, 1907/8

Cases No.	Per Cent	Condition	Healthy No.	Per Cent	Delicate No.	Per Cent	DEATHS Under 1 Year No.	Per Cent	Under 1 Month No.	Per Cent
926	74.9	Strong	721	77.8	155	16.7	50	5.4	18	1.9
311	25.1	Delicate	157	50.5	106	34.0	48	15.4	33	10.6
1,237			878	70.9	261	21.0	98	7.9	51	4.1

Source: ibid.

Table 2.19: Health of Infants and Housing, Westminster, 1907/8

Cases No.	Per Cent	Type	Healthy No.	Per Cent	Delicate No.	Per Cent	DEATHS Under 1 Year No.	Per Cent	Under 1 Month No.	Per Cent
385	31.1	Block	292	75.8	69	17.9	24	6.2	12	3.1
813	65.7	Tenement	555	68.2	186	22.8	72	8.5	39	4.7
39	3.2	Cottage	31	79.5	6	15.3	2	5.1	–	–
1,237			878	70.9	261	21.0	98	7.9	51	4.1

Source: ibid.

Table 2.20: Health of Infants and Sanitary State of Housing, Westminster, 1907/8

Cases		Condition	Healthy		Delicate		DEATHS			
No.	Per Cent		No.	Per Cent	No.	Per Cent	Under 1 Year		Under 1 Month	
							No.	Per Cent	No.	Per Cent
700	57.5	Good	547	78.1	107	15.3	46	6.5	28	4.0
359	29.5	Indifferent	246	68.5	81	22.5	32	8.9	15	4.1
159	13.1	Bad	69	43.4	70	44.0	20	12.6	8	5.0
1,218	100.0		862	70.7	258	21.1	98	8.0	51	4.1

Source: ibid.

Mrs Drake's presentation does not permit us to make exact cross-correlations, but she does add some comments about the distribution in Westminster of her categories, which make it reasonable to suggest that the 'comfortable' were largely the best housed and healthiest. Three other tables and their commentaries enable us to suggest confidently that most of the women who could afford not to work breast-fed their babies and kept their houses the cleanest. Home-work, mostly in north Soho, in tailoring, eating houses and small shops, also produced a comfortable family income and good mothering. The out-working bottle-feeders were concentrated in south Westminster amongst a population of casual and unemployed labourers in tenements.

Table 2.21: Health of Infants and Type of Feeding, Westminster, 1907/8

Cases			Healthy		Delicate		DEATHS			
No.	Per Cent		No.	Per Cent	No.	Per Cent	Under 1 Year		Under 1 Month	
							No.	Per Cent	No.	Per Cent
844	70.4	Breast	716	84.8	108	12.7	20	2.3	8	.9
31	2.6	Partly (6 months)	12	38.7	18	58.0	1	3.2	—	—
70	5.8	Partly (3 months)	35	50.0	32	45.7	3	4.3	—	—
114	9.5	Under 6 weeks	49	43.0	46	40.5	19	16.7	1	.8
140	11.7	Bottle	66	47.1	57	40.7	17	12.1	4	2.8
1,199			878	73.2	261	21.7	60	5.0	13	1.0

Source: ibid.

Table 2.22: Health of Infants and Mother's Work, Westminster, 1907/8

Cases No. Per Cent			Healthy No. Per Cent		Delicate No. Per Cent		DEATHS Under 1 Year No. Per Cent		Under 1 Month No. Per Cent	
934	75.5	No occupation	700	74.9	173	18.5	61	6.5	32	3.4
135	10.8	Home-work	94	69.6	31	22.9	10	7.4	7	5.1
168	13.6	Out-work	84	50.0	57	33.9	27	16.1	12	7.1
1,237			878	70.9	261	21.0	98	7.9	51	4.1

Source: ibid.

Mrs Drake's proof of the links between poverty and high infant morbidity and mortality were reinforced by Professor Lapage in 1910 (see Table 2.23). He showed that low rates of gain in weight correlated with the unemployment of the father. His statistics were drawn from the Manchester School for Mothers around 1909. He had about 14 cases in each unemployed/infant age category.

Table 2.23: Lapage's Survey on Infant Weight Gains, 1910

Age	Father Out of Work: Weight of Infant		Average for all Cases at Manchester School for Mothers		Average for England	
	lb	oz	lb	oz	lb	oz
At one month	6	3¼	7	4	7	8
At three months	9	4¾	10	10	10	0
At six months	10	3	12	4	14	4
At nine months	12	6¼	17	4½	16	12

Source: *Medical Chronicle*, vol. LII (1910), p. 24.

Lapage added that he had further figures which showed that the 'unemployed' group gradually fell even further behind their more fortunate cohorts as they grew older.[221]

Among the poor, only the strong and the lucky infants survived. The cumulative effects on British society of the generations of malnutrition during the foetal period and in infancy are as yet unexplored. Modern research suggests that such deprivation is associated with subsequent intellectual impairment and passivity and abnormality in behaviour. There is even clearer evidence that children deprived in infancy are more subject than their peers to defects in eyesight and hearing, and to illnesses which hinder their subsequent development. These sorts of problems are at the centre of questions about 'Hunger and Politics' which historians of the poor and working classes hitherto have overlooked.

Notes

1. B.R. Mitchell and Phyllis Deane, *Abstract of British Historical Statistics* (Cambridge, 1962), pp. 36-7; G.F. McCleary, *The Maternity and Child Welfare Movement* (London, 1935), pp. 4-5.

2. Michael G. Mulhall, *The Dictionary of Statistics* (London, 1892), p. 174.

3. Registrar-General's Reports, *PP*, 1851, vol. XL, 1861, vol. XIV, 1871, vol. XX, 1881, vol. XX, 1891, vol. XXIV, 1901, vol. XVIII.

4. M.J. Cullen, *The Statistical Movement in Early Victorian Britain* (London, 1975), pp. 32, 161.

5. See 6 and 7 Will. IV, c.86; 37 and 38 Vict., c.88; 'Report of SC on Infant Mortality', *JRSS*, vol. LXXXVI, Pt. I (1912), p. 66; Major George Graham, Registrar-General to Royal Sanitary Commission, *PP*, 1868-9, vol. XXXII, Qs. 6427-8.

6. *L*, 2 Jan. 1864, p. 18, 15 Sept. 1888, p. 530; 'Anencephalous Foetus', *GMJ*, vol. XXIX (1888), pp. 261-2.

7. Dr Henry Cooper Rose, *L*, 27 May 1876, p. 777; Robert Cory, *St Thomas' Hospital Reports*, vols. VIII (1878), p. 74, X (1880), p. 275, XXIV (1897), p. 150; Jardine in *GMJ*, vol. LXII (1904), pp. 259-60. The 'incubator' or 'artificial mother' was invented by a Parisian, Dr Arevard, in the 1880s. It came into use in Britain in 1887. It was a wooden box divided horizontally into two compartments which freely communicated with each other. The premature infant was placed in the upper compartment, above an assortment of hot water bottles and a wet sponge 'to help keep the air damp' in the lower part. The death rate of babies placed in it was 2 in 3 (*BMJ*, 12 Feb. 1887, p. 346).

8. Frank Field, *Unequal Britain* (London, 1974), pp. 10-12; S. Davidson and Reginald Passmore, *Human Nutrition and Dietetics* (Edinburgh, 1973). Cf. Davidson and Passmore for a striking difference of average bulk weight (p. 764) of babies born to upper-caste and low-caste women in India in the 1960s.

9. Cullen, *Statistical Movement*, p. 33; see also Farr to Royal Sanitary Commission, *PP*, 1868-9, vol. XXXII, Q.4461.

10. *L*, 25 Mar. 1899, p. 848.

11. *L*, 10 Oct. 1896, p. 1024.

12. *L*, 2 Jan. 1864, p. 18.

13. *L*, 15 Sept. 1888, p. 530.

14. *L*, 6 June 1903, p. 1604. For a similar situation twenty years earlier, see *L*, 18 Dec. 1886, p. 1186.

15. *Medical Gazette*, 21 Feb. 1835, p. 733.

16. T. Laycock, 'On the Sanitary Condition of . . . York', *JSS*, vol. VIII (1845), pp. 63-4.

17. Edwin Chadwick, *Report on The Sanitary Condition Of The Labouring Population Of Gt. Britain* [1842], M.W. Flinn (ed.) (Edinburgh, 1965), p. 228.

18. Dr Hugh R. Jones, 'Infants'. *JRSS*. vol. LVII (1894), p. 57.

19. E.W. Hope, 'Discussion on Infant Mortality', *Royal Institute of Public Health, Aberdeen Congress, 1900*, p. 229.

20. *L*, 15 Nov. 1902, p. 1357.

21. B.L. Hutchens, 'Infantile Mortality and the Proportion of the Sexes', *JRSS*, vol. LXXVII, Pt. I (1913), p. 86.

22. Dr Bachhoffner, Marylebone, district registrar reporting to the local Vestry, *L*, 22 Oct. 1859, pp. 415-16.

23. *L*, 18 Sept. 1875, p. 437.

24. *L*, 21 July 1877, p. 101.

25. *L*, 13 July 1901, p. 99.

26. [E.C. Wolstenholme], *Infant Mortality: Its Causes and Remedies* (Manchester, 1871), p. 21.

27. Henry Butler, *What Is the Harm?* (London, 1880) [first pub. 1864], p. 9; Dr J.B. Curvengen, *L*, 23 Mar. 1867, p. 367; J.B. Curvengen, 'Programme' of the Infant Life Protection Society, n.d. [c. 1871].

28. *L*, 4 Feb. 1860, p. 125; see also Margaret Hewitt, *Wives and Mothers in Victorian Industry* (London, 1958), for corroborative information from Manchester in the late 1860s, p. 59.

29. W.G. Lumley, 'Observations on the Statistics of Illegitimacy', *JSS*, vol. XXV (1862), pp. 221-55.

30. Jane Austen to Cassandra Austen, 17 Nov. 1798, in *Jane Austen, Letters 1796-1817*, R.W. Chapman (ed.) (Oxford, 1955), pp. 13-14. 'We had an uneasy afternoon. The Dr deciding it dangerous to go on dosing our poor baby, I went off for a Nurse & brought (under Cape's [physician] directions) an apparently nice & respectable woman with a very fine child . . . [5 Oct.] Locock [physician] spoke to me of the 'frightful' mortality among the children of wet nurses; and said the way was to make them put out their own child to a nurse. – Prayers etc. at 12' [16 Nov.] (*Gladstone Diaries*, vol. III, pp. 236, 239).

31. T.C. Haden, *Practical Observations on the Management and Diseases of Children* (London, 1827), p. 115. See also William Buchan, *Domestic Medicine* (1802 ed.), p. 3.

32. Mrs Isabella Beeton, *The Book of Household Management*, p. 1023; Pye Henry Chavasse, *Counsel To A Mother* (London, 1869), p. 16.

33. Joseph Rogers, *Reminiscences of a Workhouse Medical Officer* (London, 1889), pp. 44-5.

34. *L*, 18 Feb. 1882, pp. 280-1.

35. Haden. *Practical Observations*, pp. 122-32.

36. *L*, 12 Feb. 1859, p. 175.

37. *L*, 19 Feb. 1857, p. 201.

38. *L*, 25 June 1859, p. 637.

39. Haden, *Practical Observations*, p. 115.

40. *L*, 27 Apr. 1850, p. 513.

41. *L*, 14 Aug. 1869, p. 242.

42. *L*, 18 Feb. 1882, p. 280.

43. William Buchan, *Domestic Medicine* (Edinburgh [1784 ed.]), p. 588.

44. A.S. Taylor to SC on the Chemists and Druggists Bill, *PP*, vol. XII, 1865, Qs. 288-91; *L*, 16 July 1898, p. 159.

45. *L*, 16 Mar. 1861, p. 272, 30 Oct. 1869, p. 619, 5 Feb. 1870, p. 207, 15 Jan. 1870, p. 94; *Examiner*, 9 July 1853, p. 443; *BMJ*, 17 Apr. 1880, p. 601; *L*, 7 Mar. 1857, p. 256.

46. *L*, 30 July 1853, p. 101.

47. *L*, 10 Dec. 1898, p. 1570.

48. *L*, 2 Feb. 1839, p. 705, 30 May 1863, p. 614. There is a sketch of nineteenth-century English law on abortion in Bernard M. Dickens, *Abortion and the Law* (London, 1966), pp. 22-37.

49. 43 Geo. III, c.58; *Edinburgh Medical and Surgical Journal*, vol. VI (1810), pp. 245-7; *L*, 12 May 1821, pp. 219-20.

50. *L*, 23 July 1853, p. 89, 24 Oct. 1857, p. 425, 6 Dec. 1862, p. 627.

51. *L*, 10 Apr. 1875, 1 May 1875, pp. 521, 626.

52. *L*, 14 Jan. 1899, p. 105.

53. *L*, 26 Dec. 1857, p. 655.

54. *L*, 29 Oct. 1898, p. 1153; *BMJ*, 3 Dec. 1881, p. 909.

55. *BMJ*, 25 Dec. 1897, p. 1881; *L*, 10 Dec. 1898, p. 1651, 24 Dec. 1898, pp. 1720; *The Times*, 19 Dec. 1898, p. 14.

56. Charles Clay (Senior Medical Officer, St Mary's Hospital, Manchester), 'Statistics and Observations on the liability to Abortion', *GMJ*, vol. VI (1859), pp. 408-10.

57. *L*, 22 Mar. 1862, p. 307.

58. *BMJ*, 1 May 1880, p. 667.

59. *L*, 5 Aug. 1865, p. 153.

60. *L*, 16 May 1891, p. 1114.

61. *L*, 24 Jan. 1903, p. 251.

62. *L*, 14 July 1888, p. 80.

63. Ibid.

64. *L*, 23 Aug. 1879, p. 299; McCleary, *Maternity and Child Welfare*, p. 94.

65. William L. Langer, 'Checks on Population Growth 1750-1850', *Scientific American* (Feb. 1972), p. 96.

66. P.J. Martin, 'Observations on some of the Accidents on Infanticide', *Edinburgh Medical and Surgical Journal*, vol. XXV (1826), pp. 34-6.

67. *L*, 9 Sept. 1865, p. 293, 23 Mar. 1867, p. 367.

68. 35 and 36 Vict., c. 38; *Parliamentary Debates*, vol. cccxlii, cols. 82-91, 1082-91; *BMJ*, 9 Aug. 1890, p. 364; Hugh R. Jones, 'Infant Life', *JRSS*, vol. LVII (1894), pp. 2-6; *L*, 18 Oct. 1902, p. 1068.

69. *Truth*, 21 Mar. 1895, p. 704.

70. *L*, 10 May 1862, p. 493.

71. *L*, 16 Mar. 1895, p. 702.

72. Neville R. Butler and Dennis G. Bonham, *Perinatal Mortality* (Edinburgh, 1963), p. 193.

73. *L*, 26 Feb. 1887, p. 444. See also RC on Poor Laws, *PP*, 1909, vol. XI, p. xl.

74. Butler and Bonham, *Perinatal Mortality*, pp. 14-15.

75. T.R. Edwards, 'Law of Mortality in Each County of England', *L*, 5 Dec. 1835, p. 409; *Sanitary Review*, vol. 14 (Oct. 1858), for patterns in 1850s; *L*, 23 Oct. 1875, p. 605, for pattern in early 1870s; G. Melvyn Howe, *Man, Environment and Disease in Britain* (Harmondsworth, 1976), p. 205, for similar pattern in 1901.

76. *Medical and Physical Journal*, vol. XXVI (1811), p. 509.

77. *Edinburgh Medical and Surgical Journal*, vol. LI (1839), p. 169.

78. Mrs William Parkes, *Domestic Duties* [fourth ed.] (London, 1837), p. 362.

79. Anon., *Plain Observations on the Management of Children during the First Month* (London, 1828), pp. 10, 15.

80. Buchan, *Domestic Medicine* [1769 ed.], p. 9.

81. Ernest Jones, 'Alcoholic Cirrhosis of the Liver in Children', *GMJ*, vol. LXVIII (1907), pp. 236-7.

82. *L*, 1824, vol. II, p. 407.

83. *L*, 28 Aug. 1869, p. 34 (death of child of eight months choked on piece of ham); *GMJ*, vol. XXIII (1885), p. 332 (deaths from eating sugar and water, castor oil, rusks, arrowroot, bread); *L*, 6 Sept. 1902, p. 771 (deaths from meat pieces, ham, potatoes).

84. Anon., *Plain Observations*, p. 6.

85. *Gazette of Health*, 1 May 1816, p. 150.

86. Wilfred Blunt, *Lady Muriel* (London, 1962), p. 38; *BMJ*, 26 June 1886, p. 1246, 5 Mar. 1887, p. 515; *Medical Chronicle*, vol. LII (1910), p. 23.

87. W. Woodward, 'Infantile Diseases', *Medical and Physical Journal*, vol. IV (1800), p. 44.

88. *L*, 5 Jan. 1826, p. 540; Haden, *Practical Observations*, p. 101; Dr William Johnston, *Medical Times and Gazette*, 25 Oct. 1879, p. 483.

89. Dana Raphael, *The Tender Gift* (Englewood Cliffs, N.J., 1973), p. 67.

90. Buchan, *Domestic Medicine* [1802 ed.], p. 3; John Cheyne, *Medical and Physical Journal*, vol. XI (1804), pp. 184-5; Haden, *Practical Observations*, p. 101; McMillan, *GMJ*, vol. XXIII (1885), p. 333; Wills, *Westminster Hospital Reports*, vol. XI (1899), pp. 58-9; Barclay Ness, *GMJ*, vol. LXII (1904), p. 263.

91. *Medical and Physical Journal*, vol. XI (1804), p. 185.

92. Dr Hugh R. Jones, 'Infant Life', *JRSS*, vol. LVII (1894), p. 32.

93. Alan D. Berg, *The Nutrition Factor; its role in national development* (Washington, D.C., 1973), pp. 90-2.

94. Ronald Davie, Neville Butler and Harvey Goldstein, *From Birth to Seven* (London, 1972), pp. 71-3; Allen Clarke, *Effects of the Factory System* (London, 1899), p. 127; *L*, 8 May 1852, p. 455.

95. Davie *et al.*, *From Birth to Seven*, p. 73; Douglas and Rowntree, *Maternity in Great Britain*, pp. 152-3.

96. Charles Creighton, *A History of Epidemics in Britain* (London [1891-4]), vol. II, pp. 761-9.

97. 'Mr Coley on the Remittent Fever of Infants', *Medical and Physical Journal*, vol. XXX (1814), p. 243; Haden, *Practical Observations*, p. 165; John Roberton, 'Observations on the Mortality and Physical Management of Children', *Edinburgh Medical and Surgical Journal*, vol. XXIX (1828), p. 383; T. Herbert Barker, 'Nursery Government in its Sanitary Aspects', *Journal of Public Health and Sanitary Review*, vol. II (Oct. 1856), pp. 369-71.

98. Barker, 'Nursery Government', *Journal of Public Health . . .*, vol. II (July 1856), p. 147.

99. Anon., *The Female Instructor* (London, 1841), p. 101.

100. *Journal of Public Health . . .*, vol. II (Oct. 1856), pp. 372-3.

101. *BMJ*, 18 Dec. 1857, p. 1057, 7 Oct. 1905, p. 903. Baby shows became popular in the United States in the early 1850s and had begun in France by 1855, amidst alarm about the poor quality of conscripts for the Crimean War (*L*, 30 June 1855, p. 658).

102. *Journal of Public Health . . .*, vol. II (March 1856), pp. 57-8; *L*, 18 Oct. 1879, p. 584.

103. A. Jacobs, 'The Teaching and Practice of Pediatrics', *GMJ*, vol. LI (1899), p. 463; Ernest Roberts, *L*, 11 Apr. 1914, p. 1084.

104. *L*, 29 Oct. 1898, p. 1128; Haden, *Practical Observations*, pp. 165-7.

105. Jones, 'Infant Life', *JRSS*, vol. LVII (1894), p. 22; Haden, *Practical Observations*, p. 167.

106. *L*, 3 Apr. 1858, p. 345.

107. *L*, 14 June 1856, p. 674.

108. *L*, 28 Aug. 1869, p. 328.

109. *L*, 6 Sept. 1902, p. 711.

110. *L*, 24 Apr. 1858, p. 415.

111. *L*, 2 Oct. 1869, p. 488.

112. *BMJ*, 9 July 1881, p. 49.

113. Mrs Beeton, *Household Management* (new ed., 1880), pp. 1041-2.

114. Chavasse, *Counsel To A Mother*, pp. 9-11.

115. Herbert Preston-Thomas, *The Work and Play of A Government Inspector* (London, 1909), p. 225.

116. *Plain Observations*, pp. 27-8.

117. Esther Copley, *Catechism of Domestic Economy* (London, 1851), p. 105.

118. Chavasse, *Counsel To A Mother*, p. 11.

119. Catherine M. Buckton, *Food and Home Cookery* (London, 1883), p. 86.

120. Dr McMillan, *GMJ*, vol. XXIII (1885), p. 332.

121. *L*, 13 Feb. 1897, p. 452.

122. Buchan, *Domestic Medicine* [1802 ed.], p. 3; Haden, *Practical Observations*, p. 24.

123. *L*, 23 Nov. 1892, pp. 753-4.

124. *L*, 10 Apr. 1875, p. 520.

125. *Medical Times and Gazette*, 25 Oct. 1879, p. 483.

126. *L*, 20 June 1885, p. 1144. For the Irish, see, for example, *L*, 19 July 1890, p. 147 (Cardiff) and 8 Dec. 1894, p. 1371 (Hull); 26 Apr. 1884, p. 775 (Preston).

127. Creighton, *Epidemics*, vol. II, p. 769; *L*, 4 Aug. 1883, pp. 192-3, 16 Oct. 1886, p. 737.

128. *L*, 4 Aug. 1883, pp. 192-3; Dr Borchardt, *Liverpool Medical and Chirurgical Journal*, vol. 5 (1883), p. 401.

129. *L*, 17 June 1882.

130. *L*, 24 May 1884, p. 955.

131. *L*, 7 Sept. 1872, pp. 339-40, 2 Nov. 1872, p. 653.

132. *Liverpool Medical and Chirurgical Journal*, vol. 5 (1883), pp. 402-4. Dr Ralph Vincent's analysis, National Deterioration Committee, *PP*, 1904, vol. XXXII, Q. 12057.

133. *BMJ*, 5 Oct. 1889, p. 777.

134. Quoted in J.M. Macintosh, *Trends of Opinion About the Public Health 1901-51* (Oxford, 1953), p. 19.

135. *L*, 25 Mar. 1899, p. 851.

136. Mr Tattersall (Oldham), *L*, 8 Aug. 1896, p. 405.

137. *L*, 9 July 1881, p. 66.

138. *Westminster Hospital Reports*, vol. XI (1899), p. 59.

139. *GMJ*, vol. XXIII (1885), p. 333.

140. Alex Mair, *Sir James Mackenzie, M.D. 1853-1925* (Edinburgh, 1973), p. 44.

141. George Reid, 'Legal Restraint upon Employment of Parturient Women', *Sheffield Medical Journal*, vol. L (1892-3), p. 114.

142. Clarke, *Factory System*, pp. 87-8; Hewitt, *Wives and Mothers*, p. 126, reports a similar custom in the 1830s. *Replies of Sir Charles Shaw to Lord Ashley M.P.* (London, 1843), p. 28, reports this custom in the 1840s.

143. For comments on official import figures, see *L*, 5 Dec. 1840, p. 382, 6 Mar. 1852, p. 249; *Medical Times and Gazette*, 25 Apr. 1857, p. 426; Alonzo Calkins, *Opium and the Opium-Appetite* (Philadelphia, 1871), pp. 33-4.

144. *L*, vol. I (1823), pp. 24, 257, 10 June 1837, p. 409.

145. *L*, 6 Mar. 1852, p. 249.

146. E.F. Harrison to SC on Patent Medicines, *PP*, 1914, vol. IX, Q.2971; *L*, 23 Oct. 1909, p. 1247.

147. Mr Clarke, *Edinburgh Medical and Surgical Journal*, vol. IV (1808), p. 271; *The Times*, 12 Apr. 1844.

148. *L*, 12 Dec. 1857, p. 608.
149. Hewitt, *Wives and Mothers,* pp. 142-3.
150. *L*, 13 Sept. 1862, p. 299.
151. *L*, 18 Sept. 1886, p. 547, 27 Nov. 1875, p. 783; *BMJ*, 10 Mar. 1894, p. 540; *New Statesman,* 21 Feb. 1975, p. 238.
152. *L*, 21 May 1887, p. 1050.
153. 'Appendices to the Report of the Committee on the East India Company's Affairs', *PP*, 1831, vol. VI, p. 349; *L*, 9 Dec. 1843, p. 344.
154. *Medical Gazette*, 16 June 1838, p. 507; *L*, 23 June 1838, p. 464.
155. *L*, 5 June 1897, p. 1556.
156. A.H. Hassall to SC on Adulterations, *PP*, 1854-5, vol. VIII, Qs.5, 117.
157. *L*, 10 June 1847, p. 51.
158. *L*, 5 Feb. 1875, p. 158, 25 Dec. 1841, pp. 454-5, 7 Jan. 1860, p. 23; see also Elizabeth Lomax, 'The Uses and Abuses of Opiates in Nineteenth-century England', *Bulletin of the History of Medicine,* vol. XLVII (1973), p. 171.
159. *L*, 29 Jan. 1876, p. 183. Cf. Rowntree's confident over-simplification: 'the high general [infant mortality] rate is chiefly due to ignorance of the feeding and management of infants, rather than to causes arising out of the poverty of the people' (*Poverty*, p. 207).
160. John Sykes, *Public Health Problems* (London, 1892), p. 335; for a similar finding in Stockport in the 1890s, see *BMJ*, 6 Feb. 1895, p. 307, Jardine, *GMJ*, vol. LXII (1904), p. 261; *L*, 5 May 1900, p. 1326.
161. *L*, 3 Nov. 1888, p. 877.
162. *L*, 4 May 1895, p. 1140.
163. *BMJ*, 3 Aug. 1889, p. 255, quoted in Jones, 'Infant Life', *JRSS*, vol. LVII (1894).
164. E.W. Hope, 'Discussion on Infant Mortality', *Royal Institute of Public Health, Aberdeen Congress, 1900,* pp. 298-301; F.J. Waldo, 'Summer Diarrhoea', *L*, 19 May 1900, pp. 1427-8, 26 May 1900, p. 1496.
165. *L*, 4 Aug. 1888, p. 231.
166. *BMJ*, 19 Oct. 1889, p. 888; *GMJ*, vol. XXXVI (1891), p. 226.
167. *BMJ*, 4 Jan. 1896, p. 53.
168. *BMJ*, 8 Jan. 1898, pp. 94-5.
169. *GMJ*, vol. LXII (1904), p. 258; *L*, 25 Apr. 1903, p. 1184; McCleary, *Development of British Maternity . . . Services,* pp. 6-7; D.J. Oddy and D. Miller (eds.), *The Making of the Modern British Diet* (London, 1975), pp. 151-2.
170. *L*, 16 Aug. 1902, p. 478.
171. See H.D. Kay *et al., Milk Pasteurization* (Rome, FAO, 1953); *L*, 13 July 1901, pp. 101-2, 3 Aug. 1901, p. 311; Dr Ralph Vincent at Manchester Sanitary Association, *L*, 11 Apr. 1914, p. 1070.
172. See, for example, Marshall Hall, *L*, 9 July 1842, p. 506; Boyd Joll, *BMJ,* 22 Nov. 1884, p. 1053.
173. R.O. Millett, *Medical and Physical Journal,* vol. XII (1804), p. 52; *L*, 8 Sept. 1894. Teething powders were still being recommended by doctors in the 1950s, and still contained mercury salts, which were finally isolated as causing 'pink disease', then an important infant illness.
174. *L*, 9 July 1842, p. 506; John North, 'Practical Observations on the Convulsions of Infants', *L*, 17 June 1826, p. 366.
175. *L*, 1 May 1852, p. 436.
176. *GMJ*, vol. I (1869), p. 228.
177. *BMJ*, 22 Nov. 1884, p. 1053, Rope, 29 Nov. 1884, p. 1108, Walford, 27 Dec. 1884, p. 1318; Jones, 'Infant Life', *JRSS*, vol. LVII (1894), p. 31.
178. Edward Smith, 'English Statistics of Hooping-Cough', *Medico-Chirurgical Transactions*, n.s., vol. XXVII (1854), pp. 223-8.

179. Creighton, *Epidemics,* vol. II, p. 672; Registrar-General, *Statistical Review of England and Wales,* 1972, Part I, p. 13.

180. *Statistical Review of England and Wales*, 1972, p. 439.

181. Creighton, *Epidemics*, vol. II, pp. 673-5.

182. *London Medical and Physical Journal,* vol. XLIX (1823), p. 203; *L*, 18 June, p. 336.

183. Mrs Beeton, *Household Management,* p. 1058; Sutro, Evans, Garraway, *BMJ*, 3 Jan. 1880, p. 39, Barlow, 20 Feb. 1886, p. 374.

184. *GMJ*, vol. XXIX (1888), pp. 420-2.

185. *BMJ*, 13 June 1908, p. 1433.

186. Diary of Benjamin Newton, quoted in *Medical History,* vol. VI (1962), p. 183. F.B. Head to John Murray, 14 Sept. 1858, in Murray Papers, held at 50 Albemarle Street, London. (I owe this report to Dr Ged Martin.)

187. A.M. Honeyman, 'Folk Medicine in Dundee', *Medical History*, vol. IV (1960), p. 350.

188. *BMJ*, 27 Feb. 1886, p. 409; *L*, 16 Aug. 1845, p. 180.

189. W.S. Mitchell, 'Dr George Henderson of Chirnside (1800-1864)', *Medical History,* vol. V (1961), p. 280; *L*, 1 June 1895, p. 1416; *BMJ*, 26 Mar. 1892, p. 691.

190. Dr Joseph Carroll, *BMJ*, 2 Apr. 1892, p. 750.

191. Cecil Torr, *Small Talk At Wreyland,* second series (Cambridge, 1921), p. 59; Wilfred Blunt, *Lady Muriel* (London, 1962), p. 12; Wayland D. Hand, 'Folk Medical Inhalants in Respiratory Disorders', *Medical History*, vol. XII (1968), pp. 153-4; John Camp, *Magic, Myth and Medicine* (London, 1973), p. 51.

192. *London Medical and Physical Journal,* vol. LIII (1825), pp. 39-40; *L*, 20 Feb. 1830, p. 703.

193. *Gazette of Health* (Sept. 1817), p. 637.

194. *L*, 20 Feb. 1830, p. 703.

195. John Savory, *A Companion to the Medicine Chest and Compendium of Domestic Medicine,* second ed. (London, 1840), pp. 251-2.

196. Beeton, *Household Management*, p. 1059; *London Medical and Physical Journal,* vol. LIII (1825), p. 285.

197. William Fox, *The Working Man's Model Family Botanic Guide; or Every Man His Own Doctor,* 19th ed. (Sheffield, 1909), p. 45.

198. *BMJ*, 5 Mar. 1887, p. 515, 26 June 1886, p. 1246; *Medical Chronicle,* vol. LII (1910), pp. 19, 22.

199. RC on Poor Laws, *PP*, 1909, vol. XLI, p. 675.

200. George Newman, *The Health of the State* (London, 1907), p. 120.

201. 'Full milk' had to contain a minimum of 3 per cent of 'milk fat' and 8.5 per cent of 'other solids'. 'Skimmed milk' had to contain 9 per cent of 'milk solids'. J. Lane Notter and R.H. Firth, *Practical Domestic Hygiene*, new ed. (London, 1902), p. 153.

202. Oddy and Miller, *Modern British Diet,* pp. 148-50; Dr McVail to RC on Poor Laws, *PP*, 1909, vol. XLII, pp. 78, 81, 101.

203. *L*, 12 Dec. 1868, p. 789.

204. *L*, 1 June 1872, p. 782, 10 Dec. 1892, p. 1359.

205. *L*, 28 Jan. 1899, p. 265, 25 Feb. 1899, p. 548.

206. *BMJ*, 4 Dec. 1897, p. 1676.

207. *L*, 15 Oct. 1898, p. 1005, 28 Jan. 1899, p. 265, 25 Sept. 1909, p. 942; *BMJ*, 16 Nov. 1907, p. 1458; Helen Bosanquet, *Social Work in London 1869-1912* (1914 ed., reprinted Brighton, 1973), p. 227; Mrs Barbara Drake, 'A Study of Infant Life in Westminster', *JRSS*, vol. LXXI (1908), p. 679.

208. *L*, 2 July 1910, p. 41, 28 Feb. 1914, p. 650; *BMJ*, 21 Feb. 1880, p. 310 (Patricroft), 2 June 1883, pp. 1092-3 (Ancoats and Ordsal), 10 Mar. 1894; *L*, 25

May 1872, p. 744 (Ratcliff); Jones, 'Infants', *JRSS*, vol. LVII (1894); Physical Deterioration Committee, *PP*, 1904, vol. XXXII, Qs. 9031-3 (Miss M. Garnett, Health Visitor in Potteries).

209. RC on the Poor Laws, *PP*, 1909, vol. XLI, Qs. 42143-4, 42153-4, 47554.

210. Registrar-General's Report, *PP*, 1909, vol. XI, pp. xxvi, xxix; Report by T.H.C. Stevenson, pp. lxxvii-ix; John W. Innes, *Class Fertility Trends in England And Wales 1876-1934* (Princeton, N.J., 1938), pp. 42, 44, 124-5.

211. *Parliamentary Debates,* vol. CXXXII, cols. 906-7 (28 Mar. 1904).

212. Dr A.K. Chalmers, 'The Causes of Infantile Mortality', *GMJ*, vol. LXII (1904), p. 184; *Parl. Deb.,* vol. CXLV. col. 1905; T.H.C. Stevenson, *PP*, 1909, vol. XI, pp. xliv-vi.

213. Edgar Schuster, *Eugenics* (London [1912-13]), pp. 222-4.

214. *L*, 30 June 1855, p. 658, 9 Feb. 1889, p. 281, 15 Nov. 1902, p. 1305; *BMJ*, 12 Mar. 1904, p. 625, 26 Apr. 1913, p. 875; E.M. Little (ed.), *History of the British Medical Association*, 1832-1932 (London, 1932), p. 235. See also G.R. Searle, *The Quest For National Efficiency* (Berkeley, 1971) and John Springhall, *Youth Empire and Society* (London, 1977).

215. Bosanquet, *Social Work,* p. 253; Searle, *Quest*, p. 61; Bentley Gilbert, 'Health and Politics', *Bulletin of the History of Medicine,* vol. 39 (1965), pp. 152-3.

216. One historian who did glimpse this distinction was T.H. Marshall, 'The Population of England and Wales from the Industrial Revolution to the World War', *Economic History Review,* vol. V (1935), p. 70.

217. Stevenson, *PP*, 1909, vol. XI, pp. lxxxvi, xcvi; Glaister, *GMJ*, vol. LXII, p. 243.

218. Stevenson, *PP*, 1909, vol. XI, pp. cxxll-lll; Innes, *Class Fertility Trends,* p. 131.

219. Dr Newsholme, *L*, 10 Jan. 1914, p. 129, 31 Jan. 1914, p. 339.

220. Davie, Butler and Goldstein, *From Birth to Seven,* p. 4; Field, *Unequal Britain,* p. 9.

221. *Medical Chronicle,* vol. LII (1910), p. 24.

3 CHILDHOOD AND YOUTH

Scarlet Fever

The years between four and fourteen constituted the least hazardous stage of life. None the less, the incidence of morbidity and mortality was still enormous. The main destructive diseases were scarlet fever, measles, diphtheria and smallpox. Scarlet fever is an acute childhood disease caused by a haemolytic (blood or blood-corpuscle destroying) streptococcal infection of the throat, skin or middle ear. It is usually spread by droplet infection, but can also be carried, or remain quiescent for long periods, in clothes, dishes or bedroom dust. Occasionally it can breed rapidly in milk or food handled by an infected carrier. The normal incubation period is from two to five days. The symptoms vary, but usually the patient suffers nausea, headache and chills. A red rash, which gives the disease its name, may appear on the second day and last for about a week, when it fades, and the skin peels.

Scarlet fever varied in incidence and virulence through the century. Creighton, the great nineteenth-century student of epidemics, believed that it had been mild until 1840; thereafter its mortality rate doubled until the 1870s, when it gradually moderated again. This decline continued until its virtual disappearance in the 1920s. Throughout the period case mortality was highest among infants under twelve months old, approaching 50 per cent, falling to about 27 per cent among two- to four-year-olds. But the incidence of the disease appears to have been highest among children aged four to eight. Only 5 per cent of scarlet fever deaths were reported at ages above ten.[1]

The worst years in London after 1859 (when the diagnostic rules for registration of the disease were improved) are given in Table 3.1.

Table 3.1: London Scarlet Fever Death Rates at All Ages per 100,000

1859 — 128	1869 — 184
1862 — 122	1870 — 188
1863 — 171	1875 — 110
1864 — 110	

Source: B.A. Whitelegge, *Lancet*, 4 Mar. 1893, p. 458.

In these years, scarlet fever deaths constituted between 4 per cent and

6 per cent of the deaths from all causes in England and Wales.[2] In Great Britain as a whole, the scarlet fever death rate in 1863 was 149.8 per 100,000 and in 1874 it was 106.2 per 100,000. These rates represent almost 34,000 deaths in 1863 and over 26,000 in 1874. Thereafter the fall was dramatic, to 17 per 100,000 in 1886, amounting to a decline of 81 per cent between 1861 and 1891. Probably this decline is overstated because an increasing number of deaths formerly ascribed to scarlet fever or scarlatina were now attributed to diphtheria. But even in 1886 the 17 per 100,000 rate represents the deaths of over 6,000 persons.

The mortality was worst in the towns of Lancashire and the West Riding, London, the Black Country and the Durham and south Wales coalfields. Compared with the average rate for England and Wales of 88 per 100,000 for the 1850s Preston had a rate of 133 per 100,000, Manchester 150 per 100,000, Liverpool 151 per 100,000, Stoke 156 per 100,000, Easington 157 per 100,000, Bishop Auckland 137 per 100,000, Dewsbury 137 per 100,000 and London 94 per 100,000; while Andover had 10 per 100,000, and Ware and Swaffham, for instance, had 13 per 100,000.[3]

These figures over-simplify the situation. Scarlet fever frequently broke out in lethal local epidemics, usually associated with an infected milk supply. In 1863, for example, there were local outbreaks in Worcester, St Austell and Oxford: in Worcester scarlet fever caused 131 of the 309 deaths in the town for the year; in St Austell, 29, or over half of the 56 deaths; in Oxford, a quarter of the total deaths. A decade earlier there had been 186 scarlet-fever deaths in and around Bedford in the three years beginning 1854.[4]

Such outbreaks especially worried local sanitarians. They believed that scarlet fever hit the wealthy harder than the poor. This belief was not tested until Dr Prior investigated the outbreak in Bedford in the mid-1850s and published his results in 1869. He found that the disease had twice the case-fatality rate in the town as in the neighbouring rural parishes. Prior then classed the 186 deaths according to his 'estimated station in life'. 'Gentry and professional classes' had 19 deaths; 'trading and lower middle class', 21 deaths; and 'mechanics and labourers', 146. He then compared these with his calculations from the 1851 census report and concluded that the numbers of deaths were roughly proportional to the numbers of each class in Bedford. This was cold comfort. He remarked that 'certain rookeries escaped . . . while three of the best terraces caught it'.[5] During the normal late-summer scarlet-fever season in 1858 Dr Hall Bakewell checked the mortality for each district against the number of paupers. The two figures were always in inverse ratio:

five counties with a pauperism ratio of 54 per cent had a scarlatina ratio of 37 per cent, while eight counties with only 20 per cent pauperism had a scarlet fever mortality of 71 per cent. His correlations, Dr Hall Bakewell argued, were strong evidence for the perversity of the disease.[6]

Such findings disturbed the sanitarians' faith in the unvarying efficacy of sanitary reform. Dr Prior had noticed that the 'well-drained and ill-drained sections [of Bedford] had suffered alike'. Dr Whitmore told the St Andrews Medical Graduates Association during the epidemic of 1869-70 that the incidence of the disease and its mortality had been 'but little influenced by defective sanitary conditions'. It affected 'mansions as well as hovels'. From his experience of it in Marylebone, he confessed 'that the poorest and most destitute, who live in filth and misery . . . have suffered the least from it'.[7]

A full explanation of this phenomenon did not become available until 1885, when outbreaks of scarlet fever in Hendon and Paisley were traced to the families of dairymen. The upper classes were already known to buy more milk than the poor, and to keep the milk longer. Something of the difficulties inherent in controlling the purity of milk emerged in the report of the investigation in Paisley. I shall describe it in detail because it illustrates problems with the other milk-borne diseases which I shall discuss later. A child in the dairyman's family at Castlehead, near Paisley, caught scarlet fever. The local doctor yielded to the mother's entreaties not to send the child to the Glasgow Infirmary. She promised to keep the child 'isolated' in the house. Soon afterwards two other children in the dwelling caught it, and it broke out in five 'villas' whose occupants bought milk from the dairy. The local MOH instituted a prosecution under the Dairies, Cow-Sheds and Milk-Shops Order, issued by the Privy Council under the Contagious Diseases (Animals) Act of 1879. The dairyman admitted in court that he and his wife visited the patients (apparently they were all in one room) morning and evening, but he asserted that they did not 'touch' the children. The dairyman and his wife continued to milk the cows and served out the milk in the front shop. The servant was not told the nature of the disease and was instantly dismissed when she remarked that 'there was fever in the house'. The children gave evidence that their parents had not 'touched' them. The local magistrate brought in a verdict of 'not proven'. The relevant clause in the Order forbade 'any person suffering from a dangerous or infectious disease' or any person in 'contact' with an infected person from milking cows or selling milk. As the anonymous contributor to the medical journal lamented, such prosecutions always foundered on the interpretation of the word 'contact', no matter how conclusive the evidence about the aetiology of the outbreak. The verdict was received with 'loud cheers' in the court. Afterwards, at a special gathering at the George Hotel, his fellow dairymen presented their comrade 'with a purse of sovereigns, marble timepiece and ornaments, and also a broach and a pair of earrings for his wife'.[8]

Doctors and laymen had given little attention to scarlet fever in its early-nineteenth-century mild phase. Dr Buchan, in early editions of his household manual, told parents that there was 'seldom any occasion for medicine in this disease'. If the parents wished to reassure themselves, they could give doses of a 'scruple of nitre' and 'small doses of rhubarb' with more severe purges as the disease declined.[9] By 1830 Dr Blackmore's procedure represented the more interventionist fashion. He too believed that scarlet fever was 'mostly confined to the upper classes'. It was not a serious malady, but the doctor should act with 'decisive anti-febrile remedies [antimonial wine etc.] in the outset, and towards the end severe counter irritation on the skin [blisters, dilute nitric acid etc.], with emetics'. The ulceration of the throat could be checked by 'general evacuants' and copious bloodletting would lessen the 'unquestionable oppression of internal organs, by sanguineous congestion'. Doctors were still resorting to this kind of regimen through the middle decades of the century and apparently went on ordering it until the mid-1880s.[10]

Their efforts among the comfortable classes must have lifted the case-mortality rate and reinforced the belief that scarlet fever was most fatal among the upper classes. Case mortality in London fever hospitals during the outbreak of 1890-1 at around 7 per cent was more than twice the rate of those treated at home.[11] Many of the patients admitted would have been mortally ill and even more would have been very poor, but it was normal practice for the fever hospital to give preference to servants and nurses who had caught the disease while working for private families. During the 1850s and 1860s about one-third of the patients were indoor servants.[12] It is possible to argue that regular medical attention — and cross-infection, as the two go together — in the case of scarlet fever at least, diminished the patient's chance of survival by up to 50 per cent. Dr Stark, the medical officer at the Edinburgh North-West Dispensary, complained to his colleagues in the 1830s that he had

twice through the imprudence of parents nearly lost children by their administering spirits, or other stimulants, with a view to bringing out or keeping out the efflorescence, and heaping on clothes for fear of cold. The bad effects were . . . arrested by blood-letting, cold sponging, removing the unnecessary clothes, and giving free laxatives with antimonials.[13]

Dr Stark's patients were unfortunate: his recipe might have reduced their fever, but even more likely led to complications of streptococcal infection, middle ear, rheumatic fever and inflammation of the kidneys. This argument is strengthened by the fact that parish guardians resisted making scarlet fever a notifiable disease, on the grounds that three-quarters of their people, the poor majority, never sought medical attendance for this illness, and that notification, while it would increase doctors' incomes and increase the rates, would not persuade the poor to seek treatment.[14] If they bothered to treat the illness at all, the standard remedy was a drink compounded of maidenhair, elder-blossoms and goose-grass [*Galium Aparine*].[15]

The doctors' preoccupation with the prevalence of the disease among the comfortable classes obscured for them its persistence among the poor. An outbreak in Bristol during the summer of 1875 had a death rate that varied with the social status of the parish, from bosky Clifton at 0.3 per 1,000; Ledminster at 2.8 per 1,000; St Paul at 4 per 1,000; coming down to St Phillip and St Jacob at 6.5 per 1,000; and wretched St Mary Redcliffe at 8.1 per 1,000.[16] Also during the mid-1870s there were devastating epidemics in the coal-mining and alum-processing district of Easington in the North Riding, with about 1,000 inhabitants: 193 deaths in 1873-5; 81 deaths in 1877; 91 in 1878. Since 1851 the average scarlet-fever death rate at Easington had run at twice the national average. The investigator from the Privy Council, Mr W.H. Power, established that during 1877-9 there had been, almost incredibly, over 2,000 known cases in the district. This meant that there had been more than ten otherwise unremarked attacks to every death.[17] The comparable incidence and case-fatality rates of London and Brighton are also suggestive. Dr Arthur Newsholme, MOH for Brighton, calculated the figures for 1894: London had twice the incidence of the disease, at 4.24 per 1,000 against 1.85 per 1,000. Moreover, Brighton, presumably with a higher proportion of 'comfortable' patients, had a case-fatality rate of one in 62, against London's one in 19.[18] At Neilston, a cotton town in Renfrewshire, an outbreak in the dry autumn following the very hot summer of 1869 caused at least 169 cases, with 29 deaths, or nearly one in six. Dr Pride, who reported the outbreak, noted an aftermath that was ignored in other nineteenth-century investigations: 35 of his cases developed serious complications;

10 caught pneumonia, with 2 deaths, 20 developed 'dropsy' (probably post-streptococcal nephritis), with 4 deaths; and in 5 diphtheria ensued, with 3 deaths.[19] Among the survivors, the long-term debility must have been severe. In 1894 an exploration of the case histories of the 219 children in the Newcastle Institute for the Deaf and Dumb revealed that 44 per cent had become deaf mutes after scarlet fever, 33 per cent after 'cerebro-spinal brain fever' (meningitis) and 21 per cent after measles.[20] The reports from Bristol, London and Brighton are not conclusive about relative class incidence of scarlet fever, especially in view of the patchy nature of the outbreaks and their fluctuating virulence, even in epidemic years, but taken together they indicate that scarlet fever, like every other children's infection, probably hit the poor harder than the rich.

The communal fatalism of working-class societies, particularly in mining villages, was partly responsible for the ravages of the disease among the poor. Medical men, persuaded from the late 1860s by the strange distribution of scarlet fever through the classes that sanitary reform did not answer, plumped instead for 'isolation' of the victim. This was feasible in large houses, boarding-schools and among those lower-class families whose members they could order to a fever hospital. These activities preserved the authority of the doctors in their otherwise impotent role. They did not know that the infectious stage was the early incubation period and that it usually ended in about seven days. They erred on the safe side. At Homerton fever hospital during the 1870s patients were held for over seven weeks; at Stockwell hospital, for over five weeks. In the 1880s some MOHs insisted on an isolation period for a house-bound victim of four months: the strain provoked endless breaches of quarantine and sometimes pauperised shopkeeping and artisan families.[21] The doctors' campaign to have local authorities adopt the Notification of Infectious Diseases Act of 1889 was integral with their increasing reliance upon isolation as a prophylactic measure. But even where they succeeded notification was unsystematic and it collapsed during epidemics. Doctors hesitated to commit themselves to a diagnosis in the early 'sore throat' stage of scarlet fever, smallpox or diphtheria. Moreover they were supposed to notify only after inspecting the patient: this lost them time and money and became impossible during large-scale outbreaks.[22]

Working-class living conditions and habits affronted careful doctors. Dr Barry remarked of mining villages in the Tynemouth district, with twice the national death rate, that the villages were small and permitted too much intercourse between well and sick. Women and children gossiped at the 'pants' (public cisterns) from which they drew their water. When a child developed scarlet fever 'a special point [was] . . . made of visiting . . . so that the children get it and get it over with'. There was some sense in this, because scarlet fever rarely attacked a child twice. In 1873-4 there were 549 scarlet fever deaths; in 1878-9, 445; 1880, 112; 1882, 82. Children were always 'invited to the home of a newly deceased companion to assist in the funeral'.[23] Dr Parsons attempted to establish a free 'isolation cottage' in the mining, iron and cotton town of Atherton in Lancashire in order to diminish the infection he believed to result from 'free intercourse between households infected and . . . uninfected . . . the wearing of infected clothing at the mills and participation in large funerals', together with dirty sources of domestic water, insanitary cottages and vile common privies. Over 1876-85 the local death rate, at 1.40 per 1,000, was almost triple the national average. Measles and scarlet fever were endemic and alternated at five-yearly intervals in decimating the young population. Parsons was defeated. The parents regarded scarlet fever 'as a thing everyone ought to have and . . . the sooner it was over the better'. Once the mothers discovered they were not to be admitted to the isolation cottage with their sick children they refused to part with them. In 1885 there were 41 deaths from measles and 51 from scarlet fever among a population of 13,500.[24]

The doctors tried to clean up the milk supply, too. But here also, as the Paisley case showed, they found themselves confronting the desperate needs and dirty usages of the people. In the winter of 1895 Alfred Smith dipped a jug into a churn of milk standing at a milkman's door in the East End. He had been out of work for six weeks and had a wife and three children at home in one room. The children had scarlet fever. Smith got one month's hard labour for stealing: a crime exacerbated by the condition of his children. In the dock he was described as 'reeking of fever'.[25]

Measles

Measles is like scarlet fever in that it is highly contagious, spread by droplet infection or by touch, and becomes infectious during the first stage of the disease, three or four days before the rash appears. It is a viral illness and remains infectious until the rash begins to fade, after seven or eight days. Like scarlet fever again, it was a major killer in the nineteenth century. It first equalled smallpox in the London bills of mortality in 1804 and surpassed smallpox during the epidemic of 1807-8. It occurred throughout the year, with a peak incidence in summer, and a high case-fatality rate in midwinter when it was associated with coughs and influenza.[26] Reported cases tended to rise to epidemic levels every two to three years. In London this fluctuation occurred within a longer epidemic cycle, around every twenty years. The mortality rate from measles held up throughout the century and was slower to fall in Scotland (see Table 3.2).

Table 3.2: Measles Mortality Rate, 1838-1910 (per 100,000 living)

England and Wales		Scotland	
1838-42	53.9		
1847-52	40.3		
1856-60	42.5	1855-60	43
1866-70	42.8	1861-70	42
1876-80	38.5	1871-80	36
1886-90	46.8	1881-90	39
1896-1900	42.1	1891-1900	47
1901-5	32.7	1901-10	34
1906-10	29.1		

Source: *PP*, 1916, vol. V, p. 60; *PP*, 1914-16, vol. XI, pp. cviii-cx; B.A. Whitelegge, 'Changes in Type in Epidemic Disease', *Lancet*, 4 Mar. 1893, p. 459; C. Killick Mallard, 'The Notification of Measles', *Royal Institute of Public Health, Aberdeen Congress, 1900*, p. 275.

In 1972 there were 29 deaths recorded from measles in England and Wales and an average incidence of 2.9 per 1,000. The attacks were five times as numerous in the north, north-west and Wales as in East Anglia and the south-east. This pattern is almost identical with that of the nineteenth century. It was then endemic in mining villages where there was probably considerable opportunity for infection transfer. But it could also ravage isolated agricultural villages. Here it perhaps could 'die out', only to return after an interval of years to attack the new generation which had had no contact with it.

Measles was commonly believed to be a disease of the poor. I have figures comparing burials at the Collegiate and St John's churches in Manchester in 1812-13 which suggest that the 'middle and higher ranks' (who were buried at the latter church) were only slightly less afflicted than the 'poor', but the case-fatality rate was probably much higher among poor families and this undoubtedly impressed contemporaries.[27] We now know that measles is an especially virulent killer when it is accompanied by malnutrition. In the 1960s and early 1970s it was recorded as having a mortality rate of up to 25 per cent in the poor nations.[28]

Table 3.3: Deaths Ascribed to Measles, 1838-1911

	England and Wales	Scotland	Great Britain Total
1838	6,514		
1839	10,937		
1840	9,326		
1841	6,894		
1842	8,742		
1847	8,690		
1848	6,867		
1849	5,458		
1850	7,082		
1851	9,370		
1852	5,846		
1853	4,895		
1854	9,277		
1855	7,354	1,180	8,534
1856	7,124	1,033	8,157
1857	5,969	1,028	6,997
1858	9,271	1,538	10,809
1859	9,548	975	10,523
1860	9,557	1,587	11,144
1861	9,055	971	10,026
1862	9,860	1,404	11,264
1863	11,340	2,212	13,552
1864	8,322	1,102	9,424
1865	8,562	1,195	9,757
1866	10,940	1,038	11,978
1867	6,588	1,341	7,929
1868	11,630	1,149	12,779
1869	10,309	1,670	11,979
1870	7,543	834	8,377
1871	9,293	2,057	11,350
1872	8,530	925	9,455
1873	7,403	1,450	8,853
1874	12,235	1,103	13,338
1875	6,173	1,022	7,195
1876	9,971	1,241	11,212
1877	9,045	1,019	10,064
1878	9,765	1,372	11,137
1879	9,185	769	9,954
1880	12,328	1,427	13,755
1881	7,300	1,012	8,312
1882	12,711	1,289	14,000
1883	9,329	1,629	10,958
1884	11,324	1,440	12,764
1885	14,495	1,426	15,921
1886	12,013	681	12,694
1887	16,765	1,598	18,363
1888	9,785	1,406	11,191
1889	14,732	1,948	16,680
1890	12,614	2,509	15,123
1891	12,673	1,775	14,448
1892	13,553	2,280	15,833
1893	11,110	3,639	14,749

Table 3.3 (Cont'd):

	England and Wales	Scotland	Great Britain Total
1894	11,757	791	12,548
1895	11,491	2,063	13,554
1896	17,618	1,515	19,133
1897	12,711	2,056	14,767
1898	13,220	2,290	15,510
1899	9,998	1,599	11,597
1900	12,710	1,825	14,535
1901	9,019	1,655	10,674
1902	12,930	1,388	14,318
1903	9,150	1,133	10,283
1904	12,306	1,512	13,818
1905	11,076	1,662	12,738
1906	9,444	1,445	10,889
1907	12,625	1,153	13,778
1908	8,011	2,503	10,514
1909	12,618	890	13,508
1910	8,302	2,243	10,545
1911	13,128	923	14,051
1912	12,855	1,983	14,838
1913	10,644	1,329	11,973
1914	9,144	1,458	10,602

Source: ibid.

Measles never killed fewer than 7,000 people a year in Great Britain during the nineteenth century and in bad years like 1863, 1861 and 1874 it killed more than scarlet fever.

The pioneer medical statistician, Dr Thomas Percival, calculated in the late eighteenth century from the burial registers of the Manchester Collegiate Church and the London bills of mortality that deaths from measles among children aged two years and over had considerably increased. This growth continued in the early nineteenth century and during the first great epidemic of 1807-8 some doctors, led by Dr Alexander Watt of Glasgow, argued that the deaths were the result of the spread of vaccination against smallpox. Watt checked the Glasgow parish burial registers back to the 1790s and found that 'since the extensive practice of vaccination, ten times more children [under 10] had died of the measles than formerly'. He concluded, by some very odd logic, that 'there is some change produced in the living system by smallpox, which predisposes it to be affected by the measles in a much milder degree than when they are caught by those who have not undergone the smallpox'. Vaccination, therefore, was a destructive agent. The debate continued until 1816, at least. Sir Gilbert Blane, the naval physician epidemiologist, and physician to George IV, agreed in 1813 that the mortality of measles, as shown by the London bills of mortality, had increased by about 200 per cent over the eighteenth-century figures, but he also asserted that there was no proof that measles — or scarlet fever which also was increasing — was linked with vaccination or smallpox. He added that, given the trend of the birth rate over the period 1801-11, the total mortality was 19,000 below what it would have been had it kept pace with the births.[29] An author in the *Medical and Physical Journal* drew the full conclusion in 1816: vaccination had not increased the relative virulence of measles and scarlatina but instead it had 'enabled a larger number of children to be reared — who might be exposed to measles'. The incurred mortality from measles indeed resulted 'from the improved condition of the inferior subjects of the Kingdom'. Children who now caught measles at two years and above would formerly never have reached that age.[30]

As with scarlet fever, poor parents were stoical about measles among their children. Usually they did not bother to seek even free medical aid from a dispensary or hospital out-patients' department. As one couple in St Pancras explained to a doctor after their two children, aged ten months and four years respectively, had successively died from measles in 1862, without medical attention, the disease was too 'unimportant'.[31] Measles was accepted even to the extent that apparently there was no popular specific for it. Parents who wanted to apply herbal remedies had to fall back on the usual applications for ulcerous sore throats: infusions of white oak and white elm bark.

Early in the century Dr Horne had tried inoculation against measles among poor children in Edinburgh, 'but it did not work' and fell into disuse after about a decade of what must have been prolific destruction.[32] Among private patients, until the 1880s, doctors sought to lessen 'the violent motion or excitement of the system' by blood-letting and 'antimonial emetics'. The sore throat was treated with calf's-foot jelly.[33] In 1840 John Hiley, an Irish country surgeon at Elland in Yorkshire, was 'confidently' giving a powder 'composed of jalap and calomel in scammony and calomel, with the addition of a little ginger'. After the purging had intermitted, he gave sulphate of magnesia, nitre and antimony 'to take the edge off the inflammation'. He remarked that stupor then often set in. This required leeches to the head and 'general venesection' to afford 'sensible and immediate relief'. Vomiting he countered with general bleeding, Dover's powders and blisters to the chest. Even so, he confessed, many children sank 'from general exhaustion' and the deaths were 'many'.[34]

Treatment became rather less heroic during the 1850s, as some adventurous doctors began giving tonics and brandy, instead of resorting to venesection, purging and low diet, but most persisted with the old regimen, applying it with varying degrees of severity. By 1889 young doctors were treating the high temperature and fever with wet packs and warm baths, and dealing with the associated respiratory infections, the 'croupy cough' of measles as it was called, by 'mopping' the pharynx and epiglottis with glycerine and tannin, and giving 'large doses of chlorate of potassium'. None the less, many died. The poor, reported one doctor of the pottery towns, 'thought they could treat an ordinary case of measles with domestic remedies; consequently, when medical aid . . . [was] called in, the child . . . [was] moribund or in a hopeless condition'. The average death numbers in the towns were over 50 a year throughout the 1880s, but in epidemic years such as 1889, Hanley alone, in four months, would have over 180 deaths.[35]

Again, sanitary reform appeared to have made no difference, although the reformers seem to have been slower to realise this of measles than scarlet fever.[36] Despite their insistence on notification and isolation, there had been no considerable reduction in the mortality rate.

The working classes, at least in towns with a strong MOH like Glasgow, had gradually come to regard measles as a serious disease and began to co-operate with the sanitary authorities in isolation, fumigation and informing on neighbours 'as to carelessness in using common washhouses etc.'. But even in Glasgow, the death rate had not markedly diminished.[37]

The growing elementary schools provided reservoirs of infection which helped maintain the disease. The epidemics in Coventry in 1886, 1889 and 1894 demonstrate the pattern (see Table 3.4). School boards always resisted moves by the local MOH, weakly backed by the Local Government Board, to close their schools when disease broke out. Closure reduced the Board's normal attendance numbers and thereby whittled down their grant from the Education Department. The Department, a competitor of the Local Government Board, in turn pressed the local Boards to keep schools open.[38] As the Coventry figures show, the local authority delayed as long as possible. Indeed, the Coventry pattern can be reinterpreted to suggest that the measles would have waned regardless of whether the schools were closed or open because the virus had largely exhausted the pool of susceptible children. An attack of measles does confer good immunity. But this may be carrying the argument too far: measles, diphtheria, respiratory and other infections were endemic in schools: of 1,000 elementary schoolchildren examined in Birmingham in 1900, 355 had middle-ear infections in one or both ears.[39] Moreover, middle-ear and respiratory infections may be recurrent or chronic. This question of the relation of schooling to health merits much fuller study. Amongst other illuminations, it might supply a new understanding of parental opposition to the compulsory attendance clause.

Table 3.4: Coventry Measles Epidemics, 1886, 1889 and 1894

1886	Jan.	—	Aug.	81 cases	Schools open
	Sept.			361 cases	
	Oct. (first fortnight)			186 cases	
	Oct. (second fortnight)			111 cases	Schools closed
	Nov.			10 cases	
1889	Jan.	—	June	186 cases	Schools open
	1 July	—	24 July	629 cases	
	25 July	—	10 Aug.	218 cases	
	10 Aug.	—	1 Sept.	74 cases	Schools closed
	Sept.			17 cases	
1894	Week ending 24 Mar.			162 cases	
	" " 31 Mar.			213 "	Schools open
	" " 7 Apr.			275 "	
	" " 14 Apr.			492 "	
	" " 21 Apr.			306 "	
	" " 28 Apr.			260 "	Schools closed
	" " 5 May			134 "	
	" " 12 May			88 "	
	" " 19 May			42 "	

Source: *Lancet*, 4 May 1895, p. 1140.

Diphtheria

Diphtheria became a serious malady in Great Britain quite suddenly during 1855. Before that it was prevalent on the Continent but it was little known across the Channel and then, assuming that some outbreaks of Cynache Maligna (dog's disease) and throat distemper were varieties of diphtheria, they were seemingly rather mild.[40] In 1830 Dr Alison described such an outbreak in Edinburgh and ascribed it to 'diphtheria', 'a kind of croup . . . [and] cynache maligna'.[41] True diphtheria is caused by the bacillus Corynebacterium diphtheriae. It is spread by droplets from coughing and sneezing, by touching or clothes used by an infected person and may be transmitted by persons convalescing from diphtheria or by carriers who are otherwise healthy. Explosive outbreaks were often associated with the milk supply: the bacillus can grow in milk without altering its appearance or taste. The symptoms usually include sore throat, fever, headache and vomiting. Patches of dirty grey or yellow membrane form in the throat and gradually grow into one membrane which, together with swelling of the throat, may stop swallowing and breathing. (Diphtheria is derived from the Greek word for leather). Like whooping cough, diphtheria in the nineteenth century had a higher fatality rate among females than males.[42] The diphtheria bacillus also produces a toxin that can spread throughout the body and may damage the heart and nerves permanently. Recovery, even after a mild attack, can take many weeks.

During 1855-6 366 people died from diphtheria in Boulogne. They included several English visitors. At about the same time it appeared sporadically in Kent, Sussex, Suffolk and Norfolk and gradually spread through the rest of the country. The medical profession first began to write about it in 1857. They agreed that it was a severe form of cynache maligna and rejected the French view (the French had already distinguished and named diphtheria) that it was new and peculiar. Deaths from it were first named in 1855 by the Registrar-General, but it was classed with scarlatina until 1861 and with cynache maligna until 1869. By 1870 one student of the disease, Dr Robert Semple, remarked that 'every ailment of the throat . . . [was] fashionably called diphtheria'.[43] With this reservation about the uncertainties of diagnosis in mind, 'diphtheria and cynache maligna' were recorded as killing over 61,000 people in England and Wales between 1855 and 1869, representing an average rate of 35 per 100,000 living. About half the deaths were among children under five, and of the remainder 4/5 were aged between five and thirteen, and the last 1/5 thirteen and over. The case-mortality rate seems to have averaged about 25 per cent. By the 1890s reported diphtheria deaths in England and Wales were at the rate of 25.9 per 100,000. In London alone in 1893 there were 3,265 deaths.[44] Some contemporaries believed that these figures, because of diagnoses that were surer than the doubtful attributions which might have inflated the earlier totals, and a fall in the reported deaths from 'sore throat', 'thrush' and 'croup', reflected an actual rise in the incidence and case-mortality rate of diphtheria.[45] But the uncertainty about diagnosis throughout the period makes this conclusion speculative.

The reported incidence of diphtheria between 1855 and 1900 bewildered contemporaries. Its death rate was highest in the north Midlands, south-eastern and south-western counties, and lowest in London, the north-western and northern counties. Rural areas seemed to suffer worse than towns. The disease did not appear to be related to industrialism or to slums. The reformers' assumptions about sanitary science were further confounded by Creighton's calculation of the early 1880s that the death rate varied inversely in Great Britain with the density of population (see Table 3.5).

Table 3.5: Diphtheria Death Rates and Population Density

| | Death Rates per One Million | | |
	Dense	Medium	Sparse
1855-60	123	182	248
1861-70	163	164	223
1871-80	114	125	132

Source: Charles Creighton, *A History of Epidemics in Britain*, 2 vols. [1891-4], new ed., 1965, vol. II, pp. 740-1.

As Dr Crisp admitted in 1871, 'its spread [bore] no relation to soil, temperature, altitude, or social condition . . . yet it [was] undoubtedly contagious . . . a mystery'.[46] It was worst in winter and, Creighton asserted, more deadly in poor houses, but it hit the comfortable too. Diphtheria probably spread among the lower classes by droplet infection in schools and in overcrowded households where the victims could not be isolated. And it killed them at a higher rate because they lacked resistance.

The apparently unconnected outbreaks in comfortable households were linked with their consumption of milk. In 1887 Mr W.H. Power established such a chain in York Town and Camberley. There the incidence of diphtheria outbreak among the 'better class' was 29.3 per cent, compared with 6.2 per cent among the 'cottagers and trades-folk'. Power, working by analogy from the known fact that typhoid fever was conveyed by milk, inquired and found that the 'better class' bought more milk than the 'cottagers', that they also bought cream, and stored both. The clue to this practice came from Power's investigation of an outbreak in Farnham in the following year. His findings are given in Table 3.6.

Table 3.6: Power's Farnham Study of Milk and Diphtheria Connection

Type of Family	No. of Adults	No. of Children	No. of Families Supplied with Milk	No. of Families with Diphtheria
'Wealthier'	269	48	44	37
'Cottages and tradesmen'	145	94	50	11

Source: *Transactions of the Clinical Society of London,* vol. XXV (1892), pp. 39-40.

The wealthier families, with half the number of children, had an average of 5.2 pints of milk delivered daily, while the cottagers' families took 0.8 pints. The cottagers' and tradesmen's families consumed their milk each day. The wealthier people regularly had a remainder which they kept at least overnight and often longer.[47] Also, as I explained earlier, it was still uncommon to boil milk.

Before 1894 doctors could not cope with the disease. Calomel and other mercury preparations, in small doses every two hours, were the norm until into the 1860s.[48] The object of the treatment was to get the saliva flowing again. Sedation and isolation became standard procedure in the 1870s until antitoxin serum was introduced in 1894. Trachaeotomy (incision of the trachea to enable removal of the lesion) was known from the early eighteenth century, but I have found no evidence that doctors resorted to it in connection with diphtheria. The early antitoxins were effective only if they were administered during the first four days of the attack, when the symptoms were least clear.[49] None the less, the total number of reported deaths in England and Wales fell from 9,466 in 1893 to 7,661 in 1898, and the case-mortality rate, in London at least, from 23.6 per cent in 1894 to 14.8 per cent. This fall in mortality probably occurred largely among the upper classes because antitoxin was expensive and not distributed free; in Birmingham, for example, a notoriously bad diphtheria town, antitoxin was not provided free until 1902.[50] Thereafter the death rate was said to have fallen even more rapidly.

Before the advent of serum antitoxin general hospitals were reluctant to admit diphtheria victims. Most sufferers were under the age for admission and doctors feared, rightly, that once inside the hospital, the infection could not be controlled. Fever hospitals always had too few beds and tended to reserve them for 'more serious' diseases like typhus and scarlet fever. Only 30 per cent of the diphtheria cases notified in London in 1891 were admitted to the Fever Hospital and the general hospitals which accepted such cases.[51] The case-mortality rate in three London hospitals in the early 1890s was over 30 per cent.[52] St Bartholomew's admitted an average of 23 patients each year between 1881 and 1886, and 119 during a bad outbreak in 1890. In that year 13 other patients and 26 nurses in the medical wards caught diphtheria. As a result, the hospital revised its nursing rules: for infectious cases patients were to be put into hospital bedclothes, instead of wearing, as was usual, the clothes they brought with them; each patient was to have his personal bedpan and his own towel; and the nurses were to wash their hands and rinse them in disinfectant after touching a patient.[53]

Hospitals for Children

Hospital provision for children, especially infectious cases, came very slowly in Great Britain. The first Hospital for Sick Children (Great Ormond Street) opened in London in 1853, long after similar institutions had been established in Paris, Berlin, Vienna, St Petersburg, Turin, and even Constantinople.[54] A few dispensaries accepted child patients, but only as an act of grace. The general hospitals sometimes admitted surgical cases or medical cases of special clinical interest, but in 1843, for example, the London hospitals together only contained 136 inmates under ten.[55] The average number of deaths under ten in London at this time was 25,000.

By 1869 the Hospital for Sick Children had 75 beds. It 'relieved' 720 in-patients and 15,000 out-patients for the year. Children under two were absolutely excluded. Only 'grave' patients were admitted. By the late 1860s the hospital had built a convalescent branch at Highgate with 20 beds and 36 for chronic cases. In a typical week in the autumn of 1869, the hospital handled 1,510 out-patients (see Table 3.7).

The doors opened at 8.30 a.m. and closed at 10 p.m. A notice at the front door instructed patients not to sit on the steps of neighbouring houses, but they regularly did so, even after the crush began to ease at 9.30 a.m. The doors were closed at 10 a.m. There were two waiting-rooms. The upper one was 'long and lofty', about 16 feet wide. It contained six rows of patients 'densely full' on benches, presumably ranged across the room as in a modern bus. Patients and parents found it hard to pass between the rows, giving point to the warning on the wall against pickpockets. There was one skylight, but the 'air was very close'. The lower waiting-room was immediately beneath the first and partially underground. The one unventilated WC serving both rooms was near the door. The benches near the WC were empty: parents and patients preferred to risk losing their place in the queue by sitting on the stairs or outside in the garden.

Table 3.7: One Week's Out-Patients at the Hospital for Sick Children, 1869

369	Monday 27 September	These reflect the usual build-up from the week-end.
335	Tuesday 28 September	
258	Wednesday 29 September	
264	Thursday 30 September	This was probably the charwomen's and outworkers' afternoon or evening off.
182	Friday 1 October	
102	Saturday 2 October	

Source: *Lancet*, 16 Oct. 1869, pp. 553-4.

Each waiting-room had a consulting-room adjoining it. The rooms were small and ill ventilated. They housed the physicians, who started at 8.30 a.m. each morning, their assistants, and a press of medical students. Four mothers and their children were admitted at a time, so that the room, designed to accommodate up to six persons, usually held ten or twelve. The physician got through about 25 cases an hour. He had little time to take notes. After their 'dismissal' from the consulting-room the mothers and children congregated in a densely crowded 'covered apartment' waiting for their script to be dispensed by the two dispensers. Normally it was 3 p.m. before the crowd thinned. Most of the mothers and children had spent five hours at the hospital.

A majority of the patients belonged to 'a lower class'; but not the lowest. Like other charitable institutions, the Hospital for Sick Children exercised 'great vigilance . . . to prevent the benefits of a hospital intended for the really poor from being diverted to a class in better circumstances'. Patients received one free treatment and thereafter had to pay (the sum was unspecified; by analogy with other charities it would have been something between threepence and 2*s*. 6*d*.) for subsequent visits, unless they could produce a subscriber's letter, or a letter from a doctor, or city missionary declaring the bearer to be 'a proper object of charity'. Excluding uncounted cases of skin and head disease, Table 3.8 lists for 1868 the cases the hospital treated on a regular basis.

Table 3.8: Ailments Treated at Hospital for Sick Children during 1868

50 cases of	chicken pox
3 " "	smallpox
253 " "	measles and sequelae
160 " "	scarlatina and sequelae
18 " "	typhoid
105 " "	febricula ('slight fevers')
4 " "	erysipelas
6 " "	diphtheria
17 " "	mumps
616	

Source: Ibid.

These cases had each an average of five attendances at the hospital.[56] The ritual of abasement and mortification must have strengthened the mothers' stoicism. Certainly it testifies to their uncomplaining, helpless desperation: the numbers show that they kept coming. The ointments which they were given might have helped them treat their children's skin sores, but I find it hard to see how the children with more serious internal infections were benefited.

The hospital was a hotbed of infection. The late summer of 1869 saw a fierce outbreak of scarlatina in the neighbourhood. During the week beginning 20 October there were 238 deaths. Local doctors believed that the case mortality had jumped dramatically. Between July and October there had been over 2,000 deaths and the hospital had treated well over 4,000 victims, at the rate of 53 a day. A correspondent in the *Lancet* revealed that many doctors had seen a link between the hospital and the epidemic: 'the contagion [was] largely propagated in the out-patient room of the Children's Hospital . . . Children . . . labouring under scarlatina [were] brought to this hospital from all parts of the metropolis, and in the close waiting-room the contagion [was] readily communicated.' This is plausible. But 1869 was a bad year and local doctors in Liverpool, Sheffield and Leeds, without benefit of children's hospitals, claimed, although they pro-

duced no evidence, that their local outbreaks and case death rates were
even worse.[57]

The Evelina Hospital for Sick Children opened in Southwark Bridge
Road in 1869 with 30 beds for in-patients and provision for over 100
daily out-patients. It was the gift of Baron Ferdinand de Rothschild.
Doctors were rather suspicious of it. There had been an early row about
Christian nurses proselytising in the wards, which was partly settled by
establishing a separate Jewish section. Moreover, it was designed with a
distinct ward for whooping cough sufferers, a development reported by
medical men as a further declension into mere specialism, which they
regarded as mere narrow empiricism.[58] The severely scientific Yorkhill
Hospital in Glasgow, when it opened in 1882, still excluded children
under two, unless they were accident victims. This rule did not change
until about the turn of the century, when about 1/5 of the patients
were found to be under age.[59] In 1896 the MOH for County Durham
was still lamenting that people would not let their children be taken to
hospital because the hospitals were 'unattractive'. He thought the
people still took scarlet fever 'very lightly', but in this situation theirs
was a hard choice.[60]

The East London Hospital for Sick Children provided at least one
model for a different kind of institution. This was begun in the late
1860s in association with the Dispensary for Women which I mentioned in Chapter 1. Its building was 'tall, tumbledown, shabby-looking
. . . having nothing to distinguish it from half-a-dozen other closed tenements in the locality' except the name on blackboards set in each window. It was the first hospital in Great Britain to admit children under
two, and to allow their mothers to come in and assist with their nursing. In 1870 there were 30-40 child patients scattered over the various
storeys of the old warehouse. In two years the hospital workers had
treated over 4,600 out-patients, exclusive of home visits. The East
London was a hospital among, and seemingly at one with, its clientele.
It was one of three hospitals in the East End, compared with the 40
or so in the West End. By 1895 the hospital had grown to 102 beds,
'always full', and was handling over 30,000 out-patients a year. In 1870
the regular inmates included a dog and two puppies. In the same year
the hospital also became the first to appoint a female physician, Dr
Elizabeth Garrett (subsequently Garrett-Anderson). The hospital was
coolly regarded by the profession and the charity activists and remained
short of money and help throughout the century.[61]

Smallpox

Smallpox is a horrifying, disfiguring disease which can kill in explosive outbreaks but, compared with the diseases I have discussed, its impact in the nineteenth century has been overrated by historians. It is a highly contagious viral sickness. The virus is present in the nose and throat of the infected person, in the blisters on his skin, and in his excretions through the course of the disease which lasts three or four weeks. The incubation period of severe headache, chills, high fever and vomiting, the period of uncertain diagnosis, lasts about 7 to 12 days. There is still no known cure.

Nineteenth-century statisticians were agreed that the disease had diminished as a killer from about 1780. The Royal Commission on Smallpox in 1882 reported a decline, shown in Table 3.9, with figures based on calculations from the London bills of mortality.

Table 3.9: Smallpox Mortality Rate, 1771-1880

	Per Thousand Living
1771 – 80	5
1801 – 10	2
1801 – 35	0.83
1837 – 40	2.3
1841 – 50	0.40
1851 – 60	0.28
1861 – 70	0.28
1871 – 80	0.46

Source: Report of Royal Commission on Smallpox and Fever Hospitals, *PP*, 1882, vol. XXIX, pp. vii, 320.

These figures represent about 6,400 deaths in London in the bad years 1837-40 and almost 10,000 deaths during the epidemic of 1871-2. In England and Wales there were about 41,600 deaths in 1837-40 and 42,000 in 1871-2, amongst a population which was about 40 per cent larger.[62] In Scotland the death rate averaged 3.5 per 10,000 during 1851-60 and 1.8 per 10,000 for 1861-70 and 1.9 per 10,000 for 1871-80.[63] The last decline of the disease began in 1875 when the number of deaths fell from 1,246 in 1874 to 76 in 1875. Through the century the disease gradually left the villages and the provincial towns and concentrated in London, the great cities and the seaport towns. The num-

bers of deaths in rural counties such as Buckinghamshire, Suffolk,
Dorset and Cumberland all fell by 1/3 to ½ between 1837-40 and
1871-2, and deaths in the West Riding showed a slight fall, while
Northamptonshire, Staffordshire and Nottinghamshire all had totals
which increased by 1/3 to ½. Hampshire, with Plymouth and Southampton, rose by 300 per cent while County Durham numbers rose by
nearly 600 per cent.[64]

Smallpox also diminished by 66 per cent among children under five
and persisted among adolescents and young adults. Even so, as Table
3.10 shows, a quarter of all smallpox deaths still occurred among the
under-fives in the 1880s.

Table 3.10: Proportion of Deaths under 5 Years to 1,000 Deaths from
Smallpox at all Ages

1847 — 53	—	697
1854 — 67	—	550
1868 — 77	—	323
1878 — 86	—	238

Source: Creighton, *Epidemics*, Vol. II, pp. 571-2; B.A. Whitelegge, *Lancet*,
4 March 1893, p. 458.

It was replaced among the under-fives, as we have seen, by measles,
whooping cough and the other infections. This is especially true, as
Creighton remarked, of the 1871-2 outbreak, which was preceded by
the scarlatina epidemic of 1868-70 which removed many infants who
might otherwise have succumbed to smallpox. In between the great
outbreaks, the disease recurred in short, isolated lethal bursts every
three or four years until 1885 (in England and Wales) when it decisively
retreated, excepting a small epidemic in 1902-5. Creighton calculated
a case-mortality rate of one in six in London during the 1871-2 outbreak and one in seven during its period as an endemic disease in subsequent years. In the provinces the case-mortality rate was lower, at one
in nine, or, in the 1890s, one in ten. In general, contemporaries agreed,
the younger the patient, the greater the chance of death.[65]

Smallpox was a disease of the poor. It did have its share of victims
among the rich but, as it contracted to the great cities, smallpox increasingly became an infestation of the slums. The poor preserved
rituals which the comfortable classes had largely abandoned before the
turn of the nineteenth century. The rich had moved on to the 'anti-

phlogistic regimen', giving their isolated patient 'water pap, rice, or bread boiled with milk, good apples roasted or boiled with milk, and sweetened with a little sugar . . . barley water [and] after the pox is full, butter-milk', interspersed with the quinine, antimonials and purges ordered by the doctor.[66] The poor continued to 'roast' their patients. In Norwich in 1818 the old women who were

> the most popular practitioners among the poor . . . set the subject before a large fire, and [supplied] it plentifully with saffron and brandy, to bring out the eruption; during the whole of the next stage [the blister stage — about one week], to keep it in bed; covered with flannel, and even the bed-curtains pinned together, to prevent a breath of air; to allow no change of linen for ten or more days, until the eruptions had turned [the scab stage]; and to regard the best system to be a costive state of the bowels during the whole course of the disease.[67]

When more than one child in the family showed symptoms they were put in the one bed. 'It is a common sight . . . to see two or three children lying in the same bed', Buchan wrote, 'with such a load of pustules that their skins stick together.' The smell was sickening. The unchanged bed-linen became stiff and rasped off the scabs.[68]

The great weapon of the state and the doctors, their first confidence-building preventive discovery (during the 1790s) in combating small-pox, was vaccination. The rich readily accepted it, the poor did not. The common people's adherence to traditional practices and indifference to vaccination reflected a sober appraisal of their life chances and acceptance of the inescapability of death; theirs was an existence in which curbed hopes were safest. Their small expectations were reinforced by apathetic ignorance shading into resentment and resistance to interference from superiors whose authority derived from knowledge, practices and status outside the relationships and understandings prevailing within their stratum and neighbourhood. As Mr Smith, a medical man in Ruddington, Nottinghamshire, remarked of the poor stockingers in his town, they were 'very indifferent to medical relief in all diseases which have a determinate course'. Ruddington had experienced a smallpox outbreak in 1839. The 'middle classes and wealthy' had been protected by vaccination, but the poor had not. They were not 'against vaccination', Smith explained, 'but simply uncaring'. Their *time . . . [was] so occupied in procuring a bare subsistence, that they [did] not provide a guard against contingencies*' (original italics). Even when their children were dying, they preferred to go belatedly, to an unqualified man to 'puncture them with his needle' (inoculation) and to pay for it rather than to go to Smith for vaccination, free.[69] Dr Whitehead alleged of the poor in Manchester in 1859 that

> when a child [was] seized with fever or another severe malady, its parents [were] apt to conclude that it [had] received the 'death stroke', and from that moment they [ceased] to seek medical measures beyond their own resources, quietly awaiting the child's death.[70]

After describing how easily the poor of the Midlands abandoned efforts to obtain letters for hospitals and dispensaries, and Poor Law medical relief orders, Dr H.W. Rumsey remarked that

> a sort of fatalism is very prevalent among the poor; they have ... far less reliance on medical care than the upper classes. Some appear careless and apathetic; some resign themselves to the event; but from one or other of these causes not a few of the poorest and most degraded allow their diseases to take their own course.[71]

These reports are indications not that poor people undervalued life but that they faced reality, indeed they could not escape it, weighing their resources against the chances of obtaining a cure. And many simple people 'cared' within a frame of reference different from that of the doctors.

Vaccination prevented attacks, and eased the recovery of victims; but it was not as effective as its protagonists claimed. The opponents of vaccination were often irrational but their arguments, however extravagant, had a core of fact. The great controversy about the involvement of the state with vaccination raised fundamental issues about authority and morals. The row has its ludicrous aspects but it was, after all, a question of life and death.

The efficacy of vaccination in controlling smallpox mortality was proved by 1800. Deaths reported from smallpox within the parishes covered by the London bills of mortality fell slowly if steadily from 7,347, in the four years preceding the introduction of vaccination in 1798, to 6,560 in 1802, to 4,667 in 1806, to 5,915 in 1810. In all there appears to have been a saving of 420 lives each year.[72] Before 1798 there is some shadowy evidence that the incidence of smallpox had been rising with the increase of population. One group of careful reformers calculated a rate of 74 per 1,000 deaths for the period 1700-30 and 95 per 1,000 for 1770-1800.[73]

By 1837 doctors were able to show that unvaccinated persons were much more at risk: in London in 1836 Dr Gregory recorded 73 deaths among 193 unvaccinated victims and only 10 among 128 vaccinated sufferers.[74] The 'wealthy and middle classes' had by 1840, according to the *Lancet*, accepted the advantages of vaccination and 'invariably' had their children vaccinated before they were twelve months old.[75]

The lower orders constituted the reservoirs of the disease. Through the eighteenth century they were said to have neglected inoculation (immediate transference of the live smallpox virus). They did not actively resist inoculation and, when pressed, readily submitted to its performance by their parish surgeons but, whether from 'a supineness of character respecting disease, or insensibility to their own safety . . . or of minds whose exertion is unceasingly directed to procuring daily sustenance' they did not seek vaccination (inoculation, in theory at least, with cowpox virus).[76] Starting with the premiss that 'ignorance' on the part of the mother was the greatest hindrance to the spread of vaccination, Dr Hall Bakewell calculated, over the period 1848-54, a direct correlation between female literacy and smallpox mortality: the eleven 'best' counties, where only 30-40 per cent of women signed the marriage register with a mark, had an annual average mortality of 13.5 per 1,000 while the nine 'worst', with 60-70 per cent signing with a mark, had 22.4 per 1,000 mortality. Reasonably, Hall Bakewell inferred a lower rate of vaccination in the 'worst' counties than in the 'best'.[77] The National Vaccine Association, a charitable body established to provide vaccine for cheap vaccinations, was supplying 60,000 persons a year in London alone by 1820, but still its produce was said not to be reaching the classes for whom it was intended.[78]

After the appalling epidemic in Norwich in 1819, with over 3,000 cases and 500 deaths amounting to the worst visitation on the town since the Plague, British doctors strengthened their demand for compulsory vaccination, as on the Continent. After it was introduced in Bavaria (1807), Denmark (1810), Hesse and other German states and effectively Prussia (1818), mortality from smallpox had fallen dramatically. The mortality in Prussia, for example, had declined from an alleged 40,000 annually before 1818 to a reported 3,000 in 1826. Smallpox inoculation was prohibited and no one who had had neither cowpox nor smallpox could be confirmed, enrolled at school, apprenticed or married without producing his or her vaccination certificate.[79]

The British Parliament made its first move into state medicine in

1840, when it carried the Vaccination Act (3 and 4 Vict., c.29) for England and Wales and Ireland, directing the parish Poor Law officers to contract with the Poor Law medical officer for the vaccination of 'all persons resident'; presumably, although the Act was vague about it, the cost was to be borne by the local poor rate. This badly drafted measure was subsequently amended and extended by legislation in 1853, 1858, 1867 and 1871. The Act of 1853 made vaccination of infants compulsory before they reached three months. In 1871 a fine of 25s. or imprisonment was introduced for parents who refused to have their infants vaccinated.[80]

The medical profession opposed this linking of vaccination with the Poor Law. They rightly predicted that it would provoke resistance and make vaccination 'an object of terror'.[81] The doctors were to receive 1s. 6d. per successful vaccination from the poor rates; they wanted 2s. to be paid out of national revenue. Each poor family was to be allocated a set of vouchers valid for treatment by any doctor, the vouchers to be returned for payment through a projected National Vaccine Commission. The Commission was also to ensure that proper records were kept, so that all lymph from voucher-vaccinated children would be guaranteed 'fresh lymph for rich children', as private patients. Inoculation was to be prohibited. The government ignored the doctors.[82] They now had a new grievance against the Poor Law. Some guardians zestfully entered upon cutting local costs in their Union, too: the Stockport guardians successfully advertised for a vaccinator to work at 6d. per head and won the hatred of the local doctors; Battle Union guardians did the same, with the same result among the local medical fraternity. When the Blackburn Union sought to reduce its fees, the 15 Blackburn doctors struck for 2s. 6d. a head, but a minority began to settle for 1s. 6d., whereupon 14 of the 15 decided to vaccinate free, until this move was broken by Mr Wilding, a blackleg who undertook all the Union vaccinations for 1s. each. There were similar strikes and demands rendered unsuccessful by blacklegs in St Pancras, and St Columb in Cornwall. In many unions vaccination was to embitter relations between doctors and local authorities for a generation, and in some places, such as Wigan, and rural Cornwall, until into the twentieth century.[83]

The poor and many artisan and middle-class people who were suspicious of authority resisted Poor Law vaccination on a variety of grounds. Compulsory vaccination represented a new, and for many people, the first, intrusion into the family of state authority, in the shape of the feared or suspected Poor Law surgeon. Inoculation among neighbours, performed by a local house doctor, wise woman, preacher or itinerant quack, was a shared, understood procedure. Incision by a barely known person with superior status was neither shared nor re-assuring.[84] Some resisters held to the old humoural physiology and asserted that vaccination introduced evil humours into the child's blood. This belief was reinforced by the fact that the child was being given, everyone thought, cowpox, a 'beast's disease', and not, as in inocula-tion, smallpox, a 'human' one.[85] Other evaders, noting that vaccina-tion (and inoculation) often had nasty consequences, affirmed that it was 'better to let nature take its course', and do nothing.[86]

The dangers in vaccination began with the lymph. Until the 1890s, at least, doctors were careless about taking lymph from otherwise diseased children. This situation was worsened by two prevalent, con-tradictory beliefs about the effects of inoculation and vaccination. On the one hand, many people believed, apparently until into the 1880s, that inoculation of eczematous children and taking smallpox lymph from them both cured eczema in the victim and prevented its eruption on the child inoculated from the victim. On the other hand, 'Experienta' (a medical man) argued in 1852 that the poor objected to vaccination 'because they know their children often get ill after it with scrofula and other cutaneous eruptions'.[87] Nowadays eczematous children are the main group for whom vaccination must be deferred. Medical opinion agreed that the eighth day of infection was the best time for taking lymph, but they were divided as to how it should be done and how much should be taken. Careful doctors might not take more than three 'tubes' from a single vesicle on the same child; but impatient doctors faced with a local outbreak would try for more than four by pressing the arm to force out the drops, rather than letting the lymph ooze out. The drop which oozed out was believed to be purer than the forced material, which often included blood.[88] Some doctors preferred to use straight lymph, others mixed it with up to 15 parts water, apparently unboiled, or glycerine to preserve it and make it go further. Although they were unaware of it, and the proportion of glycerine solution was commonly too low, a 50 per cent solution of water-glycerine can kill tubercle bacilli and erysipelas streptococcus. Once they obtained it, careful doctors tried to use the lymph immediately.

The National Vaccine Association and the Local Government Board both had difficulty throughout the century in storing and transporting lymph. Glycerinised calf-lymph in the earlier twentieth century was expected to retain its potency 'for many weeks and months'; in the nineteenth century doctors believed that it began to deteriorate after

30 hours.[89] Both the usual methods of keeping and packaging lymph allowed it to dry out. The first was to hold droplets on ivory points, sometimes furnished with a screw-on cap. The other common method was to place the droplet between two plates of glass. By the 1850s some doctors half-realised that the lymph could be contaminated or 'decomposed', and several experimental packages were tried, including preserving the lymph with coal gas in closed glass phials, but the old techniques survived until the 1890s.[90] In 1900 the Sanitary Commission on Calf Lymph analysed samples from six distributors and found 'very few' to be sterile. A majority of the samples contained a 'large number of sporulating and anaerobic organisms'. Some of the distributors had failed to perform the usual post-mortem on the calf from which the lymph had been taken to make certain that the animal was not tubercular. None the less, the Commission concluded that they had found the samples 'more pure than [they] expected to find them'.[91]

Vaccinators learned on the job. The procedure was not taught in medical schools.[92] It was a lowly task, usually left to untrained assistants. When Archibald Pearson, MD Glasgow, started to practise as a parochial doctor and public vaccinator in the West Highlands in 1863, he 'got from the Glasgow Royal Infirmary two tubes of vaccine lymph'. Before he began to vaccinate he 'had to read up how this simple operation was performed, as [he] had never seen a child or adult vaccinated before'. His early efforts were often unsuccessful and he often had to vaccinate the same child two or three times before the vaccine took. The present technique involves placing a drop of vaccine on the skin of the upper arm and lightly scratching the skin with a needle. Pearson used a lancet to cut the skin. Thereafter he abandoned the lancet for a time and adopted a 'four-pronged vaccinator' but this brought no greater success rate and caused more pain than the lancet. He preferred to place the lymph on the skin, then prick two holes with the point of the lancet to the depth of an eighth of an inch deep and in diameter. By the 1880s he was set in his habits. He scoffed:

> some medical men go so far as to use a needle, and a fresh one each time they vaccinate. I have been vaccinating with the same lancet ever since I began practice — all I do is to wipe it well before beginning and after I am done.[93]

In 1859 the Privy Council issued an order providing for instruction in vaccinating method, a certificate of proficiency and register of cases. But the order seems never to have been implemented systematically.

Many surgeons cut too deeply, causing profuse bleeding which carried off the lymph: a vaccinating lancet with flanges to prevent it penetrating below the capillary blood vessels became available only in 1884.[94]

Throughout the century there was much disagreement about the technique of vaccination and, conveniently for the vaccinators, no legal or medical definition of 'successful' vaccination. Some doctors used lancets, others pronged scratchers. Some sought to make one vesicle on each arm, others were convinced that nothing less than six on each arm would serve. Others settled for a number in between. After 1871 the Local Government Board specified a minimal four insertions but made no provision for enforcing this provision. Doctors commonly only gave one insertion to infant private patients in order to please the parents, and readily issued certificates of insusceptibility after only two failures instead of after 1867, the legal three. In the mid-1850s private vaccinations of infants amounted to 10-15 per cent of children under one year. As public vaccinators were paid by the number of 'successful' vaccinations they performed, 'unsuccessful' vaccinations were almost unknown.[95] The public vaccinators were helped to this 'success' by omitting all follow-up procedures. If the child did not develop a cicatrix after eight days, the vaccinator did not want to hear about it. At 1s. 6d. to 2s. 6d. or more a head until the 1890s, and thence 5s. to 5s. 6d. vaccination was a sound source of income for Poor Law surgeons and they keenly competed for business: some paid bonuses for infants brought to them, usually twopence or a pot of beer, or a free bottle of medicine. The average town vaccinator was said to be making £150 a year (i.e. about 600 cases) from this source in 1900. Again there was no incentive for the surgeon to ensure that the vaccine had taken.[96] Surgeons who examined immigrants were unanimous that Scandinavians and Germans were better vaccinated than Britons.[97]

The National Vaccine Board by 1896 had arranged the vaccination of nearly 100,000 people 'over a long series of years' and had never reported a case as insusceptible. Yet in 1892 alone, nearly 2,000 infants in England and Wales had been so registered. By the turn of the century the local government doctors had established that above 0.35 per cent of infants were insusceptible.[98]

Surgeons had known since the 1820s at least that 'vaccine influence' underwent 'decadence' after a period of years. The statistics of admission to the London Small Pox Hospital showed a heavy preponderance of patients over 15 who had been vaccinated, presumably in infancy, as against an even distribution among the ages of unvaccinated patients.[99] By the 1880s doctors were pressing for a 'booster' at ten-yearly intervals, but this procedure was confined to private practice in the nineteenth century. (Recent routine is to give 'boosters' at five-year intervals.)[100] Poor Law guardians steadily opposed revaccination as only 'a set of jobs' which added to the rates.[101]

Given these deficiencies, it is surprising that vaccination achieved as much as it did. Not only did smallpox mortality fade, but vaccination lessened the severity of attacks. Around 1840, of 536 convict boys transported to Australia, 40 per cent of them from London, 25 per cent were pock-marked on the face.[102] By 1860 the proportions of army recruits, presumably from social strata which overlapped those of the convict boys, who were 'marked by small-pox' were:

in England 151 per 1,000;
in Scotland 102 per 1,000;
in Ireland 116 per 1,000.

The proportions of recruits who 'showed evidence of vaccination' tally roughly with these ratios:

in England 747 per 1,000;
in Scotland 790 per 1,000;
in Ireland 816 per 1,000.[103]

By 1898 the Local Government Board was able to claim that 61 per cent of infants in England and Wales had been vaccinated within the legal minimum of three months. In 1853, immediately before compulsion was introduced in 1854, the Epidemiological Society estimated that 53 per cent of babies had received protection.[104] But the proportion vaccinated waxed and waned through the century with each doctor's dedication, local resistance and the meanness of the guardians. In 1864 Bilston suffered an outbreak after the local doctors, whom a colleague described as 'lazy', refused to vaccinate until the guardians raised the payment from 1s. 6d. to 2s. 6d. Among 549 recent births only 358 infants had been vaccinated.[105] Frequently there would be a burst of vaccinating activity after an outbreak and then quiescence, particularly when the guardians showed alarm at the cost. In Reading, for instance, the number of infant vaccinations in successive years between 1854 and 1856 was 405, 275 and 231. Newmarket and Biggleswade showed similar patterns.[106]

The patchy availability of public vaccination, the timidity of the Poor Law Commissioners and their successors in the Local Government

Board, created in 1871, and the small-mindedness of local guardians, the scare about the epidemics of 1871 and the increase in the fines from 20s. and 25s. and longer gaol terms for evading the Acts all coincided in the early 1870s and all stirred the long-term opponents of 'state puncturing'. Some, like Reverend George Cardew, the rector of Helmingham in Suffolk, fought vaccination because it imposed the 'mark of the beast' and therefore was 'against Nature'. Smallpox would never leave Britain until there was 'an end of, or at least a great diminution of impurity. It . . . [was] immorality which lead to Small-pox.' Mr Cardew left unclear whether he believed that smallpox was a Divinely ordained visitation upon a profligate nation, or the result of the promiscuity that resulted from overcrowding and want of Christian virtue. Probably he thought it a mixture of both. His further objection he shared with most opponents of compulsion: that the imposition of the Act was unfair because the rich man could pay his fine for refusal, while the poor man had to go to gaol.[107]

The issue of state compulsion was closely bound with the controversy that erupted in the late 1860s against the Contagious Diseases Acts, the legislation which provided for compulsory inspection and hospitalisation of prostitutes in declared ports and garrison towns. The Anti-Vaccination League was established in 1866. Its fighters against the augmentation of state powers and intrusiveness were busy on both fronts, and were soon to be resisting the Habitual Drunkards Bill and the Medical Reform and Vivisection Bills of the 1870s. At an Anti-Vaccination League meeting at Exeter Hall in 1871 the veteran campaigner, Dr Garth Wilkinson, Swedenborgian, homeopath (he was the first editor of Blake's *Songs of Innocence and Experience*, 1839), declared that 'we are an over-legislated-for people'. F.W. Newman, another veteran proponent of polymathic unorthodoxy in, amongst other things, the pronunciation of Latin, millenialism, theology and Arabic lexicography, protested that England was 'under a despotism . . . making it the duty of every man to see that his healthy children [were] made unhealthy'.[108] 'An Englishman's house is no longer his own', Mrs Hume-Rothery, the feminist poetess, novelist and campaigner against the Contagious Diseases Acts, wrote at about the same time: 'Under favour of the odious Vaccination Acts a poor man's house may be entered by emissaries of the Medical Star Chamber to ascertain whether his children have been blood-poisoned according to law.' She saw the Acts as part of the 'unnatural dominance of females by the Male State', integral with, indeed resulting from, 'the indecent and unnatural study and practice by male practitioners of obstetric

medicine'.[109] The notable scientific name among the anti-vaccination-
ists was that of Alfred Russell Wallace. He remained a believer in miasmic contagion and denounced vaccination as scientifically unprovable
and medically dangerous. The Royal Commission on Small Pox demolished the mass of statistics he brought to buttress his argument. His
attack on vaccination was printed in the first (1898) edition of his
Wonderful Century and was silently omitted from the second (1903).
Like other liberal-radicals, the trade union leader George Howell, for
example, he hid a fundamental objection to the intrusive state under a
bushel of 'science', meaning doubtful figures and poorly substantiated
bad cases.[110]

Apart from the eczema which the campaigners and many ordinary
people believed was spread by vaccination (the present explanation is
that the child probably already has eczema, rubs the vaccination site
and scratches his other skin lesions, introducing vaccinia virus all over
the skin surface and developing generalised vaccinia), there were alleged
cases of children developing other diseases, which the anti-vaccinators
made notorious. In May 1871 there was a row at the meeting of the
Royal Medical and Chirurgical Society when Dr C.R. Drysdale, the
advocate of birth control, opponent of the Contagious Diseases Acts,
and very able diagnostician, claimed that a child of deaf and dumb
parents, to whom he had given a note saying the child was not to be
vaccinated, had, despite the note and the parents' evident agitation,
been taken to St Bartholomew's Hospital and vaccinated, and afterwards developed syphilis, 'caught', Drysdale argued, 'with the smallpox vaccine'.[111] In 1872 Mr Paxton of Sunderland became a martyr
for the cause after being fined repeatedly for refusing to have his
children vaccinated, on the grounds that the procedure was proven
dangerous: his wife had died some years before, he claimed, from
erysipelas contracted through vaccination.[112] Resolute opposition was
widespread, from Liskeard to Brighton, to Hastings, some of the East
End unions, to Northampton, Kettering, Leicester (which was in a state
of siege against the Local Government Board inspectors during 1871) to
Spalding, Keighley, Oldham, Newcastle and Middlesbrough. These were
towns with a strong lower middle and working class who had a powerful voice in the local political culture — against the state, against London, and against anonymous professional authority. The opposition
held out until into the twentieth century. During an outbreak in
Keighley in 1875, in which 208 persons caught smallpox and 25 died,
the guardians, an outfitter, draper, bolt and screw worker, builder,
farmer and currier respectively, resisted a writ of mandamus from the

Local Government Board to introduce Poor Law vaccination. They were arrested for contempt of court in 1876 and lodged in York gaol. The town, about 30,000 people, were solid for the guardians:

> It is for you, the noble Guardians
> In York Castle lay [sic] today
> To the rescue, men of Keighley
> And unite without delay.

But the three remaining guardians voted for vaccination and it was introduced. The anti-vaccinators claimed that only the vaccinated had caught the disease, while 'hundreds' of unvaccinated children had escaped.[113]

Keighley was only an extreme example of a northern town with long memories of resistance to the New Poor Law, and fights with the Poor Law doctors about vaccination and other procedures and payments going back at least to 1841. The town, again like many northern centres, was a stronghold of unorthodox treatments. In 1875 the guardians contracted the poor to an hydropathist (one who seeks to cure by external and internal application of water). The town was still holding out against compulsory vaccination at the turn of the century: in 1898, for example, under the new legislation permitting exemption, 660 parents, with 1,670 children, won their appeals as 'conscientious objectors' at a single court sitting, and such events, the *Lancet* lamented, happened 'regularly'. Leicester in 1887 had only 322 of its 4,693 infants vaccinated.[114]

Faith in the north in herbalism and other treatments reflected a deep conviction of the inviolability of each individual and his person. 'Unnecessary' surgery was trespass and it entailed retribution. As Mr J. Clayton, a medical herbalist of Middlesbrough, advertised in the *Northern Echo* in 1902:

> During the last nine years he had taken off over 200 tumours without cutting from almost every part of the body – *Cause – Vaccination* . . . because when the tumour comes off you can see the same number of holes in the part where the tumour comes off, oozing with matters that correspond to the same number of marks that are on the arm, so that it leaves no doubt on the subject . . . When the lymph travels to the liver it breeds smallpox, when it travels to the throat, diphtheria . . . to the brain . . . diseases of the mind.[115]

The return to permissive legislation in 1898 signalled an increasing recognition by both sides of the facts of the situation. In 1880 Jonathan Hutchinson, the rising authority on opthalmology and syphilis, publicly acknowledged that Drysdale and the populists were correct in claiming that vaccination did very occasionally transmit disease, including syphilis. His argument was gradually accepted by the profession, although many hesitated to make the big admission and instead took the line of the *British Medical Journal*, that it was not syphilis that was transmitted but a little-known disease called *vaccinia maligna*, thereby preserving the total value of vaccination and only emphasising the need for fresh vaccine. They supported their case with the observation that infants were naturally highly susceptible to new poisons and it was therefore 'not surprising that some of them are badly damaged by it'.[116] Meanwhile, the local evidence of the worth of vaccination grew more precise and indisuptable. In Leicester itself, during the first epidemic since that of 1871-2, Dr Joseph Priestly, the MOH, was able to show that of the first 146 cases, comprising 89 adults and 57 children, 82 adults were vaccinated and 7 not, 7 children were vaccinated and 50 not; and among the 82 vaccinated adults there were only 6 'severe' cases and 1 death, compared with 4 'severe', 3 'very severe' and 1 death among the 7 unvaccinated. Among the 50 unvaccinated children, 8 died, 22 had 'very severe' and another 22 'severe' attacks, while the 7 unvaccinated cases were all 'very mild'. The 'very mild' cases among both adults and children had all been revaccinated. Dr Priestly concluded that Leicester had by 1893 become a 'well vaccinated town'.[117] The evidence mounted through the early 1890s. During the outbreak in Birmingham in 1894, the MOH was able to produce the results given in Table 3.11.

Table 3.11: Smallpox Outbreak, Birmingham, 1894

	Average Number of Days in Hospital
All smallpox vaccinated cases	30
Unvaccinated cases	50
Cases with one mark	34
" " two marks	33½
" " three marks	29¼
" " four marks	28
" " five marks	26½

Source: *Lancet*, 25 Aug. 1894, p. 461.

And during an outbreak in Leeds in the following year Dr Cameron, the MOH, proved that there were no deaths among victims with 4-6 cicatrices, only a 2 per cent mortality among those with 2-3 cicatrices, who constituted the great majority of cases, contrasted with a 19.3 per cent mortality among the 88 unvaccinated sufferers.[118] Finally, in 1897, T.D. Acland surveyed recent outbreaks in Sheffield, Warrington, Dewsbury, Gloucester and elsewhere, and showed conclusively that, at 10 years and under, unvaccinated persons were up to 16 times more likely than vaccinated persons to contract smallpox, and at 10 and over, about twice as liable. Moreover, the vaccinated at under 30, at least, were so protected that, even if they suffered an attack, they were much more likely to survive. At Gloucester, for instance, they suffered one death compared with 192 among the unvaccinated. Over 30, the chances both of an attack and of survival tipped towards the unvaccinated, probably for want of recent revaccination and just possibly because of a higher ratio of naturally acquired immunity among these survivors.[119]

The decline of the disease remains puzzling. Vaccination undoubtedly contributed greatly, but it was incomplete in 1885 when the dominant trend became decisive; even in 1898, 33 per cent of infants in London had not been vaccinated. Moreover, the low insusceptibility rate suggests that there was very little extra natural immunity in the population.[120] Notification and isolation, which were strictly enforced in the big towns, especially from 1885, and post quarantine, also must have helped with this highly contagious disease, although they did not prevent the severe outbreak of 1902.[121] Paradoxically, isolation was especially severe in the anti-vaccination towns where proud corporations poured money into fever hospitals as a show of defiance of the London Poor Law authorities. Possibly, too, improvements in living standards helped victims withstand it better. But these speculations aside, this hideous disease was almost unique in being defeated before the twentieth century.

Physique and General Health

The standard accounts of industrial society in the first half of the nineteenth century are replete with vivid descriptions drawn from the investigative literature of the 1830s and 1840s of the morbidity, bodily deformities and shortened life expectancies among children, resulting from labour in factories and mills. The long hours, the dust, the fumes, dangerous belt-driven, badly geared, ill-protected power machinery, heavy weights, the inexorable pace of power-driven looms, the miles children walked in a day in textile mills and brickyards, and gratuitous brutality from overlookers and compeers, together overtaxed child operatives, sometimes maimed or killed them, and commonly made them old before their time.

But the factory children were a small minority of the population at risk and it is more illuminating to study their fate within the context of poor general lower-class health. Generally, the main areas of employment for the 10-14 age group in England and Wales — textiles, metal works, ships and docks, mines, potteries and brickworks, agricultural labour, 'general labour' and domestic service — occupied about one-third or 300,000 of the boys in 1851, one-quarter in 1871 and one-fifth in 1881, with agricultural labour the largest single class of employment. About one-fifth of girls, or around 170,000 − 200,000, with domestic service the largest single class after 1861, were employed between 1851 and 1871, falling to about one-sixth in 1891.[122]

The evidence about maimings from accidents and beatings in factories and mines is ghastly enough, but it is salutary to remember that contemporary medical men often argued that the health of children employed in domestic manufacture was worse. Dr Clarke of Nottingham, for instance, explained in 1809 that crippled and feeble-minded children got jobs as cleaners and helpers in local lace and hosiery factories because they were otherwise unemployable in the domestic industry. The wages they brought home, however tiny, can only have helped the family diet and comfort. He went on to contrast these children with the more miserable and unhealthy children he had known in the domestic lace and stocking industries in Northamptonshire and Buckinghamshire and in Nottingham itself. Factory lace tambours (frames on which the work was stretched) were set flexibly; home ones were fixed — usually too high; factory hosiery frames were narrow; home ones were often too wide and were usually heavier. Factories were ventilated sometimes at least, and lime-washed; domestic workers spent their days in rooms 'about fourteen feet long, ten feet broad and eight feet high', usually containing eight frames,

> at each of which one person sits at work. The door is kept closed by a lead and pull [sic]; the cracks . . . of the window are covered with paper, and the apartment warmed by a common stove, producing a suffocating sensation on entering from the external air.[123]

'Private houses' were still worse than lace and hosiery factories in the 1860s, according to witnesses testifying to the Children's Employment

Commission.[124] Domestic industry, as I shall show later, was a hotbed of tuberculosis.

Similarly in 1835, Dr Harrison claimed that the health of child textile factory workers in Preston was much better than that of their contemporaries. Children under 13, he said, were absent with illness only about four days a year, adults, about two days. These figures are sobering testimony to the endurance of the children and the necessity which kept them on the job; none the less they are weakened by Harrison's failure to mention the turnover of employees and the numbers who had dropped out. Harrison's account, like nearly all reports on industrial health in the nineteenth century, is also vitiated by the short time-span (3½ years) of his observations. Over a period of years, as Dr Reynolds affirmed in 1914, 'cotton dust can . . . injure by mechanical irritation of the air passages, setting up a bronchitis asthma'.[125]

Even so, for every witness to the Children's Employment Commission of the 1860s who had been damaged by the damp, dust, long hours and 'dreeness' of her or his work, two others chirpily claimed to be perfectly fit. As always, it is the stoical low expectations of the workers which colour the whole. Mary Walker was 21 in 1862 and had been employed as a fustian cutter in Lymm since she was ten. She worked from 6 a.m. to 9 p.m. Fustian-cutting shops were then outside the Factory Acts. The 'little ones' (10 and upwards) got 'very tired', she said. Fustian is undyed twilled cotton cloth straight from the mills, 'stiffened' with flour paste. The cloth was also lime-washed in order to remove grease stains. Mary Walker explained:

> There's not much dust [flue] made at cutting, but before we cut, we card [brush] each length, and that makes a dust, partly the stuff that comes off and partly the lime; I don't suppose that's very good for us, but I don't know that we are liable to any particular disorder of chest or lungs. We often have colds, but that comes from the drafts when we have the windows open.

The two local surgeons, Simpson and Bennett, both testified that fustian cutters were 'very subject to bronchitis etc.'.[126]

Harrison, the Nottingham surgeon, also argued that maiming factory accidents were much less frequent than similar accidents which happened elsewhere. Again, he might well have been right, and it is salutary to recall that up to 3 per cent of boys transported to New South Wales in the 1840s, few of whom were likely to have been factory lads, were described as having 'post traumatic lesions involving the hands' visible enough to merit mention in their official description. Another 1 per cent showed permanent scars from burns and scalds.[127] Leonard Horner's Factory Inspectors' reports on 2,000 textile factories in Lancashire over the summer six months in 1844 show an accident rate of about 9 per cent, mainly 'lacerations of the extremities' and 'contusions and bruises to trunk and extremities'. But only two of the 90 accidents to children were reported to have resulted from 'unfenced machinery'; most came from 'carelessness'. We must remember here that 'unfenced' had a very narrow legal meaning. Again the figures are complicated by the deaths and accidents happening to children under 13 in the factories, forbidden by law from working but 'playing' there, presumably accompanying their parents or elder siblings who worked at the mill.[128] The pattern of amputations of fingers and bruises to arms, body and legs kept up into the 1860s at least: the 'out-patients' book' at the Birmingham General Hospital showed an overwhelming preponderance of such injuries. Or at least these were the injuries for which parents and employers sought attention for child employees.[129] Jane Grosvenor was 17 and worked in a brickyard at Stourbridge in 1863. She told the Children's Employment Commission that she 'cut [her] finger off two months ago at the press under which the clay is put'. The stump of her finger had gone stiff and was, Jane Grosvenor said, 'in the road'. She 'must have it taken off to the bottom if she [could] get a recommendation ['lines'] to the hospital but she had been unable to get a letter'.[130]

In the metal trades, with comparatively high accident rates, there were 1,114 notified accidents in 1868. But only four of these involved 'young persons'. Under the 1844 Factory Act reporting of accidents seems to have been rigorous, within the legal limits of what had to be reported, at least: small mishaps were listed and investigated; but after the 1867 Act 'Accidents' were only reported if they caused the victim to lose one day's work, or two days in the iron industry.[131] The printed reports of the Factory Inspectors are just the starting point: they provide little sense of the relative severity of accidents in the various industries, and their impact on the victim through time, which only detailed local research can provide.

As the case of the fustian cutters indicates, some of the child workers most at risk were in industries outside the Acts. The children in agricultural work, unlike their urban fellows, were said not to suffer from accidents from machinery or vehicles, but they had to endure very long walks to their work and were often wet to their middles all day. They frequently reported strained backs, blistered hands and chilblains.[132]

These conditions must have been exacerbated by their poor nutrition and housing. Country children rarely drank milk; the farmers would not sell it and it was not a normal 'charity' to give milk away.[133] The water supply in many villages was as poor as in the great towns and its badness persisted longer. At Bideford in 1871, the water was 'tainted by sewage and pigs' styes'. The sewage from the village ran down from the rows of working-class cottages to the beach, where it swept 'around the Quay' on the River Torridge. The cottages were 'sodden'; the walls were 'wet with filth'. Typhoid had raged there for the previous three years, with a mortality of 82 per 1,000, but the local medical officers had been afraid of the local shopkeepers and lodging-house keepers and had refused to report the place as unhygienic or to declare any dwelling unfit for occupation.[134] At nearby Appledore, also in 1871, the drinking-water was polluted with sewage and typhoid was endemic. One hundred cottages had no privies and over a mile of the sea shore was 'solid with sewage and refuse'.[135] Burton Latimer in Northamptonshire had a population of 1,200 in 1872. During the spring of that year the endemic enteric fever had turned virulent: one-sixth of the population caught it and there were 12 deaths. The wells were sunk in shallow porous ground and were thick with 'debris from cesspools, pigstyes and refuse holes'.[136] Market Weighton, at the foot of the Yorkshire Wolds, 'had some kind of epidemic every year' up to the mid-1880s. In 1885 it had been enteric fever. As elsewhere, the wells were shallow and polluted from the cesspools.[137] Linslade in Buckinghamshire provoked a similar report in 1895.[138]

Some of the political and economic causes of rural dirt and ill health emerge in *Truth*'s report on the Vale of Ryedale in the North Riding in the mid-1890s. The valley was headed by the village of Helmsley, from which all the sewage and rubbish went straight into the Rye. Every village down to Vale had endemic typhoid. During the visitation of 1895, more than ten villages recorded cases, with eleven deaths. Helmsley itself had had another ten deaths. There had been several attempts over the years to improve the sanitation of the village, but each threatened to increase the rates and had been successfully resisted. Since 1877 the town beck, the main water supply, had been dredged once, when the swamp and rubbish had been piled against the walls of the nearby cottages and reached the window sills. During the typhoid outbreak immediately preceding that of 1895, when 50 people had been attacked, there had been complaints about the house drains. Three local councillors had been deputed to inspect such house drains as existed. They reported that all were 'perfect' except those of the vicar, the doctor and the bank manager. This trio had jointly lodged the original complaint. Other observers said that theirs were the only carefully maintained drains in the village. The chairman of the district and parish councils was Lord Feversham, who owned most of Helmsley and the Vale. He was also president of the rural sanitary authority. His fellow councillors were small farmers and tradesmen, his tenants, as were the local MOH and Inspector of Nuisances. After the 1895 outbreak the Local Government Board finally sent an inspector to survey the village, but upon his arrival it was discovered that his inquiry and report were to be 'private'. The inspector reported to Lord Feversham, who announced that the typhoid had emanated from an infected dairy and not from the beck. Most cottages in Helmsley were 'tumbledown shanties', without drains or 'even the most elementary conveniences of common decency'. People usually relieved themselves on the edge of the beck. It was a local rule that no cottage could be erected in any part of the town 'to such a height that the roof [could] be seen from the terrace of Lord Feversham's mansion a mile away'.[139] The evidence about Selby Stamford, New Jerusalem in West Riding. King's Norton in Warwickshire, Tamworth and Bettws-y-Coed provides similar stories.[140]

Children from these dark smelly places commonly displayed what one country doctor described as the 'chronic catarrhal condition'. They walked to their work in the fields or to school and spent the day with wet, cold feet. The results show in the entry for 28 April 1899 in the logbook of Wadenhoe elementary school in Northamptonshire. 'Several children very poorly, work disturbed by the continual coughing.' Country children also shared disabilities more commonly associated by historians with their city cousins. Of 150 children examined at Grimbury School in Oxfordshire in 1898, one-fifth had 'defective eyesight'.[141]

Beyond the work and regional situation, the deprivation that generally afflicted working-class and pauper children, still about 75 per cent of the whole in 1910, shows, among other indicators, in their size relative to that of their more fortunate peers.[142] In 1835, in Preston, the average height of 197 'young persons' in factory work said to be aged 14 was 4 feet 7 inches. The measurements were reported to be 'distorted' by the slightly larger sizes of the girls.[143] Convict transportees recorded as fourteen-year-olds in 1840 averaged 4 feet 6 inches for boys tried in London, 4 feet 7¼ inches for boys tried elsewhere in England, and 4 feet 7½ inches for boys from Scotland.[144] The British Association anthropometrical survey of 1878-83 covered 45,000 children. Boys at English public schools aged 11-12 averaged 4 feet 7 inches, the same height as the Preston factory 14-year-olds of four decades earlier. But male 11-year-olds at English industrial schools in the 1870s survey averaged only 4 feet 2 inches.[145]

There were class differentials in weight too. Dr Charles Roberts carried out a survey in 1873, the results of which are given in Table 3.12.

Table 3.12: Comparison of Boys by Average Weight in Pounds, 1873

Age Last Birthday (Alleged)	London Charity School ('well fed and plenty of exercise')	Factory Report 1835	Factory Report 1873	'Agricultural' Children	Public and Middle-Class Schools, ('highest standard of our English race')
9 years	51.63	51.76	58.72	60.02	61.98
10 "	54.53	57.00	62.74	65.29	67.20
11 "	58.32	61.84	67.92	71.01	74.19
12 "	62.80	65.97	71.06	75.00	78.98
Number of observations:	1,770	160	2,958	800	1,210

Source: *Lancet*, 21 Aug. 1875, pp. 274-5.

Roberts's figures show a gradual improvement over the generation between 1835 and 1873 and a greater physical robustness among rural children.[146] Moreover, candidates aged 14 to 20 *accepted* (there are no figures reported for the whole class of applicants) for the Post Office in London showed a gradual increase in height and weight over the period 1876-1903 – at age 14, for example, from an average rise of 190 pounds to 229 pounds.[147] But the class differentials continued into the twentieth century. In 1904 the Reverend W. Edwards Rees reported to the Physical Deterioration Committee the findings of a survey of 42,000 children in Salford, roughly equally divided between school-attenders in a 'poor working class quarter', schools of a 'medium sort' and schools in the 'better quarter'. Thirteen-year-old boys at the poor John Street school averaged 4 feet 5 9/35 inches tall and weighed 65 pounds; their peers at 'best' Rugby Street were 5 feet 1 3/5 inches tall and weighed 98 pounds. Over all, boys of thirteen at the 'medium' schools were 4 feet 7 7/10 inches tall and 68½ pounds, and those at 'better' schools, 4 feet 9 1/3 inches and 79½ pounds.[148] In 1913 500 boys and 500 girls aged 13 were measured in Manchester (see Table 3.13).[149]

Table 3.13: Height and Weight of 13-year-olds in Manchester, 1913

	Average Height	Average Weight
Girls in 'poor class' schools	4 feet 6 inches	75 lb
" " 'medium class' "	4 feet 6 inches	77 lb
" " 'good class' "	4 feet 9 inches	83 lb
Boys in 'poor class' schools	4 feet 4 inches	70 lb
" " 'medium class' "	4 feet 6 inches	73¾ lb
" " 'good class' "	4 feet 9 inches	82 lb

Source: *Lancet*, 17 Jan. 1914.

In the early 1950s girls (no social class appears to have been specified) in Edinburgh aged 13.5 years averaged 5 feet 1 inch in height and weighed 98.8 pounds, and boys 5 feet and 92.6 pounds.

The relationship between deprivation and physical size was first explored in about 1908-9 by Dr Mackenzie and reported by Alfred Mumford. He distinguished tenement dwellings by the number of rooms per family and correlated this information with the average height and weight of the children of the family to show that the meaner the dwelling, the smaller the child. Mumford's explanation derived from the prevailing medical belief in fresh air and ventilation as prime agents of development. Fresh air was free and ventilation could be enforced cheaply; whereas other improvements in living conditions involved dangerous questions about redistribution: 'the more densely packed the home, the less the fresh air and stimulus for growth, and, no doubt closely allied, the less the food supply, the clothing, and the amount of rest for recovery from the fatigues of the day'.[150]

Mackenzie's figures express in a concentrated way the disparities between ranks within the poor and, together with the other figures I have given, they provoke speculation about the increase in the size of children in this century, and why the age of the menarche has almost certainly decreased over the same time-span. Most authorities agree that improved nutrition is mainly responsible, but other complex factors must be involved as well, even fresh air perhaps, especially as these changes involved the rich as well as, or even more than, the poor.

Table 3.14a: Loss of Pounds in Weight of Children According to Size of Tenement: That is, Pounds Below National Averages

Ages	6	7	8	9	10	11	12	13	14
Group I single room	3.1	4.0	6.6	6.7	8.5	9.4	13.2	16.0	21.3
Group II two rooms	2.3	3.7	6.0	5.0	7.5	9.0	13.0	15.0	20.0
Group III three rooms	1.4	1.1	2.6	2.0	3.2	4.6	6.6	11.2	10.5

Table 3.14b: Loss of Inches in Height of Children According to Size of Tenement: That is, Inches Below National Averages

Group I single room	2.2	2.0	2.5	2.8	3.3	3.5	4.3	4.2	4.7
Group II two rooms	1.6	1.8	2.1	2.7	2.7	2.7	3.5	3.6	4.1
Group III three rooms	0.1	0.7	0.3	0.6	0.6	0.8	2.4	1.8	2.7

Source: Alfred A. Mumford, 'Imperfections in Physical Growth as Hindrances to Social Development', *Child-Study*, vol. 3 (1910), p. 93.

School Health

The spread through the lower classes of regular school attendance after 1870 created new reservoirs of infection, as I noted earlier with measles, and exposed new aggregations of deprivation and debility. At Pirbright, for example, diphtheria, which had been endemic since 1881, swept through the school and the siblings at home each time the school opened; and the epidemic declined when the school closed.[151] Since 1877 in Coggeshall, the incidence of attacks was 50 per cent greater among the 7- to 12-year-olds who were enrolled at school, than amongst the non-enrolled. Among 12- to 15-year-olds, school-attenders had an incidence of diphtheria three times that of non-attenders. At nearby Radwinter, 76 per cent of persons who suffered the first attack in a hospital were school-attenders aged between 3 and 12. In each town the disease raged worst in the seedy, more overcrowded and ill-ventilated schools in the poorer districts.[152] In the London School Board area, diphtheria deaths between ages 3 and 10 were decreasing between 1861 and 1870. The total for the decade was 4,805. Thereafter deaths increased, with a sudden jump in 1881-5, to 4,019 and another jump as regular attendance extended, to 6,870 in 1891-5. Parents did not take 'sore throat' very seriously. Mr Shirley Murphy complained that children 'commonly go to school with diphtheria if they can walk'.[153] Dr Wellington Lake, the MOH of Guildford and Woking, began in 1895 to inspect the children's tongues and throats at the beginning of each term. He excluded from attendance every suspicious case. Diphtheria did diminish, but it remained endemic: Dr Lake 'carefully cleansed . . . the tongue depressor . . . after the inspection of each child's throat . . . in a basin of hot water'. Boiling water, changed for each inspection, would, he remarked, have been 'theoretically' safer, but it was impractical.[154]

The Education Act raised the problem of children unable to pay the required fees, and who had too little food and clothing to allow them to attend. In London in 1887, 13 per cent of the enrolled children, or over 50,000, were having their fees remitted. Some School Boards, including the London one, began in the late 1870s to issue boots and clothing.[155]

Provision of school meals to 'necessitous' children began in the mid-1870s at Roosdown in Devon and in Forfar under the aegis of local philanthropists like Sir Henry Peek and Dr James Campbell. Their schemes were probably copied from the pioneering school meals system in Brussels. The children were supplied with a bowl of soup each day for ½d. or 1d. The scheme was self-supporting. Teachers were reported as testifying that the 'health . . . and afternoon staying power' of their pupils who were 'usually half-starved', had 'perceptibly improved'.[156] A similar scheme was organised by the Rev. W. Moore Ede throughout Tyneside. By 1884 he was feeding 6,000 children on each school day. Moore Ede had begun by requiring one penny from every child but had been compelled to allocate many dinners gratis. By the mid-1880s Penny Dinners were being provided in Birmingham, in Bristol and, under the sponsorship of the Charity Organization Society, in London. The COS, in particular, was keen on the penny payment 'self-supporting' 'non-demoralizing' principle.[157]

In this, the COS was unduly optimistic. The 'really deserving cases' could hardly manage ½d. and the Penny Dinner Society in Birmingham, for instance, had to come down to ¼d. in 1886.[158] School Boards and teachers everywhere, to the vexation of the COS, regularly allowed free eaters to join the queues. This cost structure did not allow room for superfluities. The Bristol dinners were mostly 'wheat puddings' and 'vegetable soup', with 'a little meat' twice a week.[159] Moore Ede's recipe for 117 dinners on a weekly 'meat day' in 1884 was:

> 1 oxhead and a half (11½ lb meat and bone)
> ham bones (1s. worth)
> pea flour (7 lb)
> rice (6 lb)
> onions (4½ lb)
> potatoes (7 lb)
> bread to go with soup (14 lb)

The whole cost 9s. 1d. He supplied the dinners and, as an indicator of the amount of water that went into the soup, he was left with 44 quarts. These he sold to the parents at ½d. per quart. On other days Moore Ede varied the menu with rhubarb pudding, rice with treacle and jam pudding. The children were allowed second helpings, presumably free.[160] The ¼d. soup in Birmingham contained meat in the form of ½ lb dripping to every 1¼ dinners, that is, every 11 gallons. Sometimes 2 lb of 'meat scraps' were added (despite the protests of the local Vegetarian Society). But the children preferred the soup 'light', that is, made only with peas and lentils. 'The very poor . . . cannot and will not eat meat; and the longer they have been on the edge of starvation, the less meat they can eat.'[161] By the winter of 1888, nearly 45,000 children at 48 London Board schools were dependent upon such meals.[162] In the following year the COS calculated from returns made by teachers that the children receiving meals constituted only half the number who 'habitually attended in want of food'.[163]

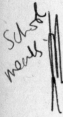

Agitation for legislation to enable municipal corporations to subsidise school meals from the rates continued through the 1890s but the 'socialistic' Education (Provision of Meals) Act of 1906 was passed only after the uproar which Gorst, Lady Warwick and their allies were able to provoke about 'National Deterioration' in 1904. By 1908 only 39 local authorities had sought and received authorisation from the Board of Education to spend money on school meals.[164] And only the London Education Committee took their opportunity seriously. They provided better-quality meals and refused to charge for them.[165] More typical was the Gateshead Council which in 1900 reluctantly levied a ½d. rate for school meals in winter. This move was fought by the town's doctors led by Dr A.P. Arnold and the former radical *Newcastle*

Daily Chronicle as 'only another step in the direction of the wholesale pauperisation of the people and the encouragement of thriftlessness'. It was less drastic than that. In December 1910, 728 children were receiving breakfast consisting of porridge, half a pint of milk and a bun. The porridge was heavily salted to discourage gluttony, the milk was the cheapest, and the buns were cheap stale ones.[166] By 1914 some doctors, at least, were agreed that school meals had not made up nutritional deficiencies.[167]

The children's preference for 'light soup' was not solely the result of their difficulties with unwonted protein and fat. Many would have been unable to masticate the meat scraps. The children's teeth were appalling. The projectors of the Dental Hospital of London in 1859 declared that a quarter of the permanent teeth of the 'lower orders' aged between 6 and 15 were 'decayed'.[168] In 1892 two dentists, Fisher and Cunningham, examined the teeth of 1,985 schoolchildren at Sutton in Surrey. They reported that only 527 had 'sound dentition'. The teeth of the poor, they explained, were 'commonly green . . . standing in irritated and receding gums'. The poor never cleaned their teeth; occasionally they picked them with a dead match.[169] The results of an inspection of 1,000 Board schoolchildren in central London were even worse; only 137 had 'sound dentition'. The examining dentists recommended over 1,300 fillings and, true to the art in the days before conservative dentistry, over 1,000 extractions, three-quarters of them 'temporary' teeth.[170] Of 729 boys in Board schools in Dunfermline in 1908, aged 7-10, only 5 per cent had 'sound teeth', and 20 per cent had up to one-fifth of their teeth 'bad'.[171] One-quarter of the recruits for the Navy during the Anglo-Boer War were rejected because of bad teeth.[172] Outside London, school dental services were almost unknown. Occasionally, as in Liverpool, conscientious teachers and doctors advised parents to take their child to a dental hospital, or even to a private dentist, but the parents ignored them and there was, as one doctor lamented, 'no follow up'.[173] In Scotland in 1909 Dr McVail reported that the poorer the locality, the poorer he found the teeth. 'Toothbrush drill', which had entered some English elementary schools, had yet to come to Scotland.[174]

The eyesight of Board schoolchildren was as defective as their teeth. In London in 1896 Dr Brudenall Carter found that 61 per cent of 8,125 children lacked 'normal vision'.[175] Among 588 Govan children in 1901, only 55 per cent had 'full vision'. Of the remainder, almost a half had 'less than half . . . vision', and nearly all of the 45 per cent 'complained of headaches and pain in the eyes on reading'. Those with

defective vision were concentrated in the lower divisions of each standard.[176] Dr Wright Thomson found that 25 per cent of children in
Glasgow charity schools in 1907 had 'functionally defective eyes', compared with 3 per cent in an 'outer middle class school'.[177] In 1914 over
4,500 among 32,000 Birmingham children were found to have 'defects
of vision', 'squints', or 'corneal ulcers, opacities etc.'. (The national
incidence of squint among children in 1965 was 3 per cent, but it was
still most common among social Class V.[178]) In those surveys which
differentiated by sex, girls had about a 33 per cent worse rate of impaired vision, possibly resulting from nutrition even more deprived than
that of the boys.[179] It would be worth investigating whether there were
markedly more girls than boys in the lower standards. The method of
testing mostly used was Snellen's 'distant types'. This was an unglazed
white card with nine lines of letters. The reader was stationed 20 feet
away.[180] Presumably, reading difficulties and anxiety worsened the
response rate among children in the lower standards; and I have found
one indication that girls were more inhibited in their answers than
boys. Octavius Sturge, physician to the Hospital for Sick Children in
the 1880s, remarked that of 18 cases of 'school anxieties' he had
treated in 1884, including fears of 'caning, examinations . . . etc.', 17
were girls.[181]

The children were not helped by the design of their schools. Complaints about the bad lighting of schoolrooms were frequent. During the
winter of 1913-14 the light was so dim in Cumberland schools that
doctors from the Board of Education could not see to test the children's
sight.[182] Teachers worsened the childrens' trials by regularly using blue
chalk on the blackboard. Sewing classes proceeded inexorably, 'even on
the darkest days'.[183]

The hearing of many children, especially those in the lower standards, was defective too. Their hearing was tested by holding a 'loud
ticking watch' near one ear, while the investigator blocked the other
with the palm of his hand, and the child kept her eyes closed, as
ordered. The questions were whispered: 'rabbit' or 'robber', 'snake' or
'sneak'. Doctors found it 'hard to get answers'. As Dr McVail explained,
the children were 'stupid' and 'the cause was wax'.[184] Forty per cent of
elementary schoolchildren in Scotland were alleged to have been
reported as showing 'defective hearing' in 1903-4.[185]

Some national deteriorationist-eugenist doctors built the association between poor eyesight, bad hearing and slow learning into an
axiomatic explanation. In Glasgow in 1909, for example, Dr Hugh
Wright Thomson examined 52,000 Board schoolchildren. He found

that 35 per cent had defective vision, one-half of which, and here the great physician Sir Thomas Oliver quoted him authoritatively, ' "was due to mental deficiency aggravated by malnutrition" '.[186]

The sheer amount of bodily infirmity in the common schools alarmed medical contemporaries, and drove them to make even larger, ever more gloomy — and self-fulfilling — investigations. Their criteria of defectiveness remained vague and all-embracing; the incidence of various defects was reported to vary enormously between towns, and doctors. None the less, the reported total amount of defectiveness remained appalling by present standards. In 1890 Dr Francis Warner led an investigation under the auspices of the COS of 50,000 London Elementary and Poor Law schoolchildren.

In Stockport in 1909 the MOH inspected nearly 4,000 children, equally divided between the sexes. His object was to weed 'out the . . . feeble minded degenerates' to protect them from 'being injured and being an injury to the community'. Eight per cent had 'bad teeth'. Another 2,340 or 59 per cent were 'notified for various defects': nearly 600 for 'dirty heads', 800 for 'mouth breathing', 300 for 'heart diseases and anaemia', and 125 'totally excluded from school', including 18 with 'discharging ears', 65 with 'ringworm and skin diseases', 10 with 'chest troubles', 5 'glands in neck', 14 'eye diseases', 12 'infectious diseases', and 1 'tubercle'.[187] This was a fair cross-sample. In two much larger communities, Manchester and Birmingham, in 1912 and 1913, the doctors found 'many thousand cases of skin disease', a 1 per cent rate of 'anaemia', a 5 per cent rate of 'malnutrition', 0.5 per cent of 'defective hearing', and 16 per cent of the total with 'enlarged tonsils,

Table 3.15: Warner's 1890 Study of 50,000 Elementary and Poor Law Schoolchildren

'Feeble-minded or mentally exceptional'	234
'Epileptic, or a history of fits during school life'	54
'Crippled, maimed, deformed'	239
'Cases presenting bodily defects of various degrees of importance'	5,851
'Cases presenting some defective action or ill-balance of parts of the body, indicating deviations from the normal nerve-state'	5,487
'Children pale, delicate or thin'	2,003
'Eye cases (squint, not opthalmic)'	1,473
'Children that appear to require special care'	817

Source: Helen Bosanquet, *Social Work in London, 1869-1912* (1914, reprinted Brighton, 1973), p. 198.

adenoids, or glands'.[188]

Upper-class children suffered from poor eyesight and headaches, too. But the incidence was much smaller than among their Board school peers. Mr Buxton used Snellen's types and the 'astigmatism fan' to test the sight of 2,493 boys 'in the upper and middle classes in grammar and private schools and [in] private practice'. Over 63 per cent registered a perfect pair of 6/6's, and another 12 per cent were 'good'. Another 7.5 per cent were fair '6/9 both', while 5.0 per cent were 'bad' at 'under 6/9' and 12 per cent 'very bad' at 'minus 6/12'.[189] These grammar-school boys had spectacles prescribed for them: the 1890s was the decade of the spread of middle-class children's glasses and the emergence of the bespectacled swot. Board schoolchildren whose sight and hearing were found to be defective were also recommended for spectacles, ear washes and dental care. But their parents had to turn to private practi-tioners for them, so few working-class children received them. More-over, Board schoolchildren, unlike upper-class schoolchildren, were usually tested only with the Snellen chart. This measured only myopia or long-sightedness and not astigmatism. This means that the figures for sight defects among working-class children are understated, as com-pared with their grammar-school peers; and probably their defects, as the result of years of neglect and debility, were worse.[190] None the less, upper-class children with ear trouble did not fare much better under treatment. In the 1890s the standard procedure was, in 'catarrhal cases', to 'breathe into the ear', and in severe cases, the doctor applied 'blister-ing fluid, leeches and incisions' together with a mixture of 'atropine, morphine and cocaine' ladled into the ear.[191] Private schools also began to check their pupils' health on admission and, especially girls' schools, to reject unfit applicants. 'Swedish' exercises became fashionable in private schools from about 1891. Edwin Chadwick, that visionary authoritarian, had been advocating compulsory 'drill' in factory schools since 1861. His ambition was to transform callisthenics from being a mere therapeutic ancillary (as it had been since at least the 1840s) into a mechanism for improving the nation. Medical spokesmen first called for military-type drill in schools, conducted by Guards' officers, in 1870.[192]

These procedures developed partly out of concern about 'over-pressure', which had arisen in the 1880s. 'Educational fanatics', prop-onents of competitive examinations and book-learning to the exclusion of sport, had captured the private schools and were destroying the manhood and womanhood upon which the future of the Empire depended. Dr J. Martin told the BMA meeting at Cardiff in 1885:

Children had to pore over their lessons until ten, one and twelve at night. Next morning the child could not eat its breakfast, and there followed headaches, vomiting, nervous debility, brain fever, St Vitus's dance, curvature of the spine, heart disease, myopia, and in some cases convulsions and death.

In Germany, Martin added, where the fanatics had also triumphed, '30-40 per cent of girls had curvature of the spine'.[193] Solitary, sedentary reading also led to solitary vice, the Rev. R. Ashington Bullen, a school chaplain, warned in 1886. And solitary vice, with its concomitant excitement of the nervous system, led to insanity. The indisputable increase in lunacy and immorality in the nation was the direct result of 'the system of competitive examinations'.[194]

'Brain pressure' affected elementary schoolchildren less, the COS explained, because they were less academically ambitious or, as Dr Octavius Sturge explained, they and their parents were 'less careful and observant and more happy-go-lucky than the rest of us'.[195] But equally, the COS reformers argued, 'any work' was 'more or less burdensome' to ill-cared-for, ill-nourished, ill-clad children whose overcrowded, undisciplined and noisy households allowed them insufficient sleep. In 1899 nearly all of the 20,000 Board schools in England and Wales made returns on the numbers of their pupils in employment. Of their two million or so pupils, 144,000 'full timers', comprising 110,000 boys and 34,000 girls, worked (see Table 3.16).

Most boys worked in shops — over 76,000 of them; 19,000 did 'odd jobs as messengers etc.'; 15,000 sold newspapers; and 6,000 were in 'agriculture'. The girls were generally employed in laundry work, basket-making and minding babies. Among the exceptional cases was a boy

Table 3.16: Board Schoolchildren in Employment, England and Wales, 1899

Hours Worked per Week	No. of Children
10-20	6,268
20-30	27,000
30-40	9,778
40-50	2,390
Over 50	750

Source: *Lancet*, 13 May 1899, p. 1309.

who was an undertaker's assistant, who got 1s. a week for measuring corpses. One boy aged six peeled onions for 20 hours every week; he got 8d. Another six-year-old delivered milk for 21 hours for 2s. A boy of 10 worked 72 hours as a farm labourer for 3s.; a 12-year-old spent 78 hours each week in a druggist's shop for 5s.; and one greengrocer's assistant aged 12 started at 2.30 a.m. six days every week, and went for his day's schooling at 9.30. A 'nurse-girl' of five spent 29 hours on the job for 2d. and food.[196]

The children's home life would hardly have allowed them the sleep necessary to help them through their school and work hours. Over-crowded dwellings, two or three siblings to a bed, the prevalence of itchy skin and noisy respiratory infections all contributed to broken sleep and listless, exhausted waking hours. In 1908 Alice Ravenhill published the results of a survey (among teachers?) of reported hours of sleep among English elementary schoolchildren (see Table 3.17).

The agitation for rate-supported school medical inspection and care began in the late 1870s but failed before the lethargy of the Local Government Board, the opposition of ratepayers, the doctors and the COS. The three latter argued that school clinics would only be pallia-tive and that the real way to national health lay through leading 'indo-lent, incompetent mothers' to adopt 'total care'. This involved finding one's self-respect through the independence created by work and cleaning up, under supervision.[197]

Inspection was only worth while if it remained under professional medical control, distinct from, but ancillary to, the state and state purposes. Only doctors could determine the defects in sight, hearing and physique that marked out the mentally deficient and thereby rendered them incapable of 'becoming . . . normal citizens'. When the Psychological Committee of the BMA reported in 1889 on a survey of elementary, industrial and district pauper schools, the members lumped together as social deficients cases with 'signs of . . . nerve weakness or defect', apparent 'defective . . . nutrition', 'mental dulness', 'cranial abnormalities' and 'disease or defect of eyes'. It was to support crea-tures such as these that the middle classes were, as one academic eugenist complained, being 'taxed out of existence'.[198] The medical profession knew, better than any set of laymen, the disabilities in child-ren produced by the unhealthy conditions under which the poor lived and the 'reckless early marriages' encouraged by 'charity'. Better than any other group, the medical profession could advise the state on the introduction of legal bans to early and reckless marriage and, as Dr C.N. Gwynne put it, 'the imposing of other restraints that might be deemed

Table 3.17: Hours of Sleep among English Elementary Schoolchildren

Age	Standard Hours (according to Alice Ravenhill — middle-class routine hours?)	Average of 6,180 Returns from Elementary Schools
3–5	14.00	10.90
6	13.75	10.60
7	13.00	10.50
8	12.50	9.90
9	12.00	9.50
10	11.50	9.40
11	11.50	9.25
12	11.00	8.90
13	10.75	8.00

Sources: *Child-Study*, vol. I (1908), p. 119; Dr Rees to Physical Deterioration Committee, *PP*, 1904, vol. IX, Q.4418.

advisable'.[199] The growth of state power, epitomised in medical inspection of elementary schoolchildren, enabled the doctors in the latter part of the century to progress from seeking to control the sick person and his family ambience to claiming to set standards for the whole society.

The threatening social implication of the profession's claims to improve the environment, whether thoroughgoing authoritarianism or thoroughgoing redistribution, or both, had to be, and were, implicitly curbed and obscured by the profession's counter-assertions about the class-specific nature of defective nutrition, 'nerve weakness' and poor eyesight, and their fundamental origins in moral incapacity. Throughout the nineteenth century, but more especially during the decades around the turn of the twentieth century, environmental factors, mechanistic-fundamentalist explanations and assumptions about heredity in classes and individuals were inextricably mingled in medico-political discussions.

When the London Education Committee moved to avail itself of the provision in the Educational (Administrative Provisions) Act of 1907 to establish school clinics, the COS and the doctors were outraged. School clinics 'would take employment from local general practitioners'. If clinics had to come, let every local doctor participate in them and have his share of the rates.[200] The proponent of school clinics, Rev. Stewart Headlam, argued that the abolition of waiting time would mean that more children would be inspected and treated. The overall cost of hospital treatment, when the parents had the time to take the child, worked out at 5*s*. 8*d*. per head. Headlam claimed that 12 clinics could handle 131,000 children for £20,000, or about 4*s*. a head. The BMA condemned the scheme and forbade its members to join.[201] The Education Committee had proposed to operate its clinics as adjuncts to the big teaching hospitals, paying the hospitals for their services. Charing Cross undertook to treat 1,000 cases of 'refraction', 300 'skin cases', and 1,000 'throat and ear' cases a year. The London said they were willing to treat 15 aural and 15 opthalmic cases on four days each week. Spokesmen for the other hospitals said they had to 'protect the general practitioners'. Four other specialist hospitals offered to help. Altogether, the Education Committee found that it could place 460 new cases each week, or 20,000 each medical year. Then the Committee discovered that the participating hospitals intended to reject any supervision or audit from the Education Committee's doctors or officials. This implied that the hospitals planned to turn the students loose on the clinic children. The scheme was dropped.[202] By 1914 some clinics, especially opthalmic services, were operating in the provincial cities.[203] But a great chance to launch an integral school health service was lost. The move would have improved medical education, too. In 1900 there was teaching in paediatrics in only three hospitals in Britain. In one leading medical school, Glasgow, attendance at lectures and clinical instruction in diseases of childhood did not become compulsory until 1914.[204]

The fact that, relatively, so many children survived infancy to school age and to enter working life proves their fortunate genetic endowment; and it raises major questions about human genetics and population dynamics in history which I am incompetent to discuss. That reparable disabilities of sight, hearing and skin infections among the survivors were permitted to go untreated because of selfish professionalism illustrates how easily such professionals can disserve individual potentialities and vitiate natural communal advantages.

Notes

    1. Charles Creighton, *A History of Epidemics in Britain* (London [1891-4]), vol. II, pp.726-7; Henry Ashby, 'Some Points In The Pathology of Scarlet Fever', *Medical Chronicle,* vol. III (Oct. 1885 – Mar. 1886), p. 183; Hugh R. Jones, 'The Perils . . .', *JRSS*, vol. LVII, p. 11; Benjamin W. Richardson, *Clinical Essays* (London, 1862), p. 56.
    2. Richard J. Reece, 'Scarlet Fever: Also Called Scarlatina', *West London Medical Journal,* vol. IX (1904), pp. 263-8.
    3. *PP*, 1916, vol. V, p. 60; *PP*, 1914-16, vol. XI, pp. cviii-cix; Creighton, *Epidemics,* vol. II, p. 727.

4. *L*, 6 Feb. 1864, p. 163.

5. C.E. Prior, 'A Contribution to the History of Scarlatina', *L*, 23 Oct. 1869, p. 570.

6. *BMJ*, 11 Dec. 1858, pp. 1034-5.

7. *St Andrews Medical Graduates' Transactions* (1870), p. 45; R. Thorne Thorne, *The Progress of Preventive Medicine during the Victorian Era* (1888), pp. 30-3; B. Lumley in *L*, 20 May 1882, p. 854.

8. 'The Outbreak of Scarlet Fever at Castlehead Paisley', *GMJ*, vol. XXIII (1885), pp. 278-81.

9. William Buchan, *Domestic Medicine*, 1769 ed., p. 291; cf. 'Remarks on the Angina and Scarlet Fever of 1778', in *Memoirs of the Medical Society of London*, vol. III (1792), pp. 356-7.

10. Edward Blackmore, 'An Illustration of a Fatal Species of Scarlatina Lately prevalent at Plymouth', *Medical Gazette*, 24 Apr. 1830, pp. 114-15; Henry Daly, in *Medical Times & Gazette*, 3 Mar. 1855, p. 218; Report of BMA discussion of scarlet fever in *L*, 21 Aug. 1886, p. 350.

11. Creighton, *Epidemics*, vol. II, p. 730.

12. Charles Murchison, 'Scarlet Fever', *L*, 25 June 1864, p. 725.

13. *Edinburgh Medical and Surgical Journal*, vol. XLVI (1836), p. 371.

14. *L*, 20 Aug. 1892, p. 439.

15. O. Phelps Brown, *The Complete Herbalist or the People Their Own Physicians* (London, 1867), p. 209.

16. *L*, 20 Nov. 1875, p. 746.

17. *BMJ*, 20 Mar. 1880, p. 459.

18. Arthur Newsholme, 'A National System of . . . Registration of Sickness', *JRSS*, vol. LIX (1896), p. 2.

19. David Pride, 'Notes of a Scarlet Fever Epidemic', *GMJ*, vol. I (1869), pp. 440-1.

20. *L*, 8 Sept. 1894, p. 567.

21. *L*, 6, 13 Apr. 1867, pp. 424, 467 (for outbreaks at Eton and Harrow); 13 Nov. 1875, p. 712; *Medical Times & Gazette*, 11 Mar. 1882, p. 265.

22. *L*, 19 Jan. 1895, p. 171.

23. *L*, 26 Apr. 1884, p. 773.

24. *L*, 30 Oct. 1886, p. 841.

25. *Truth*, 5 Dec. 1895, pp. 1395-6.

26. Creighton, *Epidemics*, vol. II, pp. 650-1.

27. William Henry in *Medico-Chirurgical Transactions*, vol. IV (1814), pp. 442-4.

28. Alan D. Berg, *The Nutrition Factor; its role in national development* (Washington, D.C., 1973), p. 4; Barbara Gastel, 'Measles: A Potentially Finite History', *Journal of the History of Medicine and Allied Sciences*, vol. XXVIII (1973), p. 35.

29. Sir Gilbert Blane, *Medico-Chirurgical Transactions*, vol. IV (1813), pp. 466-72.

30. *Medical and Physical Journal*, vol. XXXIII (1816), pp. 419-20.

31. *L*, 27 Sept. 1862, p. 349.

32. P. Macgregor, *Medico-Chirurgical Transactions*, vol. V (1814), pp. 437-41.

33. Dr Ferguson, 'On the Epidemic Measles of 1808', *Medical and Physical Journal*, vol. XXI (1809), pp. 364-6; James Foulis Duncan in *Dublin Journal of Medical Science*, vol. XXII (1843), pp. 29-31; John Webster, *London Journal of Medicine*, vol. 2 (1849), p. 1064; 'Measles Epidemic in Pottery Towns', *L*, 26 Jan. 1889, p. 192.

34. *L*, 22 Feb. 1840, p. 786.

35. *L*, 26 Jan. 1889, p. 191.

36. *L*, 8 Dec. 1888, p. 1143, 17 July 1909, p. 160.

37. 'Epidemic of Measles in Glasgow', *GMJ*, vol. XXXI (1889), pp. 277-8.

38. *L*, 19 Feb. 1887, p. 387, 14 May 1887, p. 1001.

39. James Miller, *BMJ*, 21 Dec. 1907, pp. 1772-3.

40. Robert Hunter Semple, 'On Diphtheria, And the Diseases Allied to it, which may be mistaken for it', *St Andrews Medical Graduates' Association Transactions* (1870), p. 199; Farr, *Vital Statistics* (London, 1885), p. 323.

41. *L*, 27 Feb. 1830, pp. 734-5.

42. Creighton, *Epidemics*, vol. II, pp. 740-1.

43. *St Andrews Medical Graduates' Association Transactions* (1870), p. 199.

44. *L*, 14 July 1894, p. 89.

45. D. Biddle, *L*, 14 July 1894, p. 108.

46. *St Andrews Medical Graduates' Association Transactions* (1871), p. 105.

47. *Transactions of the Clinical Society of London*, vol. XXV (1892), pp. 39-40; *L*, 15 May 1875, p. 703; Thorne Thorne, *L*, 14 Mar. 1891, p. 587, and *Progress*, p. 45. Dr J.B. Russell also argued that the high mortality in 'better-class houses' resulted from their possessing internal sewerage systems, which worked badly (*L*, 1 June 1878, p. 805).

48. *L*, 8 Feb. 1862, p. 164.

49. *L*, 29 Dec. 1894, p. 1537.

50. Richard T. Hewlett, *L*, 14 Apr. 1900, p. 1093, 19 July 1902, p. 178.

51. *L*, 8 Oct. 1892, p. 855.

52. *Transactions of the Clinical Society of London*, vol. XXVIII (1895), pp. 68-9.

53. *St Bartholomew's Hospital Reports*, vol. XXVII (1891), pp. 262, 279.

54. *L*, 30 Mar. 1850, p. 389.

55. *L*, 22 Mar. 1851, p. 331; Lomax, 'Opiates', *Bulletin of the History of Medicine*, vol. XLVII (1973), p. 172.

56. *L*, 16 Oct. 1869, pp. 553-4; Thomas Archer, *The Terrible Sights of London and Labours of Love in the midst of them* (London, n.d. [? 1870]), pp. 76-8.

57. *L*, 2 and 9 Oct. 1869, pp. 484, 513, 530.

58. Archer, *Terrible Sights*, pp. 83-6.

59. Edna Robertson, *The Yorkhill Story: the History of the Royal Hospital for Sick Children, Glasgow* (Glasgow, 1972), p. 66.

60. *L*, 12 Dec. 1896, p. 1710.

61. Archer, *Terrible Sights*, pp. 62-73; *Truth*, 19 Dec. 1895, p. 1506; V.A.J. Swan, 'The East London Hospital for Children', *Medical History*, vol. VIII (1964), p. 136.

62. *Medical and Physical Journal*, vol. VII (1802), p. 487; Creighton, *Epidemics*, vol. II, p. 615; Report of RC on Smallpox And Fever Hospitals, *PP*, 1882, vol. XXIX, pp. vii, 320.

63. *PP*, 1896, vol. VII, Royal Commission on Vaccination, p. 632.

64. *L*, 6 Jan. 1872; Creighton, *Epidemics*, vol. II, p. 616.

65. Creighton, *Epidemics*, vol. II, pp. 571-2, 622; B.A. Whitelegge in *L*, 4 Mar. 1893, p. 458; *L*, 11 Feb. 1871, p. 206.

66. John Savory, *A Companion to the Medicine Chest, and Compendium of Domestic Medicine* (1840), p. 237; George Hilaro Barlow, *A Manual of the Practice of Medicine*, second ed. (London, 1869), pp. 670-1.

67. John Cross, 'A History of the Variolous Epidemic . . . in Norwich', *Edinburgh Medical and Surgical Journal*, vol. XVII (1821), pp. 116-17; Creighton, *Epidemics*, vol. II, p. 577.

68. Buchan, *Domestic Medicine*, 1769 ed., p. 256; *L*, 20 Apr. 1839, p. 173.

69. *L*, 27 June 1840, p. 504.

70. *L*, 30 Apr. 1859, p. 447.

71. SC on Medical Poor Relief, *PP*, 1844, vol. IX, Q.9144; for similar com-

ments on the poor of Dublin, see Dr Speer in *Dublin Hospital Reports*, vol. III, p. 195.

72. *Medical and Physical Journal*, vol. XXVI (1811), p. 509.

73. *Medical and Physical Journal*, vol. XIV (1805), p. 279.

74. *British Annals of Medicine*, 10 Feb. 1837, pp. 194-5.

75. *L*, 30 May 1840, pp. 338-9.

76. 'Memorial of Medical Committee, Norwich', *Medical and Physical Journal*, vol. XIV (1805), p. 279.

77. *BMJ*, 11 Dec. 1858, pp. 1034-5.

78. *London Medical and Physical Journal*, vol. XLIV (1820), p. 534.

79. [Robert Gooch], 'Vaccination', *Quarterly Review*, vol. XXXIII (Mar. 1826), p. 550; *L*, 28 July 1827, p. 558, 17 Apr. 1852, p. 391.

80. *L*, 25 Apr. 1840, p. 164; *Once a Week*, 4 July 1863, p. 36; Ann Beck, 'Issues on the Anti-Vaccination Movement in England', *Medical History*, vol. IV (1960), p. 311.

81. *L*, 30 May 1840, pp. 340-1.

82. *L*, 9 May 1840, pp. 235-6.

83. *L*, 3 Oct. 1840, p. 70 (Stockport), 12 Dec. 1840, p. 424 (Battle), 8 May 1841, pp. 237-8 (Blackburn), 15 Aug. 1840, p. 754 (St Pancras), 19 Sept. 1840, p. 941 (St Columb). There were other open clashes at Clutton, in Somerset, Dover and elsewhere. The wrangle continued throughout the century. See, for example, *L*, 20 Jan. 1900, p. 177 (Wigan) and 12 July 1902 (St Germans).

84. W.H. de Lannoy, 'Small-Pox at Dover', *L*, 25 Oct. 1834, p. 177.

85. Ralph H. Major, 'Think Before You Vaccinate: An Item of Historical Interest' (actually written by Rev. George Cardew), *Journal of the History of Medicine*, vol. VI (1951), pp. 125-6.

86. *L*, 30 May 1840, p. 339.

87. Edward Crickmay, Laxfield (Suffolk), *BMJ*, 25 Sept. 1880, p. 534; *L*, 28 Aug. 1852, p. 208.

88. Archibald Pearson, 'Twenty-one Years' Experience of Vaccination', *GMJ*, vol. XXII (1884), p. 200.

89. *L*, 10 Apr. 1830, p. 45; L.J. Spencer, 'Smallpox', *Encyclopaedia Britannica* (fourteenth ed.), 1924.

90. *L*, 10 July 1852, p. 40.

91. *L*, 28 Apr. 1900, p. 1236.

92. *Once a Week*, 4 July 1863, p. 36; A.J. Pepper in *L*, 11 Sept. 1909, p. 767.

93. *GMJ*, vol. XXII (1884), p. 200; see also Sir Benjamin Ward Richardson, *Vita Medica: Chapters of Medical Life and Work* (London, 1897), p. 15.

94. *L*, 17 Dec. 1859, pp. 627-8; *BMJ*, 12 July 1884, p. 71.

95. *L*, 26 Nov. 1859, p. 548, 9 Feb. 1889, p. 391, 13 Feb. 1889, p. 749.

96. *L*, 5 June 1858, p. 559; *Once a Week*, 4 July 1863, p. 38.

97. *L*, 3 Dec. 1853, p. 531.

98. *L*, 8 Aug. 1896, p. 401.

99. *L*, 10 Apr. 1830, p. 45.

100. Thorne Thorne, *Progress*, p. 9.

101. *L*, 8 Jan. 1870, p. 55.

102. B. Gandevia, 'Some physical characteristics, including pock marks, tattoos and disabilities of convict boys transported to Australia from Britain c. 1840', *Australian Paediatrics Journal*, vol. I (1976), p. 10.

103. *L*, 18 Oct. 1862, p. 416; *BMJ*, 23 Jan. 1869, p. 79.

104. *L*, 6 Sept. 1902, p. 695; *Transactions of the Epidemiological Society of London for 1855*, p. 8.

105. *L*, 7 May 1864, p. 539.

106. *L*, 1 May 1858, p. 441; cf. Herbert Barker in *Journal of Public Health and*

Sanitary Review, vol. I (1858), p. 69.

107. Major, 'Think Before You Vaccinate', pp. 125-6.

108. *L*, 24 June 1871, p. 863.

109. Mrs Hume-Rothery, *Women and Doctors or Medical Despotism in England* (London, n.d.) (c. 1871), pp. 2-5.

110. Herbert Preston-Thomas, *The Work and Play of a Government Inspector* (London, 1909), p. 170; George Howell, Diary, 19 Jan. 1877, Howell Collection Bishopsgate Institute. Other Liberal-radical opponents of the Vaccination Acts included: Thomas Burt, John Bright, C.H. Hopwood and P.A. Taylor. *Newcastle Daily Chronicle*, 29 Dec. 1880, 30 Sept. 1887, 15 Oct. 1897.

111. *L*, 13 May 1871, pp. 649-52.

112. *L*, 2 Nov. 1872, p. 659.

113. *L*, 8, 29 Jan. 1870, p. 55 (Northampton), 2 Feb. 1889, p. 335 (Kettering); Ian Dewherst, *Gleanings from Victorian Yorkshire* (Driffield, 1972), pp. 87-90 (Keighley); *Newcastle Daily Chronicle*, 24, 28 Dec. 1880. For a general discussion of 'anti-statism', see Henry Pelling, *Popular Politics and Society in Late Victorian Britain* (London, 1968), esp. Chapter I.

114. *L*, 8 Oct. 1898, p. 960, 22 Sept. 1888, p. 585.

115. *L*, 12 July 1902, p. 126. This cast of mind was also strong among certain aristocratic opponents of vaccination, Lords Dysart and Clifton, for instance. Cf. Dysart, in *Newcastle Weekly Chronicle*, 30 Apr. 1887, and James Stansfeld to W.E. Gladstone, 3 May 1886, complaining about Clifton. Gladstone Papers, B.L. 44497 f. 97.

116. *BMJ*, 19 June 1880, p. 910.

117. *Medical Chronicle*, vol. XVIII (1893), pp. 152-3.

118. *L*, 4 May 1895, p. 1140.

119. *Saint Thomas's Hospital Reports*, vol. XXV (1897), pp. 66-8.

120. *L*, 6 Sept. 1902, p. 695.

121. J.C. McDonald, *'The* History of Quarantine in Britain During the 19th Century', *Bulletin of the History of Medicine*, vol. 25 (1951); William Hanna, *Studies In Small-Pox And Vaccination* (Bristol, 1913), pp. 7-10.

122. Calculated from statistics in B.R. Mitchell and Phyllis Deane, *Abstract of British Historical Statistics*, (Cambridge, 1962), pp. 12-13 and Geoffrey Best, *Mid-Victorian Britain 1851-1875* (New York, 1972), pp. 112-13.

123. *Edinburgh Medical and Surgical Journal*, vol. V (1809), pp. 197-8.

124. See evidence of Thomas Adams and Emma Frost, 'Lace-finishing', Children's Employment Commission, *PP*, 1863, vol. XVIII, pp. 93, 193.

125. *Edinburgh Medical and Surgical Journal*, vol. XLIV (1835), p. 428; *Medical Chronicle*, vol. LX (1914-15), p. 148.

126. Children's Employment Commission, *PP*, 1863, vol. XVIII, pp. 16-18.

127. Gandevia, 'Physical Characteristics', pp. 3, 49.

128. 'Factory Inspectors' Reports', *PP*, 1846, vol. XX, pp. 5, 20; *PP*, 1852-3, vol. XL, pp. 48, 55.

129. Children's Employment Commission, *PP*, 1864, vol. XXII, p. 147.

130. Ibid., Q.683.

131. 'Factories Inspectors' Reports', *PP*, 1868-9, vol. XIV, pp. 16-17. See also Oliver MacDonagh, *Early Victorian Government* (London, 1977), Chapter 4.

132. Children's Employment Commission, *PP*, 1867, vol. XVI, Qs. 128-34, 181.

133. Pamela Horn, *The Victorian Country Child* (Kineton, 1974), pp. 168-9.

134. *L*, 4 Mar. 1871, p. 31.

135. *L*, 18 Mar. 1871, p. 391.

136. *L*, 14 Dec. 1872, p. 860.

137. *L*, 14 Feb. 1885, p. 310.

138. *L*, 26 Jan. 1895, p. 247.

139. *Truth*, 21 Nov. 1895, pp. 1266-7, 5 Dec. 1895, p. 1381, 26 Dec. 1895, p. 1588.

140. *Truth*, 20 June 1895, p. 1507 (Selby); *L*, 23 Apr. 1870, p. 597 (Stamford); *L*, 19 Jan. 1889, p. 140 (New Jerusalem); 3 June 1882, p. 927 (King's Norton); *Truth*, 19 Sept. 1895, p. 670 (Tamworth); *L*, 27 Aug. 1898 (Bettws-y-Coed). The astonishing account of the Latimer Cottages in Suffolk, the site of 'The Last Epidemic of Plague in England 1906-1918', as described by David van Zwanchberg, shows that living conditions in some small isolated villages had scarcely changed since the seventeenth century (*Medical History*, vol. XIV (1970), p. 72).

141. Horn, *Victorian Country Child*, pp. 173-9.

142. E.H. Phelps Brown, *The Growth of British Industrial Relations* (London, 1959), pp. 52-4.

143. James Harrison, *Edinburgh Medical and Surgical Journal*, vol. XLIV (1835), pp. 425-6.

144. B. Gandevia, 'A Comparison of the Heights of Boys Transported to Australia from England, Scotland and Ireland, c. 1840', unpublished distributed paper, 1975, Table I.

145. Physical Deterioration Committee, *PP*, 1904, vol. XXXII, p. 3.

146. *L*, 21 Aug. 1875, pp. 274-5. See also Charles Roberts, 'The Physical Requirements of Factory Children, *JSS*, vol. XXXIX (1876), pp. 684-98.

147. *PP*, 1904, vol. XXXII, Appendix IXA, p. 19.

148. Ibid., Q.4446.

149. *L*, 17 Jan. 1914, p. 206; see also on this point, A.A. Mumford, 'Medical Inspection', *Medical Chronicle*, vol. LVII (1913), p. 67.

150. S. Davidson and R. Passmore, *Human Nutrition and Dietetics* (Edinburgh, 1973), pp. 690-1; Alfred A. Mumford, 'Imperfections in Physical Growth as Hindrances to Social Development', *Child-Study*, vol. 3 (1910), p. 93.

151. *L*, 7 July 1883, p. 21.

152. Thorne Thorne, *Progress*, p. 42; *L*, 7 Mar. 1891, p. 59.

153. *L*, 21 Jan. 1899, p. 184.

154. *L*, 20 Aug. 1895, p. 1000-1.

155. Helen Bosanquet, *Social Work in London 1869-1912* (1914, reprinted Brighton, 1973), pp. 231, 237; Gillian Sutherland, *Elementary Education in the Nineteenth Century* (London, 1971), p. 38; *L*, 10 Jan. 1885, p. 76, 26 Jan. 1895, p. 234.

156. *L*, 15 Dec. 1883, p. 1067, 31 Jan. 1885, p. 233.

157. Helen Bosanquet, *Social Work*, pp. 244-5; F.W.D. Manders, *A History of Gateshead* (Gateshead, 1977), pp. 204-5.

158. *Truth*, 2 Apr. 1885, p. 525.

159. *L*, 19 Apr. 1884, pp. 71-2.

160. *L*, 7 June 1884, p. 1052.

161. *BMJ*, 28 Jan. 1888, p. 214.

162. *BMJ*, 23 Nov. 1888, pp. 1170-1.

163. Helen Bosanquet, *Social Work*, pp. 250-1.

164. *BMJ*, 4 Apr. 1908, p. 831, cf. Dr Eichholz at Physical Deterioration Committee, *PP*, 1904, vol. XXXII, p. 478; Bentley Gilbert, 'Health and Politics', *Bulletin of the History of Medicine*, vol. 39 (1965), pp. 152-3.

165. *L*, 27 Nov., p. 1640; 18 Dec. 1909, p. 1843.

166. Manders, *Gateshead*, pp. 204-5.

167. *L*, 24 Jan. 1914, p. 263.

168. Richards in F.N.L. Poynter (ed.), *Medicine and Science in the 1860s* (London, 1966), pp. 281-2.

169. *L*, 17 Sept. 1892, p. 677.

170. *BMJ*, 26 Mar. 1892, p. 676.

171. *BMJ*, 28 Mar. 1908, p. 755.

172. *L*, 17 Mar. 1900, p. 814.

173. *BMJ*, 11 Dec. 1877, p. 1754.

174. *GMJ*, vol. LXXII (1909), p. 186.

175. *L*, 25 July 1896, p. 254.

176. *L*, 17 Aug. 1901, p. 492.

177. *BMJ*, 14 Sept. 1907, p. 628.

178. *L*, 9 May 1914, p. 1352; R. Davie, N. Butler, H. Goldstein, *From Birth To Seven* (London, 1972), p. 90.

179. *L*, 27 Dec. 1902, p. 1770.

180. Dr McVail in *GMJ*, vol. LXXII (1909), p. 183.

181. Octavius Sturge, 'School Work and Discipline As a Factor In Chorea', *L*, 3 Jan. 1885, p. 9.

182. 'Annual Report of Chief Medical Officer of Board of Education', *L*, 7 Mar. 1914, p. 701.

183. Sir John Gorst to Physical Deterioration Committee, *PP*, 1904, vol. XIV Q.11872; Dr E.W. Hope, *L*, 4 Jan. 1914, p. 263.

184. *GMJ*, vol. LXXII (1909), pp. 184-5.

185. Sir John Gorst to Physical Deterioration Committee, *PP*, 1904, vol. IX, Q.11872.

186. *L*, 25 Sept. 1909, p. 907.

187. *L*, 23 Oct. 1909, p. 1247.

188. *L*, 28 Feb. 1914. p. 638; 9 May 1914, p. 1352.

189. *L*, 27 Apr. 1895, p. 1048.

190. *BMJ*, 20 Jan. 1894, pp. 151-2; T. Jefferson Faulder in *L*, 2 July 1910, p. 21-3; E.W. Hope in *L*, 24 Jan. 1914, p. 263.

191. Dr Atkin, at Sheffield Medico-Chirurgical Society, *BMJ*, 11 Nov. 1893, p. 1052.

192. *BMJ*, 24 Feb. 1894, p. 438; *GMJ*, vol. XXXVIII (1892), p. 44; *L*, 7 Sept. 1861, p. 234, 10 Oct. 1840, p. 86, 5 Nov. 1870, p. 650.

193. *Truth*, 6 Aug. 1885, p. 208.

194. Rev. R. Ashington Bullen, *Our Duty As Teachers* (London, 1886), p. 14.

195. Bosanquet, *Social Work*, pp. 243-4; *L*, 3 Jan. 1885, p. 9.

196. *L*, 13 May 1899, p. 1309.

197. *Medical Times and Gazette*, 4 Jan. 1879, p. 14; *L*, 4 Feb. 1899, p. 330; Bosanquet, *Social Work*, p. 257.

198. Mumford, *Medical Chronicle*, vol. LVII (1913), pp. 66-7; *GMJ*, vol. XXXII (1889). p. 206; Ferdinand C.S. Schiller, *Eugenics & Politics* (London, 1926), pp.13-19.

199. C.N. Gwynne, Presidential Address at Sheffield Medico-Chirurgical Society, *BMJ*, 19 Oct. 1889, p. 877.

200. Bosanquet, *Social Work*, p. 263.

201. *L*, 4 Dec. 1909, pp. 1699-1700.

202. *L*, 31 July 1909, pp. 313-14.

203. *L*, 24 Jan. 1914, p. 263.

204. Robertson, *Yorkhill Story*, pp. 34, 101.

4 ADULTS

In this and the following chapter I raise questions about particular maladies — tuberculosis and heart disease, for example — and about institutional developments in the Poor Law system, the hospitals and the medical profession, which ramify beyond 'adults' and 'the old'. I had not intended to stray beyond the fences but the evidence proved unexpectedly massive and multifarious. There is also a larger reason which I have pursued from the outset, namely, that the social history of health and ill health must consider the interactions between patients and doctors, the chronology and geography of innovation and resistance, and the differing impact of illness and medical procedures upon sick people in various social classes. Seen from this standpoint, seemingly disparate elements — the behaviour of wealthy valetudinarians, the rise of the medical profession and the financial crisis in the hospitals — emerge as interlinked forces and I have tried to convey, perhaps at too great length, this fundamental cohesion.

1. DIRT AND DISEASE

Towards the end of the nineteenth century veterans of the sanitary movement could look back on their work and see that it was good. Their promise, as proclaimed in 1842, for instance, in Edwin Chadwick's report on the *Sanitary Condition of the Labouring Classes of Great Britain* that improved sewage disposal, greater ventilation and better medical services, among other reforms, would lessen epidemic disease, lower the death rate and increase life expectancy, was being fulfilled. It is difficult now to recapture the visionary quality of their early programme or to comprehend the dirt, decay, disease and desolation they confronted, let alone understand the minds of their opponents, but the sanitarians' achievements, however misapplied, piecemeal and belated and, in the outcome, overestimated, bettered the life chances of every person in Victorian Britain. Tables 4.1 and 4.2 show how the death rate for Great Britain fell.

In general, between ages 10 and 34, females died at a higher rate than males, although the rates for females at the reproductive ages were lower than those for males, suggesting that childbirth was less dangerous than heavy work. After the over-all mortality rate began to fall during the late 1870s female mortality diminished at a quicker rate than that of the males, leaving the males with the higher death rate.[1] This decline is related to the faster diminution of tuberculosis among young adult females, a development I shall discuss later.

Table 4.1: Death Rates per 1,000 in Different Age Groups, 1838-1912, England and Wales

Year	Age Groups — Males and Females											
	10—14		15—19		20—24		25—34		35—44		45—54	
	M	F	M	F	M	F	M	F	M	F	M	F
1838	5.3	5.8	7.4	8.2	9.9	9.3	10.7	10.6	13.4	13.0	19.1	16.4
1842	5.0	5.3	6.9	7.9	8.9	8.7	9.3	10.0	12.0	12.2	17.2	15.3
1847	5.5	5.9	8.0	8.4	10.8	9.9	11.0	11.7	14.5	14.4	20.5	18.1
1852	5.2	5.4	6.9	7.8	9.2	8.8	9.8	10.2	12.4	12.3	18.0	15.3
1857	4.7	4.6	6.4	7.1	8.4	8.4	9.2	9.5	12.0	11.8	17.3	14.8
1862	4.4	4.6	6.2	6.8	8.2	7.8	9.2	9.4	12.4	11.7	18.1	14.8
1867	4.0	3.9	6.0	6.4	8.4	7.8	10.0	9.5	13.6	12.0	19.1	15.6
1872	4.1	4.0	6.0	6.2	8.7	7.6	10.3	9.3	14.0	11.8	19.4	15.1
1877	3.5	3.6	4.9	5.1	7.0	6.3	9.1	8.2	13.7	11.3	19.7	15.3
1882	3.2	3.3	4.6	4.7	5.9	5.9	8.2	7.9	12.6	11.0	19.0	15.0
1887	2.9	3.0	4.2	4.2	5.4	5.4	7.3	7.0	11.9	10.3	18.7	15.2
1892	2.6	2.7	4.0	4.0	5.2	4.7	7.1	6.7	12.1	10.3	19.8	15.5
1897	2.4	2.4	2.6	3.4	4.8	4.1	6.4	5.6	10.8	8.9	17.7	13.7
1902	2.2	2.3	3.3	3.1	4.6	3.9	6.2	5.3	10.4	8.4	17.8	13.4
1907	2.0	2.1	3.0	2.9	4.0	3.4	5.5	4.6	9.0	7.4	16.1	12.4
1912	1.8	2.0	2.9	2.7	3.6	3.2	4.8	4.0	7.9	6.3	14.6	11.1

Source: B.R. Mitchell and Phyllis Deane, *Abstract of British Historical Statistics* (Cambridge, 1962), pp. 34-43.

Table 4.2: Death Rates per 1,000 in Different Age Groups, 1860-1912, Scotland

Year	Age Groups — Males and Females									
	10—14		15—24		25—34		35—44		45—54	
	M	F	M	F	M	F	M	F	M	F
1860-2	5.2	5.2	8.7	7.6	10.3	9.6	12.4	11.5	17.3	14.4
1870-2	5.4	5.8	9.3	8.5	11.2	10.4	14.0	12.4	20.0	16.1
1880-2	4.3	4.7	7.1	7.0	8.9	9.2	12.5	11.2	19.4	14.9
1890-2	3.5	4.0	6.5	6.2	8.3	8.8	12.2	11.6	20.8	15.8
1900-2	2.8	3.2	5.0	5.1	7.5	7.1	11.7	10.0	19.5	15.6
1912	2.3	2.4	4.0	3.9	5.6	5.3	8.7	8.2	15.8	12.6

Source: ibid.

Life expectancy also increased. Between 1838 and 1854 the average age at death for males in England and Wales was 39.9 years. It became 41.9 by the early 1880s and was 44 by 1890. Over the same period female life expectancy increased from 41.9 to 45.3 to 47. The vital statistician, Noel Humphreys, calculated in the 1880s that 70 per cent of the females and 65 per cent of the males lived their increased years between the ages of 20 and 50.[2] These general figures tell us little about the actual effects on various classes in the community, but in one rare analysis, Mr Farrow, the MOH for Leek, used his knowledge of his community to assert in 1894 that while the mean duration of life for gentlemen and professional men had remained stationary at the 60 or so years that Chadwick had calculated for the class in the 1830s, 'shopkeepers and tradesmen' had increased their years from 30 to 36 between the 1850s and 1890s, 'artisans', from 26 to 31, and 'silkworkers' from 22 to 30. Over all, the mean age at death in Leek, presumably for males and females, had risen from 24.8 to 32.9.[3]

Filth and Nuisances

The gains during the years after 1870 have obscured the fragile immobility in the mortality rate through the preceding four decades. Sanitary reform, among an overwhelmingly young urbanising population, was just holding the line. The mushroom suburb of Croydon had no sewerage system for its 13,000 inhabitants and only 'rudimentary' drainage in 1848. Its growing streets, lanes and courts were outside the jurisdiction of any existing Board of Highways. Among the poor courts there was one privy to every three crowded houses. The excrement of the children was scattered about the courts and yards. The privies of the town were clustered over the open ditch which ran through the centre.[4] The average age at death in the boom town of Dudley (population around 40,000) in 1852 was said to be 16 years and 7 months; nearly 70 per cent of the population was said to have died before 20 (on arithmetical grounds it must have been more like 40-50 per cent). There was no piped water supply: the people took water from the canals. In some parishes, like St John's, this meant a walk of two miles. The community here was always short of water and did not wash. Only the very respectable had an earth closet or midden. The rest relieved themselves in the fields, while 'the back streets, courts and other eligible places are constantly found strewed with human excrements'. Here, as elsewhere, one of the great divisions between the respectable and unrespectable was where and how one relieved oneself, and whether parents taught their children to relieve themselves in the house or yard in a closet or pot, or simply sent them outside to the nearest lane or field. 'Primrose' in Dudley was 'a sort of long street in St Andrew's district', with eight pigsties built against the houses. Even 'respectable people and tradesmen' kept pigs. In 1856 the local Board of Health sought to ban pigs within the city limits, but the town revolted in the interests of, as a public meeting declared, 'the liberty of the subject'. The local Board appealed to the General Board of Health, who tactfully decided that, while the local Board could rightfully make such a regulation, it could not enforce it.[5]

The population of Gateshead tripled to over 25,000 between 1811 and 1851, but it remained concentrated in the medieval core of the town because nearby land was not released for subdivision until the 1850s. Pipewellgate, the centre of the Irish immigrant community, had three privies for its 2,000 inhabitants in 1843, together with 181 tripe shops and 'numerous piggeries'. The town also contained 31 slaughterhouses, all 'offensive', and 'several inches deep in blood, offal and dung'.[6] The town had no formal system of scavenging. Here the pigs undoubtedly helped. Utterly objectionable though they were to reformers, pigs were efficient, reasonably healthy disposers of wastes and gave good value in cash and calories. In the short run, by analogy with contemporary pig-keeping communities in the Pacific Islands, and nineteenth-century Ireland with its death rate consistently lower than Great Britain's, pigs probably curbed the death rate more than reformers. Moreover, whenever pigs were banned the people went in more heavily for less hygienic poultry, as in Paddington during the 1860s.[7]

Reading, with 378 pigsties in 1847 among 2,500 houses and courts containing about 17,000 people, had virtually no drainage and was 'overwhelmingly dependent' on open privies. The illness rate was said to be high, 'but never catastrophic'. Even in the mid-1870s, after successive onslaughts of fever, Winchester with over 15,000 people had only one sewer, serving the Barracks. Excepting the college and the female convict establishment, which boasted dry earth closets, the rest of the town's sewage went into huge, ancient cesspools. The town's water, from one central well, was discoloured and smelly. Typhoid fever was endemic.[8]

The Search for Legislative Remedies

The great clean-up effectively began when the central government carried the Health of Towns Act of 1848 to enable local authorities in England and Wales to raise funds on the rates to establish drainage schemes and water-supply systems. There are excellent accounts of

nineteenth-century public health legislation by M.W. Flinn, Royston
Lambert and Oliver MacDonagh, and I need only provide the briefest
framework here.[9] The two-tiered system of central government permissive legislation and local government implementation, created at the
outset, continued through the century. Nuisance Removal Acts of
1855, 1860 and 1863 were carried successively, like other public
health measures, to try to make the local authorities act, to close gaps
in the law and to extend the clean-up to rural parishes. The Public
Health Act of 1848 gave the central health authority the first feeble
powers of compulsion over the localities, and these powers were made
clumsily workable by the Sanitary Act of 1866. This meant that the
government for the first time seriously tackled the problem of the
actual initiation of reform. The Act of 1866 enabled any ten inhabitants to requisition the Privy Council to instruct the local authority to
act against a nuisance. In 1872 another Public Health Act enabled local
bodies to borrow more easily from the government, while it prescribed
uniform sanitary machinery throughout Great Britain and the appointment of a minimum staff. This Act and that of 1875 finally consolidated the great mass of nuisance, public health, infectious diseases,
sewers, slaughtering houses and water-supply legislation for England
and Wales. The legislation was to stand for 60 years. The Scottish law
had been consolidated in 1867.

Progress was exceedingly slow and piecemeal. Local initiatives, then
as now, were easier to praise in the abstract than to carry through. And
local initiative did not always entail reform. Radical and Tory populists
joined to fight 'centralization' and 'despotism'. 'Centralization', according to the main resolution of a citizens' meeting in Leeds against the
Health of Towns Bill in 1848, was 'dangerous and unconstitutional . . .
[because it] would remove all control over the public expenditure of
the borough from the local authorities, and vest it in the hands of the
central commissioner in London'.[10] Old Corruption lingered in men's
memories, and it would not receive its quietus until its last flourish at
the Crimea. The Whig ministry of 1830 had promised to end corrupt
patronage and employ 'nothing but consideration of ability . . . in their
selection of public servants': yet they had appointed a gang of notorious
incompetents, headed by the President of the Royal College of Physicians, to advise on the cholera outbreak in 1831. Men with experience
of the disease in India were passed over. The incompetents, whose
advice proved worse than useless, each got £500 a year.[11] 'Despotism'
would come in the form of outside experts and officious local busy-
bodies. They would, as the Tory *Patriot* explained, be creatures of

central ministerial patronage, puppets worked by the overbearing, impractical Mr Chadwick, not officers subject to parliamentary or municipal control.[12] Ratepayers throughout the kingdom exploited the provision in the Act of 1848 requiring a two-thirds majority for its adoption to fend off proposals which threatened to increase local rates and hence give non-ratepayers benefits they had done nothing to deserve, thereby implicitly transferring property, and which also promised to subject ratepayers to interfering outsiders. Moreover, adoption of the Act cost about £1,000-£1,200 in legal fees, and each successive amendment or innovation would cost the same.[13]

By late 1853 only 164 places had adopted the 1848 Act. Many towns, like cholera-ridden Newcastle, for example, had instituted a totally ineffective local act to forestall imposition of any compulsory clauses (for places with high death rates) or move to adopt the central Act and establish a local Board of Health. The Birmingham corporation spent £10,000 of ratepayers' money to obtain a local act as a preventive. The larger Scottish towns used the same tactic against the threat of the Scottish Police and Improvement Act.[14] In general, the poorer the place, the more likely it was to adopt the 1848 Act and, being poor, the less possible it was for the local authorities to implement it. London, whose local authorities successfully excluded her from an equivalent to the 1848 Act, remained in insanitary and legal chaos while conflicting vestries, boards of guardians and commissioners for sewers wrangled over their respective jurisdictions and perquisites.[15] By 1865, of 570 localities under the Public Health Act and Local Government Act of 1858, with populations varying from 214 to 200,000, 50 had no inspectors of nuisances; 153 had one; 16 had two; and four had three. Bristol, with 154,000 inhabitants, and Sheffield, with 200,000, had each only one, while some small places with under 800 had two, which suggests that some of them were 'jobs'. The ratepayers in 111 of the towns, with populations between 20,000 and 200,000, had not availed themselves of the opportunity to appoint a MOH. The London boroughs, with over three million people in their jurisdiction, had only 47 MOHs between them.[16]

In the face of deep popular resistance, the law necessarily was weak and local magistrates readily connived at resort to loopholes and imposed light penalties upon inescapable convictions. After all, their property might be attacked next. In 1853 six people were conducting horse-slaughtering and gut-manufacturing establishments in a densely populated neighbourhood in Green Street off the Blackfriars Road. One of them, R. Trotman, a bone-boiler, had on his premises a 'large quantity' of bones boiled and unboiled, and 'animal matter'. He was summoned by an inspector of nuisances instructed by the parish authorities after complaints from nearby 'householders'. The bone heap in Trotman's yard was as 'high as the police court'; the heap was said to have been there ten years. The complainants alleged that the 'very offensive smell' caused the cholera which was endemic in the neighbourhood. Counsel for the defendant argued that the magistrate had 'no jurisdiction to interfere with a nuisance *like this*, if it were a nuisance, *which had existed for more than 30 years*. The only remedy was by indictment.' The magistrate said he could not 'interfere'; moreover 'nothing had been brought forward to show that there had recently been any increase of the nuisance'.[17] Similarly, in 1854 another unlearned and resistant magistrate acquitted George Bull, a butcher of Broadway, Westminster, when he was charged with keeping pigs within 40 yards of dwelling houses. Bull's counsel successfully argued that pigs kept for slaughter were not within the meaning of the Nuisance Acts, which used 'keeping' in the sense of 'retaining and breeding up'.[18]

Even after the improved Sanitary Act of 1866 landowners and their lawyers found evasion easy. The central difficulty was compensation and the costs of initiating reforms. This entailed a redistribution from the public purse which nineteenth-century legislation would entertain only in relation to diseased cattle and, during the last quarter of the century, house property. Magistrates decided that the 1866 Act did not permit them to order that dung pits be provided with covers, because it was unclear who should pay for them. Dung heaps were private property: even when they were legally declared nuisances there was no provision in the Act for their compulsory seizure and sale, or the costs of carting away to be charged against their owner. Owners or occupiers could only be ordered to abate a nuisance by the 'best practicable means'. The prosecution in any subsequent action had to prove that the best practicable means had not been used. Magistrates commonly held that 'practicable' in the case of a trade, a business, or a process emitting effluvium excluded diminution of normal income from the trade or process. Moreover, in country parishes, where inspection was virtually non-existent, the occupier or owner could meet an order to abate a nuisance with either a token clean-up, or by 'agreeing' to abate it and then doing nothing.[19]

Defending counsel's favourite means of defeating serious charges under the Nuisance or Local Acts was to manoeuvre the complainants into alleging that the nuisance was injurious to health. In strict law the complainants did not have to prove this, but their inability to do so always impressed magistrates. Prosecutors and complainants did have to prove that a nuisance was an annoyance and detrimental to comfort; but again, if the prospects looked bad, the defendants could always produce a last-minute witness to swear that he loved the smell and had never seen any rats. In 1848 Mr Gore was prosecuted by the parish officials of St Luke's under a 'laystalls' provision in a local Act for keeping dustheaps in Hadfield Street, off the Goswell road. His 'golden mounds' were up to 14 feet high and overtopped the nearby houses. One heap comprised 'dry rubbish', the sweepings from cellars, old iron, etc. The other was composed of 'wet muck', the sweepings of Smithfield and Newgate markets, and brewery refuse: cabbage leaves, dead animals, spent brewing grains, decayed potatoes. The 'sulphuretted hydrogen' generated from the mounds was pervasive for up to 400 feet away. The value of the nearby houses had depreciated. Gore produced a team of scavengers who all swore that they were perfectly health and that working on the heaps gave them hearty appetites. Dr Guy and Mr J. Ryan, from King's College Hospital, swore that the 'heaps were not injurious to health' and that they and their colleagues had seen 'no more sickness around the heaps than elsewhere'. The jury found Gore guilty.[20]

As late as 1889 a bench of magistrates in Birmingham refused to make an order to close polluted wells. The prosecution proved that the water was polluted but failed to prove that it had damaged the health of those who drank it. In 1890 a High Court judge finally ruled that 'nuisance' was incorporated in the term 'offensive trade' and thereby made convictions easier to obtain.[21]

The want of compensation hit the poor and nourished their suspicions of intruding sanitarians. Before the Act of 1867 and 1875 there was no provision for compensation for articles destroyed during disinfection. Such payments as there were had been *ex gratia* and apparently depended upon the humanity of some local official. The seizure and burning of beds, bedding and clothing in infected households during cholera or typhus outbreaks added to the terrors of the disease.[22] The Scottish Act set an effective limit of £50 for 'damage' which apparently had to be proved in court. The English Act of 1875 allowed local authorities to compensate for such seizures, but the section (308) was said in 1881 never to have been used. Moreover, compensation could only be considered if the claimant was not 'in default'.[23] Disinfection became even more terrible after new fumigation techniques were developed in the mid-1880s. The house was closed. The wallpaper was stripped and burnt. Then either steam at 260°F was applied for 30 minutes to furniture, clothes, bedding etc., heaped in an iron 'steam chamber', or 'hot air at $230°$ F was applied in the chamber for five hours, while the rest of the house was suffused with chlorine or sulphurous acid gas for 12 hours. The local authority was not liable for damage, except through proven 'negligence'. Until 1890 the local authority had no responsibility for the family excluded from their dwelling during fumigation. After the Infectious Diseases Prevention Act of that year the authorities were supposed to provide shelter. But two years later virtually no local authority had obeyed the Act.[24] The fumigation of clothes posed a special difficulty for working-class people: most had only one set. This, a doctor remarked in the *Lancet* in 1895, was the 'large problem' in disinfection and its evasion.[25]

The rich, dwelling as single families in large houses, could retire to a set of rooms and privately arrange the fumigation of the remainder. Only in proud anti-vaccination towns, like Leicester, were there free isolation hospitals to which whole families, rich and poor, could go 'voluntarily' while their homes and contents were disinfected at the public expense.[26]

Difficulties about the will to increase expenditure, the machinery of implementation and the hardships that implementation entailed fettered sanitary reformers throughout the age. This is a vast, largely unexplored subject which the existing celebratory accounts of sanitary progress do not touch. Yet detailed local studies could tell us much about attitudes to local and central authority and explain much that is obscure in the history of sanitary reform itself, not least the effects of such comparatively large investment on the local economy and local employment.

Food and Drink

One clear lesson is that, among the working classes and the poor, all choices were dirty ones. Take meat. The crucial point is not *how much* meat the lower classes got (the old issue between the 'standard of living' debaters), but its quality. Meat at ruling prices was sold in at least four grades: first to third, and then 'inferior'. First-class meat was about one-third dearer than 'inferior'.[27] But below 'inferior', there was an enormous trade in cheap offal and old and diseased meat. In the countryside, before the 1850s, bullocks' heads and ox-cheeks were 'never seen', a sheep's head had to be 'bespoken weeks' before the sheep was killed and sheep's pluck 'cost too much' for agricultural labourers' families. Within the family, both rural and urban, into the mid-1860s, wives who were not delicate or who did not go out to work

were said 'never' to eat meat.[28] Throughout the century there was no
effective control on the quality of meat at the point of slaughtering: no
cheap and effective way had been found of marking approved meat or
rendering bad meat unfit for sale. Street vendors of food, unlike other
hawkers, remained unlicensed until at least 1912.[29]

Bacon seems to have been the meat most commonly eaten by the
working classes and poor. It was cheaper than other meats, could be
cut and purchased in smaller portions, and it kept better. The habit of
keeping a pig and of slaughtering it privately meant that the meat could
be traded among neighbours. In 1895 Dr Thomas Oliver, a pioneer
investigator in this field, recorded bacon as the only meat regularly
consumed by Tyneside coal-miners, English navvies, semi-skilled engineers and Sheffield steel-grinders. He also found one widow in Newcastle
who ate bacon 'in very small amounts'.[30] Bacon came cheaper than
normally – and tastier – when its fat had turned yellow and it had
begun to smell. It was cheapest when it showed black spots (anthrax).
Food poisoning was not uncommon and deaths occurred occasionally:
the relatively low incidence of such afflictions resulted from the fact
that meat, as Dr Oddy pointed out, 'remained a flavouring rather than
a substantial course'.[31]

Pigs were especially prone to the disease of anthrax because butchers
kept them in their slaughter-yards to consume unsaleable offal. Irish
pig-keepers had a special trade in 'measle' bacon. The keeper pulled
open the pig's mouth, thrust a stick under the tongue and, if the stick
brought out worm larvae with it, the pig was sent to the public market:
no Irish family would eat 'measly meat'.[32] In 1902 butcher Harris of
Clerkenwell suffered his second conviction for selling bad meat. He had
pork that was 'suppurating and decomposed', and veal that was 'green
and slimy'. Harris claimed that the meat was only 'muggy' and would
be 'alright [when] it was wiped'. (Here Harris presumably is referring
to the standard practice of rubbing bad lean meat with fat, in order to
'polish' it.) He got four months' hard labour.[33]

The ordinary people's dependence upon the cheapest bits of sheep
and cattle also caused difficulties for their would-be protectors. Heads,
tails, kidneys, tongues, hearts, livers and skirt were the staple of the
local markets and street sellers. Yet often the prosecutor had to 'produce' a whole carcass before he could obtain a conviction for selling
bad meat. Moreover, as inspection of slaughterhouse and meat improved in London during the 1860s, butchers took to killing outside
the metropolis and bringing in the dismembered portions by train. In
1857 a young veterinary student, J.S. Gamgee, found the carcasses of

three oxen and two sheep at Copenhagen Fields Market each 'a dusky red' and the oxen 'all pleuropneumoniac'. He secured the otherwise unsaleable lungs, the only part which obviously shows pleuropneumonia and took them to the authorities at the Mansion House. But Gamgee found that he could not secure an order forbidding the sale of the rest of the carcasses without presenting the carcasses or even a part of the meat normally for sale.[34] In 1863 a veterinarian estimated that over £1,200,000 worth of sheep died annually from disease in England and Wales, and that one-fifth of the carcasses were sold to butchers. The rest was fed to pigs.[35]

Beef always became cheaper during outbreaks of animal disease. In mid-1861 farmers were getting 2*d*. per pound for the meat of diseased beef and sheep; 'they were pleased to get it'. If the animals were destroyed by order of the local Boards of Health the owners got nothing. In 1857 a Bill to control the sale of diseased meat, with the aim of preventing the spread of cattle plague, had been thrown out once the plague abated.[36] At around 1½*d*. per half pound retail (the average wholesale price for good-quality meat at Smithfield Market in 1861 was about 6½*d*. per pound) the common people were paying less than half the prices charged in the West End.[37] Trollope noted in the mid-1860s that a gentleman-clergyman's family, with three children, might buy three pounds of meat a day at 9*d*. per pound, working out at £40 a year, or nearly two-thirds the annual income of a moderately skilled, fully employed artisan, and equal to the income of one-quarter of the working population in 1906. The Reverend Mr Crawley had £130 a year.[38] None the less, as surveys before 1900 showed, working people were prepared to allot to meat up to one-quarter of the 60 per cent of their total income that they spent on food.[39]

The first successful prosecution in London for selling bad meat came in February 1861. Mr Firmin had five 'rotten' sheep in his shop. They were so wasted with disease that instead of weighing the usual 80 pounds they were each only 18-25 pounds. Firmin sold them to street salesmen for 2½*d*. per pound. Dr Letheby, the food analyst and MOH for the City of London, asserted, as the traditional stance of the law required him to do, that such meat, if ingested in 'a partially cooked state' would produce either 'low fever or violent vomiting and purging', although he could not prove it. Firmin's counsel, employed by the Butchers' Association, led evidence from several salesmen that the meat was safe because the disease was always 'hidden when the meat became frozen'. The Butchers' Association was outraged when the court reversed its usual stand and fined Firmin £10.[40] Assumptions that food was likely to be 'half-cooked' and warnings against this practice continue through the century.

After this success seizures and convictions became more frequent, in London at least. The trade in poor meat was a very big one. Cheap meat was not simply the staple of the indigent. When a farmer found disease among his herd his first move was to sell the animals to a butcher. A Blandford farmer-butcher sent 300 pounds of bad beef to Bermondsey in April 1861.[41] During the first week of November in 1862 the City of London inspectors seized over 4,500 pounds of meat and 73 head of game and poultry. In 1865, during the cattle plague, the market was 'flooded': over 9,000 pounds and 128 quarters of beef were seized in one week in November. Next year 340,820 pounds were seized and destroyed in the City markets, in addition to 'game, poultry, fish and venison'. (There are no figures for the total amount of dead meat supplied to the London markets in the 1860s, but in 1859, as a rough guide to the proportions involved, over 7,800 tons were sent to Newgate and Leadenhall Markets.[42]) By 1908 the inspectors in Manchester were destroying annually as 'unwholesome' over 241,000 pounds of meat, 247,000 pounds of fish, and over 5,000 rabbits, in addition to 'great quantities of vegetables . . . fruit and poultry'. Seventy-two shopkeepers were cautioned in 1907 for holding bad food, but only two prosecutions were launched under the Public Health Act. Each delinquent was fined £7: by this time fines of this magnitude were possibly a considerable deterrent.[43]

From 1857 at least there had been half-hearted attempts at legislation to control the public sale of diseased meat, usually framed to block the entry of foreign meat when cattle murrain broke out on the Continent. But these moves failed each time as the murrain abated. In London until the Public Health Act of 1875 most prosecutions seem to have been made under the Nuisance Acts. The problem of private small slaughtering for sale remained intractable. As long as milking cows were housed within the town limits there was private slaughtering. The Strand was a traditional site for cellar dairies and until the late 1850s at least it was a well known slaughtering and distribution centre for cheap meat.[44] In 1860 Dr Letheby swooped on irregular slaughtering houses in the City of London and seized half a ton of bad meat. Calves found in slaughtered cows were sold as 'slink veal'.[45] The bulk of our evidence is from London but this is probably because the authorities were more active. There are indications that affairs were no better in the country. When the cow at the Spalding workhouse developed symptoms of 'milk fever' in 1885 the guardians sold it to a local butcher for

£5. A girl died in Ashby de la Zouche in 1884 after eating a decomposing calf's liver. Her mother had bought it from a butcher, together with a calf's head, for 9*d*, 'far below the ruling price'. The butcher had purchased the calf from a farmer for £1.5*s*.0*d*. because the calf was 'a bit amiss' with pleuropneumonia.[46]

Increased sanitary surveillance at the public market induced butchers to boil down their bad meat. During the last three months of 1860 Dr Letheby had seized over 17 tons of meat and 500 rabbits at the City markets. But he was convinced that a great deal of bad meat had got through, and he noted among the bad meat very little fat. This, he asserted, was sent for boiling down 'in the manufacture of butter', as an adulterant. Other suspect meat was sold directly for sausage-making or for rendering into meat extract.[47] In Leicester in 1885 a butcher was fined £25 for using putrid meat to make brawn. It was his second offence. The business must have been large and profitable enough to make the usual fines of £5—£10 bearable. Ruffin and Co. of Bermondsey were also fined £25 in 1898 for possessing 44 barrels of stinking livers intended for meat extract. The same firm probably was the anonymous one convicted of a similar charge in 1866.[48]

Had the wealthier ratepayers been more directly threatened by bad meat they might have acted more decisively to end it; but as long as they had access to top-quality cuts they did not move to block the lower classes' access to such offal as they could afford. At the end of the 1870s, 689 districts in England and Wales had bye-laws, at least, governing the slaughter and public sale of meat. But 205 did not.[49] From the beginning of that decade some reformers looked to cheap tinned Australian meat as a replacement for inferior local meat but it turned out that the poor did not like the stringy tasteless stuff, or the spongy, bloody lumps that appeared in the shops after the frozen meat trade developed in the 1880s. In 1871 and 1872 the inmates of two workhouses rioted against being served Australian meat.[50]

Fresh fish was generally unavailable to both rich and poor outside fishing villages until the 1850s, when power was supplied to fishing boats and the railways helped distribution. Even salt fish was too dear for the working classes. Consignments of fresh fish were auctioned in large lots and this, together with difficulties of handling and inevitable high wastage; led most shopkeepers to avoid it.[51] In the great towns until the 1880s 'third day fish', mackerel with a 'horrid stench' at six for a shilling, for example, were the only fish available to the poor. Fried fish shops, using offal fish, piper or dab, or hake or codfish which had gone off, spread during the 1880s. Tinned fish came in during the same decade, but it was comparatively expensive (even Boots' 'special salmon' which was half the average price at 4½*d*. a tin), and expensive enough, as were other tinned foods, for poor families not to possess a tin-opener as a normal piece of equipment.[52]

One main item of diet, bread, varied enormously in quality. Wealthy people, farmers and others who ate bread baked at home were said to be relatively free of the 'indigestion and its consequent calamities' usually traced to eating baker's bread.[53] As Samuel Palmer warned his fellow artist George Richmond, when advising him to get wholesome bread: 'Consider what a responsibility you incur for aluming up your children's entrails every day to an iron rigidity.'[54] Alum was a traditional adulterant of flour and bread. During the first forty years of the century when brown bread was despised (rightly, as it was tough, sour and gritty), alum was included to whiten the loaf, although it had long been illegal. It was also added to bind the rice flour, itself an adulterant, and the poor-quality spring wheat flour used to make cheap bread.[55]

Reformers believed the cheaper the bread, the more alum it contained. But Dr John Snow showed by analysis that the opposite was true. Fashionable Regent Street shops sold very white bread with over an ounce more alum to every loaf than in cheap shops in the East End.[56] The adulteration of the cheaper bread really began with the flour: 17 of forty samples seized in Newcastle in 1872 contained rice flour. Indeed this grade of wheat flour, and oatmeal or barley meal, adulterated with sawdust, had the special trade name of 'Jonathan' in the North of England.[57] After Arthur Hill Hassell provided, in microscopy, the first sure means of detecting and legally proving adulteration, the law developed through a series of measures in the 1860s and was consolidated in the Sale of Food and Drugs Act of 1875. Analysis was still far from unchallengeable in the courts and defence counsel were quick to find loopholes, such as making the prosecution prove that the seized bread was intended for sale, but effectively alum and sawdust disappeared from bread after 1875. As bread continued to be a basic food for the people into this century this improvement represented a major gain.[58]

This advance was brought about less by the adulteration Acts than by changes in the structure of the industry and in baking methods. Until the 1870s bread production in London and the large towns was dispersed among a multitude of small, competitive, primitive bakeries. The typical bakehouse oven was built in a cellar under the roadway. The mixing troughs and kneading boards were in an uncleaned, vermin-infested basement. Bakers worked through the night and it was normal to lock them in, to prevent their stealing, or drinking, while unsupervised. The usual temperature in the basement was 80° to 110°F. Some bakehouses had a privy under the stairs, but in even less capitalised concerns the men relieved themselves on the coal-heap. The men used both hands and feet while kneading the dough, sweating as they worked. They washed in the water used for the next batch of dough. A journeyman had to be on the job for an 18-20 hour shift for most days and towards the weekend he was expected to stay at the bakehouse 'nearly two entire days in succession'. The average wage was 17s. a week. Bakers were notorious consumptives: while compositors were counted to spit blood in the ratio of 12½ per 100, bakers had a ratio of 31 per 100.[59] They were a 'pale-faced, flabby, anxious-looking race'. On Friendly Society tables they constituted the fifth worst risk, with an average claim of 178 weeks of sickness during their working life, which usually ended at 40. In 1859, while the builders waged their famous strike for a nine-hour day, the bakers courageously, and amidst considerable public sympathy, struck for 12.[60] This strike failed, as did another major one in 1872, when the men offered, in return for the 12-hour day and an extra 3s. a week, to withdraw all men from 'dishonest', that is, adulterating and light weighing, shops. This strike failed, too.[61] The prominence of demands for abolition of night baking among the Chartists and during the Paris Commune becomes less curious when we begin to realise the conditions which bakers endured and the shameful stuff they made. The employment in night baking of persons under 18, who constituted a large minority of the 50,000 or so in the English trade, was forbidden under the Bakehouse Regulation Act of 1863. This Act also provided for the washing of bakehouses at six-month intervals. But inspection of bakehouses did not become effective until 1883 and bakers were still an exploited group outside the protection of the anti-sweating laws until 1910, at least, when bakers were still working an average 85½ hours a week.[62]

The 'cutting bakers' shops' in the poorer streets sold bread 1d. or 2d. lower than the usual price, which, in the 1850s and 1860s, was around 7d. per four-pound loaf. The cheaper bread had more water than the normal loaf. The dough was 'mixed thin', that is 96 loaves to the sack of flour instead of the usual 90, and then only three-quarters cooked, to keep the steam in. Observers reported that babies suffered particularly when fed on it.[63] Such bread lingered until the twentieth century, but the invention of the kneading machine and Stevens's process for making aerated bread in the 1860s, together with the gradual capital growth of the industry and forcing out of the smallest bakers, steadily enlarged opportunities to buy more uniform, better-quality bread. Peak, Frean and Co. set the new pattern of large-scale, hygienic, mechanised baking in tins in 1860. They could turn out a complete bake every 1½ hours, compared with the small hand-baker's 3-5 hours.[64]

Other staple parts of the people's diet remained dubious for longer. The Chinese coloured their tea with Prussian blue (ferric ferrocyanide, lime sulphate and turmeric). Foreign buyers and English tea-drinkers with expensive tastes liked the look of it.[65] Ordinary cheap tea often was sold mixed with hawthorne and elm leaves and dried used leaves added, but by 1861 sampling revealed that most tea was 'genuine'. After 1875 tea was tested by the customs department, under the provisions of the Sale of Food and Drugs Act of that year; by this time the tests were mostly superfluous because large-scale adulteration of tea for the British market had ceased.[66] Presumably the spread of proprietary packaging and chain stores during the 1880s also furthered quality control. Pickles were coloured with copper salts until into the 1890s. Customers were said to prefer a good 'bright' colour and would return the bottle if it were not green enough.[67]

The addition of substances injurious to health was also prevalent in the confectionery trade until the mid-1850s. Children's sweets, in shops in both rich and poor districts, were coloured with copper carbonate, lead carbonate, copper arsenate and lead chromate, and chocolate was enriched with Venetian lead (red iron oxide). The frequent outbreaks of vomiting after children's parties were not simply, as was said at the time, the nemesis of gluttony. But after some notorious cases and the anti-adulteration campaign of the mid-1850s, and, coincidentally, with the take-off in the English confectionery industry from an output of 8,000 to 25,000 tons per annum between 1855 and 1862, the practice died away.[68]

The adulteration of beer and spirits sold for public consumption had much more serious implications for health and behaviour. Concerned doctors first noticed what they alleged to be a huge increase in the importation of nux vomica (strychnine – in small repeated doses an hallucinogen) and cocculus indicus (the dried seed of the *Anamirta Cocculus*, from the East Indies – another bitter poison which can act convulsively on the central nervous system and induce 'confusion') in 1830, soon after the Beer Act opened the way to the spread of beer-shops kept by struggling proprietors. As one critic remarked, 30,000 pounds of nux vomica and 12,000 pounds of cocculus indicus could not possibly all be used in medicine or the destruction of vermin. Heavy penalties were provided for the use of these drugs in brewing, but writers of manuals on brewing, Child and Morrice, for example, openly described their use. For a 'strong-bodied porter' Morrice recommended 3 pounds of cocculus indicus to every 10 quarts of malt: 'it gives an inebriating quality which passes for strength of liquor'. Small brewers and beer-shop keepers could not afford to sell beer unless they diluted it with water. The added narcotics compensated for the dilution of the alcohol.[69]

The imports remained at about the 1830 levels until the 1870s. In 1865, for instance, 9,400 pounds of cocculus indicus were brought in, enough to adulterate 120,000 barrels of beer according to the usual brewers' recipes. By 1868, 119,168 pounds were being imported, sufficient, the *British Medical Journal* asserted, to adulterate three-fifths of all British ale, porter and stout. A special class of 'brewers' druggists' had developed to serve the trade. They specialised in selling 'black extract' to brewers although, to evade the law, the 'black extract' ostensibly was made for sale to tanners.[70] Before the late 1870s analysts could not determine the presence of narcotics in beer or porter and curiously, the Excise seems to have taken no interest in the problem. Both nux vomica and cocculus indicus entered Britain duty-free. A rise in the price of hops after 1860 led some brewers even to experiment with strychnine in bitter beers as a near total substitute.[71]

Workmen liked adulterated beer. Pure beer, they said, just went down and they 'felt nothing of it'. Yet adulteration with these hallucinogens doubtless explains some at least of the bizarre degradation, brutality and murder that pervaded Victorian lower-class life. In 1866 the Commissioner of Inland Revenue reported that 'acts of violence and crime are especially prevalent in those counties where adulterated beer is known mostly to be found'. Adulteration could help explain the puzzling variations in the pattern of arrests for drunkenness between the very high rates for seaports and mining counties and the much lower rates for inland manufacturing towns.[72] But it must also be said that seaport drinkers had access to the stronger export beers and mining communities the world over are heavy drinkers. For reasons probably connected with changes in the licensing laws and the decrease of small beer-shops and with Gladstone's changes in the excise in 1880, adulteration of beer with noxious substances died away during the 1880s. By 1896 a parliamentary committee of inquiry could report that common salt remained as the only major adulterant. It still appeared in up to four times the legal 50 grains per gallon.

The problem with spirits was mainly dilution with water. Capsicum and sulphuric acid were added occasionally, and more frequently, it was alleged, unrectified corn spirit, but presumably the higher initial alcohol content made watering easier than with beer. Until 1879 there was no legal definition of proof spirit content for retailers. Thus, in 1875 a glass of gin in one shop might contain 50 per cent proof spirit, in another 76 per cent. But 17 years after 1879, one-quarter of all samples were on average 27 per cent below the legal proof level.[73]

As control of adulteration strengthened, tampering contracted to the two mass-consumption perishables, milk and butter. The milk started in bad surroundings and thereafter got worse. Until the 1860s, in London, and elsewhere until the twentieth century, milking cows were kept crowded in yards, cellars or closed sheds within cities and towns. The standard feed was brewers' grains and distillers' wash. This gave the milk a distinctive taste and the cowsheds a distinctive 'offensive smell'. Dairymen believed that the more immobilised, by crowding, the cow was kept, the less food she consumed and the more milk she gave. Until 1862 in London and 1879 elsewhere, there was no law requiring cowsheds to be regularly cleaned. The Acts were permissive on the local authorities, and were rarely enforced. In St Pancras in 1857 1,400 cows were held in 141 sheds with an average of 230 cubic feet per animal. A year later the London MOHs calculated that London had 846 cowsheds housing almost 12,000 cattle; in Manchester City, Dr Niven found in 1896 176 cowsheds, of which 127 had less than 600 cubic feet per stall.[74]

Disease was rampant. Until the Metropolitan Local Management Amendment Act of 1858 dairies were jointly run as slaughterhouses. Beasts *in extremis* were quickly dispatched as meat, so disease could not be calculated. But as an indication of the proportions involved, one man who kept a shed of eight cows admitted in 1858 that over the preceding 12 years he had lost 230 animals from lung disease. In 1869 about 44 per cent of the cowsheds in St Pancras and about 44 per cent of the beasts in them were afflicted with foot and mouth disease. But milking proceeded and only two beasts were slaughtered. At Manchester in 1896 41 per cent of the cows slaughtered at the *abbatoir* were tubercular, as were 49 per cent of those slaughtered in Glasgow *abbatoirs* in 1903. The tubercular bacillus had been isolated by Koch in 1882 but the Adulteration Acts had not been amended to cover bacilli. So analysts, looking for water or other adulterants to milk, never bothered with tuberculosis. It was also difficult, time-consuming and ultimately expensive to test: it took up to four weeks for the bacillus to germinate in an infected guinea-pig. The government did not begin to tackle the problem until 1913, when the Tubercular Order provided compensation for the slaughter and disposal of tubercular cows.[75]

The dilution of milk with water, which preoccupied doctors and legislators, might have been less destructive. But the water in the milk was dirty, for it usually came from the water butt for the cattle or the farmyard pump – 'the cow with the iron tail'. When in 1885 Dr Phillips, the MOH for Balsall Heath in Worcestershire, wanted to stop an outbreak of typhoid fever which he had traced to a milk-seller, he found he could not legally prevent the man selling milk, but he could and did close the man's water pump. Dairymen added water first to make the cream rise quickly, so that they could skim it before delivery. Once in the shop or among the local roundsmen it was diluted further. In 1856 Mr Hodson Rugg, who studied London's milk supply, claimed to have calculated that even on a conservative estimate of 25 per cent dilution, Londoners were paying £475,000 annually for the water, a sum equal to the aggregate income of the London water companies.[76] Rugg must have been exaggerating, for his estimate works out at around 5s. per head per year, but his calculations, which contemporaries accepted, give some notion of the pervasiveness of adulteration.

Adulteration of milk first became a legal offence in England and Scotland in 1860, but few local authorities adopted the legislation. None the less this Adulteration of Food and Drink Act disturbed London dealers sufficiently to alter the prevailing colour of their milk from blue to yellow, by the addition of yellow ochre to disguise the water.[77]

The government set minimum proportions for fats and solids in the Adulteration Act of 1872. But seasonal variations in the nature of milk and loopholes in the law continued to baffle analysts and would-be prosecutors. They had to prove that the vendor adulterated the milk himself or had express knowledge of its adulteration by another. Defending counsel also exploited the endless complications about the procedure for taking samples and giving due warning to the seller. Even after conviction, magistrates were generally sympathetic to the milkman. In 1890 a vendor in the parish of St George's Square was found to have kept two pails of milk under the counter: one was 'heavily watered' for sale to children; the other was for 'regular customers'. The seller sold some watered milk to a boy, and then noticed an inspector outside. She took back the milk, poured it out and filled the can with good milk. The magistrate refused to convict. Fines were also derisory: in York in 1888 the going rate was 20s. for 33 per cent water and 10s. for 30 per cent water.[78]

None the less adulteration of milk diminished through the 1880s

as the law became more widely enforced and in big cities large com
panies emerged to handle the growing market and the transport of milk
by rail. In Manchester from 1875 to 1889 23 per cent of milk samples
were adulterated; in 1889-90, 7.5 per cent and in 1893-4, 4.9 per cent.[79]
On the other hand, the milk was also older, about three or four days in
London at the turn of the century. Suppliers took to adding formalin
or boracic acid to stay and to hide fermentation. And handling, despite
the invention of the steel milk churn and better refrigeration, was still
rough and ready. In 1903, 32 per cent of samples in Finsbury contained
'pus' and 40 per cent 'dirt'. In 1910 Dr Vernon, an authority on tuberculosis, reported that 20 per cent of milk samples and 10 per cent of
butter contained 'living tubercle'. In most working-class homes, short of
pantries and cupboards, people had nowhere to store milk and butter.
The favourite place was near the stove, ready to put in the tea.[80]

Butter was adulterated with animal fats, arrowroot, farina and
potato starch. Dutch, French and German butters were much the worst.
Swedish, New Zealand and Australian much the best. Irish butter contained too much salt and up to 30 per cent water (5-14 per cent was
normal in quality butter). Working people preferred the strong salt
butters: they were up to 3*d*. cheaper than mild butters and would keep
for up to five months through the winter.[81] Adulteration with margarine or starch was almost impossible to detect and prove, so prosecutions were rare.

Yet the diet of the great bulk of the people was improving. As
adulteration diminished, the output of milk and milk products rose
between 1870 and 1900 by an estimated 33 per cent, a rate of increase
only exceeded by that of poultry and eggs.[82] The production of pig-
meat went up by 10 per cent. The increase in consumption was not
evenly distributed between the classes: Dr Oddy argues persuasively
that those at over 30*s*. per week increased the quality and quantity of
food they purchased, while those under that income still ate badly,
especially the women and children. By 1913, there is evidence, for
Glasgow at least, that the cut-off level was 20*s*. regular income a week.
Over all, working-class families in 1905 consumed less than two pints
of milk and 1½ pounds of meat a week. But even this might have been
a distinct improvement on the situation in the first two-thirds of the
century.[83] The relative decline in consumer expenditure on alcoholic
drinks after the mid-1870s (itself probably a symptom of improved
diet), coupled with the rise in real wages, must have left more working-
class housewives with more money for imported butter, bacon, jam,
dairy products and fruit, quite apart from the newly available mass-

produced consumer durables, boots, clothing, bedding and cooking utensils.[84]

There was one other staple and filling foodstuff which was beyond adulteration, which kept well, was easily prepared, palatable and filling, and which was nutritious, especially in the otherwise rare vitamin C, although much of this could be lost by ageing or prolonged boiling. This was the potato. Its prominence in workhouse dietaries suggests that it was cheap throughout the century, and every report mentions its substantial part in the diet of the ordinary people. But its virtues, especially its immunity to adulteration, meant that it remained beyond the ken of official investigation, and we know tantalisingly little about it. Presumably, the palatability and ease of cooking of the potato ensured that as the buying power of housewives increased they bought even more and perhaps better-quality potatoes. Working people still obtained inadequate proteins, fats and iron, and their calorie intake for adults, at around 1,200-2,000 between 1880 and 1914, is lower than present standards by one-third, but it remains, on Dr Oddy's showing, an improvement.[85]

Water Supply: Uses and Abuses

The provision of a safe water supply was the other main requisite for survival. The increase of population and urbanisation, together with the spread of water-borne sewage disposal systems, brought the water problem to crisis point during the early 1840s. At the same time Edwin Chadwick produced his magnificent, visionary plan for an integrated water supply, self-cleansing sewer and drainage system for London. The story of the political, financial and engineering difficulties which beset Chadwick's scheme has been well told by Dr R.A. Lewis and Professor Oliver MacDonagh.[86] I want only to add some points germane to the relation between water supply and health.

For most of the nineteenth century piped water was a dear commodity, only intermittently available to the poorer classes, and it was dirty. The story of the supply in Edinburgh is representative of the difficulties of growing cities. Before 1818 the inhabitants depended upon their own pump wells. These produced so much water that the surplus was allowed to run down the High Street. In 1818 the town authorities surrendered their rights to a joint-stock water company from Crawley, which introduced piped water. The comfortable classes installed water-closets, and left off using their pump wells. The water ceased to flow down the High Street. A shortage of water developed, apparently during the 1820s, and in order to save water for those who paid for it, the company's public wells from which the poorer people derived their now sole supply lost their second and third service pipes and were restricted to one nozzle. By 1847 the inhabitants of two-fifths of the dwellings, about 27,000 in numbers, rated at under £4, had no piped water and were dependent upon queuing at the public wells. Landlords of taverns dispensed small amounts of water gratis to those who bought liquor from them. Landlords of 'respectable' tenements put in a small cistern on each floor, but this remedy failed because the company, by the 1830s, was supplying water either for only a few hours daily or only every second day during the spring and summer. By 1842 the company was supplying an amount that worked out at only one gallon per inhabitant per day, among a total population of 166,000. Edinburgh's annual summer drought continued until 1860, at least.[87]

At Middleton in 1848 ratepayers opposed a petition for the creation of a local Board of Health as the first step to receiving a water supply. The local wells for the 5,700 inhabitants were 'abominable'. Most people bought water from carriers, who charged a minimum of 8d. per weekly load for even the smallest cottages and 1s. 3d. on washing days. People hoarded this valuable stuff and used it repeatedly until it was fit only to wash the floors.[88]

When Loch Katrine water was brought to Glasgow in 1857 those whose houses were not connected to the mains could get it only if they spent 5s. for a key to one of the public taps.[89] The rate for connected houses in small towns in the south of England during the 1860s was reported to be between 1s. 6d. and 2s. per 1000 gallons, with a further levy of 6d. in the pound valuation as an annual connection fee. Some companies, like that in Aberdeen, charged 6d. extra on the normal connection fee if the water was supplied inside the house.[90]

Not surprisingly, occupiers and owners of small property were hesitant about buying piped water, while ratepayers like those in Liverpool between the 1850s and 1890s thwarted proposed capital works schemes which would lift the rates while benefiting mainly the poor and the factory proprietors.[91]

Moreover, the pattern of domestic consumption subserved the comfortable classes more than the poor, quite apart from in WCs, because the comfortable classes kept horses. Stables were notoriously ill-drained places which had to be washed and swept regularly. The author of the article on 'sanitary science' in the 1860s edition of *Chambers Encyclopaedia* estimated that each day every adult needed 8 pints of water for 'drinking and cooking', 16 gallons for 'cleansing', and 9 gallons for 'sewage', but then added that each horse drank 8-12 gallons daily and needed 3-4 for grooming. The existence of stables in a town also raised the costs of scavenging.[92]

The question of the distribution of the actual burden of taxation and the relative benefits accruing to different classes from its spending remains almost unexplored, but there are some grounds for supposing that the occupiers of cottage property themselves paid for more than they got. The authorities at Barnard Castle instituted new water supply and drainage works in 1852. For this purpose they obtained local powers under the Public Health Act of 1848, at a cost of £116. A full local Act would have cost £2,000. The water and sewerage works applied only to cottage property. The costs of installing a WC and connection to the main was 2¼d. per week, of which 1¼d. was to be paid by the tenant. 'House property', which apparently formerly received water from the polluted Tees, was now connected to the new superior supply, but does not seem to have been charged for the general works. Moreover, 'house property', under the new local powers, was relieved of the highway rate and 'the land' from contribution to the general district rate.[93] The question is extremely complicated, as even this sketch of the machinations in one small community shows. But fundamental questions are involved about local politics and thousands of pounds of expenditure and the well-being or ill-being of millions of people. Not least, a study of such episodes might show that the opposition of the small ratepayers and the unenfranchised to improvement proposals did not arise simply out of bloody-minded ignorance, as alleged by contemporary propagandists like Charles Kingsley and Chadwick.

By 1860 the ratepayers in most towns were fairly well served. The second great cholera epidemic of 1853 and the spread of the notion that cholera was water-borne had led to unprecedented public investment and construction. Most of this activity was conducted under local Acts, like the Metropolitan Water Act of 1852, carried before the cholera, but the cholera ensured that these measures did not remain dead letters. In London in 1850, 270,581 houses had water supplied; in 1856, 328,561; and the total average gallonage allowed per house per day went up from 160 to 246. By 1856, nearly all the 'separate dwellings', that is, about 100,000 of them, were connected. In Liverpool the number of households paying the special extra rate for WCs and baths had jumped to about 6,000. The wealthier inhabitants of Greenock paid 1s. in the pound to the private company for their continuous 'delivered' water, while the poorer paid 6d. for corporation water obtained from public taps. The consumption of water in Glasgow doubled between 1840 and 1859: during this time about 8,000 new baths and 16,000 new WCs were installed. There was no extra rate for these in Glasgow: 'even working men . . . installed WCs'.[94]

Among the comfortable classes the 1850s and 1860s were the decades of the fastidious revolution. The soap excise was removed in 1853. The wholesale price fell by one-third while consumption jumped: in 1841 nearly 76,000 tons of soap were produced and in 1871 over 150,000 tons. Consumption per head almost doubled between 1841 and 1861 and probably almost doubled again by 1891, to reach 14 pounds per person a year.[95] The middle years of the century were also the years of growth in the scented toilet-soap industry, when Pears, Knights and others began to expand. Cleanliness in its new sense of ablutionary prophylaxis, rather than John Wesley's original neatness of apparel, had moved closer to godliness. Respectable people now not only dressed differently from the labouring classes, but must have smelt different.[96]

During these years the notion of cleanliness began to encompass the moral and social order. Fastidious upper- and middle-class improvers began to carry the gospel of cleanliness to the dangerously insalubrious classes. Lord Shaftesbury believed that 'the amount of political . . . discontent . . . existing among the masses' was directly related to their insanitary conditions of life. Moreover, 'fever might break out in some noxious and remote district; but when at length it came to desolate some contagious and wealthy region, then they began to see the consequence of this intolerable evil'. In 1853 the Bishop of London, C.J. Blomfield, warned in a pastoral letter that it was 'certain that persons immersed in hopeless misery and filth [were] for the most part inaccessible to the . . . gospel'. Among F.D. Maurice's first concerns at the new Working Men's College in 1854 were lectures on God's laws and man's, as they affected health and disease. Thomas Hughes began his teaching at the College with lectures on cholera and social order.[97]

The Ladies Association for the Diffusion of Sanitary Knowledge, led by Mrs M.A. Baines, and numbering among its patrons Lord Shaftesbury, Monckton Milnes and Charles Kingsley, was launched in London in 1858. It specialised in distributing tracts. By 1861, it had distributed nearly 140,000 tracts on 'the power of soap and water'. Its sister body in Manchester issued ornamental information cards suitable for hanging on walls, 'Cottage Dwellings' and 'Clothing and Cleanliness' among them.[98] Shaftesbury helped launch the public wash-house movement in the mid-1840s, after one had been successfully created by Mrs Catherine

Wilkinson, 'a poor woman', in Liverpool in 1842. The 1850s was the
great decade for the building of such institutions by local philanthropists and corporations. Doctors, who were probably washing themselves
more often, began to complain openly during the mid-1840s that their
poor patients stank. Mr Liddle of Whitechapel remarked that the linen
of the poor smelt even after they had washed it. He could smell a poor
patient approaching the foot of the stairs of his house, he said, and had
begun necessarily to keep his door open while he treated such a patient.
The linen smelt of 'wash', the stale urine in which it had been doused,
while the poor were notorious for washing only the exposed parts of
their bodies. They worked and slept in the same clothes for weeks
at a time. The entry fee for the new public baths, 6d. at the City Road
and much the same elsewhere, was still high even for the 'middling'
classes. Some charities gave soap to deserving families, but they had
insufficient water to use it in washing themselves.[99]

The spread of piped water among the comfortable dirtied the
environment of the poor. Chadwick believed that the sale of sewage
retrieved in water-carried schemes would help amortise the costs of
installation. He himself had shares in several such companies. But in the
short run Chadwick's scheme did not eventuate this way. Human excrement proved unprofitable as agricultural manure. It was costly and
difficult to gather from the pipe system, and to transport. The sanitary
engineering was clumsy. The sewage passed untreated into the rivers
and estuaries. Dr Rumsey told the National Association for the Promotion of Social Science in 1868 that Britain's rivers had 'become much
worse in the last thirty years . . . since sewage came in'.[100] (The word
'sewage' was invented in the 1830s (*Oxford English Dictionary*) but it
became a vogue word in the later 1850s (*Blackwoods* (1859), p. 228).)
By 1857 250 tons of faecal matter was put into the Thames daily. The
River Tame in Birmingham was 'black' with the sewage of the town and
of Bilston upstream by the late 1850s, less than twenty years after the
sewage system was built. Yet the river remained the main source of
water for Birmingham. The inhabitants of Maidstone were forced to
rely again on old wells providing only 20,000 gallons a day of extremely
hard water because the Medway had become unusable by the late
1850s. The 'upper parts' of Basingstoke were drained and sewered into
the Loddon and the canal, the source of drinking-water for the people
in the 'low part'. In 1884 a woman tried to drown herself in the Irwell
at Manchester. She was fished out alive but died five days later,
poisoned, the doctors said, by the water she had swallowed.[101] Ten
years after the permissive Pollution of Rivers Act of 1876 only two

corporations had fully adopted it. There had been only 56 legal cases to
enforce its provisions and only 26 of these had succeeded: 19 of the 56
cases had indeed been prosecutions, apparently for breaches, against
sanitary authorities, the very authorities to whom the implementation
of the act was entrusted. Moreover the prosecutions had mostly been
brought in the interests of manufacturers, not citizens seeking potable
water, because the streams had become too filthy to use in industry. It
was cheaper for each local authority along the river to 'pass it on', as
the contemporary phrase went.[102] When in the early 1860s the corporation of Bristol was finally shamed into building a sewer for the lower
part of the town with its 80,000 inhabitants, it ended the sewer at the
city boundary.[103] Domestically, the aldermen and respectable members
of sanitary committees were less directly affected than one might
imagine. Their possession of servants made it possible for them to have,
without any personal exertion or noticeable expense, filtered and
boiled water or, later in the century, water with Condy's Crystals added.

During the early 1840s the going rate for a load of human and
animal sewage and household refuse carted away by farmers for manure
was 2s. 6d. This constituted 'a considerable part of the rent' for dwellers in the poorer courts. The pattern of dealing was unpleasant because
the farmers only collected the loads during the winter and spring and
left it to accumulate in the courts while they were busy at harvesting
and other jobs during the summer. It was bad luck that guano became
available as a cheaper, more manageable fertiliser during 1847. It did
not need to be pumped. Thereafter the market for human manure
collapsed. A few men with much capital and perseverance, like the Earl
of Essex, at Watford, continued to use it, but even he could only make
a profit from it at a maximum price of 1¼d. per ton. Enterprises such
as the Native Guano Company, set up to process sewage into manure,
staggered on into the late 1870s, but they proved neither efficient nor
profitable. No one knew how to disinfect and deodorise sewage cheaply
and effectively.[104]

Some of it was sold for addition to brick-making clay, with one part
refuse to five parts clay, until the practice was stopped in 1886, in
London at least. One brickfield at Streatham in 1885 'cast sickening
and pestilential odours for nearly a mile around'. The brick-maker was
prosecuted for creating a nuisance. Several members of the Wandsworth
Board of Works, the sanitary authority for the district, appeared as witnesses for the defendant, together with their surveyors and inspectors
of nuisances. All swore that the brickfield was salubrious. One Board
member owned extensive small-house property built with the defend-

ant's bricks; Labouchere's *Truth* reporter thought this was simply 'corrupt', but presumably the Board member and his colleagues also had an interest in maintaining a market for their refuse.[105]

Had the sewage market developed, it is conceivable that sanitary improvements would have spread less tardily through the poorer districts. As it was, the labouring classes in their cheap, low or unrated dwellings, loomed as an unmitigated encumbrance on the rates and a drag on sanitary progress. While the respectable citizens got WCs the poorer classes continued with unsewered privies and middens. Birmingham still had 30,000 pan privies and middens in backyards in 1898. There the men who implemented Chamberlain's improvement scheme had found it easier, during the preceding 20 years, as did improvers elsewhere, in Bradford for instance, to 'level' bad houses than sewer them.[106] One wonders who benefited from the areas of prime building land which these and similar schemes made available. One vestryman of St Luke's, London, made £8,000 out of clearances in Golden Lane carried out under the Artizans' Dwellings Act. A close examination of rate books, council minutes and parish plans, property sales and census returns, the local press and that untapped gold-mine for this sort of information, *Truth*, would give British local history writing the bite that, with a few splendid exceptions like the work of Professor H.J. Dyos and Dr J.R. Kellett, it currently lacks.[107] In Cardiff in 1858 the high north district, housing 'gentry, professional men and respectable tradesmen', was drained and paved; the east district with 'a few tradesmen, respectable mechanics and labourers' was paved but not, apparently, drained; the south, Bute Town, around the docks, was unpaved and undrained. Its courts, occupied by 'labourers', were 'frequently flooded with foetid water and cesspool soakings'. At Keighley soapsuds from the upper town mingled with the midden sewage of the lower to form an 'abomination'. The South Staffordshire Water Company finally connected all of Quarry Bank in 1882. The town was 'inching forward', the MOH reported. But the inhabitants still had no regular removal of their night soil.[108]

Some places suffered from being pioneers in sanitary reform and the heavy initial borrowings that some early schemes entailed. Nottingham had sewers for water-borne disposal, but even in 1902 these were only connected to houses 'in the better streets'. A pail system had been introduced for the rest of the town in 1868, to replace middens, but the cheap pails were wooden, and leaked. Steel pails with an effective top, though long available, only supplanted them gradually from 1901. The 'leaks' often occurred, with the resulting fouling of the nearby yard and lanes, because penny-pinching corporations in the 1890s, like Wirksworth, in Derbyshire, levied a fixed charge for each removal of the pail or emptying of the closet. The owners waited until the privy was overflowing before paying the removal charge. Gravesend, among the large towns, was still wholly dependent upon cesspool and well water in 1909.[109]

Even after local corporations moved to compel the installation of WCs, things could go awry. Reigate made such a bye-law in the mid-1890s, but after 'small builders and owners of cottage property' captured the town council, the bye-law was amended to remove the provisions for compulsory flushing. So numerous dwellings had WCs but no water connected to them. Maidstone and King's Lynn acted similarly. There was also a sound practical objection to compulsory flushing: in places like Liverpool where the water supply was cut off each day in the summer, the houses were invaded by sewer gas. This problem was not solved until the invention of a cheap sewer trap in the 1880s.[110]

Connection to the water main was still no guarantee that the WCs would be properly used and sweet. Weak bye-laws and inadequate and shoddy plumbing issued in a great deal of nastiness. Until 1862 cisterns storing water for domestic use and the WC cisterns were connected by direct pipe, because it had hitherto proved impossible to feed them effectively otherwise. In that year Mr N. Rigby, 'a bricklayer', and otherwise uncelebrated, published the first workable method of separating them.[111] He must thereby have saved more lives than many a sanitarian notable, and deserves a place in history. However, the favourite, most economical, place for the generally uncovered domestic cistern was directly above the WC and it remained so in cheaper housing at least into the 1880s. In 1887 in Dalry, an Edinburgh suburb comprising houses built since 1860, inhabited by 'well to do' artisans, an inspection of 558 cisterns supplying 870 families revealed the following: 193 were clean; 365 were 'dirty and some very foul'. Only 91 were covered. Twelve contained dead mice.[112]

At Worthing the corporation pump did the double duty of bringing the town's piped water and raising the town's sewage through the same valves and outlets.[113] The standard cheap WC in the 1870s and 1880s was the tin 'long hopper'. It corroded quickly, blocked easily and never flushed fully. Of 1,747 houses inspected in 1885 by the Jewish Sanitary Committee for the East End, 1,621 (90 per cent) had WCs which were broken or 'could not flush'. A visitation of 5,000 houses in Folkestone in 1893 revealed 2,000 WCs with inadequate flushing, leaking joints and bad ventilation. Until the early 1890s the standard

amount of water allowed for flushing was an inadeuqate two gallons.
Water companies and owners fought the increase for years. Flushing
with a buck was, they said, 'more economical' and the system did
not freeze. In 1886-7 more than half the houses of London still did not
get water on a constant supply basis; and vestries still lacked, and many
did not want, the power to order the connection of the water supply
to the WCs.[114]

Throughout the century drains were laid which did not flow, joints
were made which did not meet or were not concreted, materials were
used, crumbling brick, over-thin lead, and lightweight tin sheet, which
did not last. The City and Guilds Institute introduced courses in plumbing in 1887, to help a trade that had, as one teacher of plumbing confessed, 'sunk to a low ebb'. In 1890 an inspection of 3,000 houses in
London revealed only 36 (1 per cent) 'free from defects in plumbing
and draining'. But by 1899 still only about 20-25 men were taking the
course.[115]

Housing

Considerations about who got what from sanitary reform are also pertinent to the question of overcrowding. Fundamentally, overcrowding
was the result of population increase outrunning the increase of housing
stock and the consequent huddling of poorer communities, especially
immigrant Irish, into the cheapest accommodation they could find. Perhaps it was beyond the compass of the national economy, as it certainly
was beyond the practical imagination of the governing classes, to provide sufficient housing for the population at rates which the bulk of the
people could afford. However, 'improvement' exacerbated the problem.
In 1841, 655 people, two-fifths of them Irish, were living 24 to each
house in Church Lane, St Giles. 'Improvements' to Oxford Street in the
mid-1840s razed the accommodation of thousands. By 1848, 1,095
people were living 40 to each house, two families to every room, in
Church Lane. Of every 100 born there, 46 died at under two years.[116]
Under the Glasgow City Improvement Act of 1865, the city was
enabled to borrow £1¼ million, at a rate which started at 6*d*. in the
pound and had reduced to 2*d*. in less than ten years. The city bought
up 'quietly' £1 million worth of property for demolition. Equally
quietly, it quickly sold £400,000 worth 'at a profit'. The poor were
'moved 500 at a time', it is not clear where. Private builders were
permitted to build on some of the land at 500 years' lease. Other
'moderate' land was reserved, with pre-emptive right, for rental at 22½
years' purchase. Edinburgh copied this scheme, beginning in 1867.[117]

Chamberlain's scheme for Birmingham in 1876 involved the razing of 4,000 back-to-backs, containing 18,000 people. The houses, sceptical contemporaries remarked, were not notably insanitary, nor was there 'excessive' overcrowding. Chamberlain proposed to spend £2 millions on the project.[118] The more one ponders the economics of the plan, even allowing for contemporary hyperbole, the odder it becomes.

Lord Shaftesbury had tried unsuccessfully since 1853 to have workable provisions inserted in railway Bills to compensate people displaced by railway building. The provisions that did belatedly enter the legislation were easily evaded and reasonable compensation was rarely paid. Weekly tenants, in particular, had no legal standing whatever. Compensation for heads of households displaced by improvement orders under the Artizans' Dwellings Act was not effectively provided for until two amending Acts were passed in 1879.[119] In one representative year, 1873, over 10,000 houses were reported as demolished for railway construction in the United Kingdom, displacing a reported 57,000 people.[120] Londoners possibly suffered worst. As the MOH for Westminster explained in 1874, they could be forced to move beyond practicable walking distance from their employment because the rentals of unaffected houses nearby could rise by up to 50 per cent in expectation of the increased density of occupation. But the effect of sudden railway expansion must have been almost as severe in smaller communities. The Great Northern demolished a reported 250 homes and displaced a reported 1,500 people in Derby (total population around 70,000) in 1876. Extensions to the Post Office in Newcastle, which the 1879 legislation did not cover, drove an estimated 1,879 people out of their houses in 1890. Most could not pay the higher rents demanded elsewhere and ended up in cellars.[121] Between 1853 and 1873 the Charity Organization Society calculated from the railways' reports to Parliament that about one million people had been unhoused by them. This figure is a gross underestimate. It misses the massive dislocation caused in London before 1853 and, as Dr Kellett shows, the railways dishonestly minimised their figures. Probably the one million, which counts only heads of households, should be multiplied by four. And railways caused only a part. The greater proportion of displacement, as Dr Kellett suggests, was caused by street, housing and sanitary improvements. In another sense, as a proportion of the total population existing between say 1853 and 1900, the four millions or so is small enough to permit the argument that the railway companies and local improvers could have afforded to pay more for their resettlement.

Decisions about improvement schemes were made amidst crosscurrents of scandalous rumour, prejudice and private interest which are now all but irrecoverable. But as I suggested earlier, if we try to trace their bases we find that popular resistance to apparently admirable schemes becomes more comprehensible. When the contracting firm of Burleigh and Plowden failed in the 1880s, the mortgage brokers discovered that the contractors' books recorded payments of £200 to Knowles, the town surveyor of Accrington, 'for assistance rendered in connection with the contract', and £200 to Whittaker, the town clerk, 'for services rendered'.[122] Such outlays were probably necessary ways of cutting through the mass of local bodies with overlapping powers, vestries, lighting and paving commissions and corporation subcommittees which infested local government. Rev. Samuel Barnett complained in 1880 that a large part of his Whitechapel parish had been condemned in 1875 under the Artizans' Dwellings Act of 1875 and Torrens Housing Act of 1868, but nothing had been done. 'There were too many local authorities to whom reference was necessary before action could be taken.' The delay and confusion also enabled sharpers to make money along the way. Six sites cost the ratepayers effectively £30,000. Weekly tenants were compensated at the rate of £1 for each year of their past tenancy; a large traffic in old rent books had developed. Leaseholders also received 'abnormally high compensation'. The high compensation encouraged owners and leaseholders 'to get their property into bad order', because compensation promised more than the proceeds of a forced sale, due to proximity to condemned housing, of property in good order.[123]

In the rare instances where tenants showed some desire for improvements and had the vote, they could still be rendered politically impotent. Even in 1885 the London Court of Common Council refused to permit secret ballot: one leading opponent of the suggestion, Mr Deputy Fry, said he 'liked to hear people voting for him'. In one ward of Chelsea vestry with 3,000 voters, the election, not advertised, was held in an obscure mission hall. To meet the requirement of the Act, one announcement of the poll was posted 30 minutes before. It was placed on the inside door, upside down. Two 'outsiders', property owners, were elected, with 22 and 20 votes respectively. The market price of a municipal vote in Oxford in the 1870s and 1880s was 2s. 6d. (the price for a parliamentary one was 15s.). After the Parish Council Act of 1894, local landowners throughout the country were said to have stacked the councils with their tenants at will and employees. At Castle Combe, the election was followed by a diphtheria epidemic. Critics attributed the outbreak to the insanitary state of the place but 'influences [were] at work . . . calculated to stop the Parish Council doing anything'. R.C.K. Ensor recalled the 'cruel disillusionment' that set in when reformers found that the parish councils, with an upper rate limit of 6*d*., had no real spending power.[124]

The Great Clean-Up

Despite all, the clean-up did 'inch forward'. The rate accelerated as local bye-laws became tighter after the 1875 Act and the local MOHs finally gained both security of tenure and ancillary staff, again under the 1875 measure. Energetic doctors and their inspectors were freer of harassment and possible dismissal by their corporations. The stock of housing seems to have grown sufficiently to allow the laws against over-crowding to be enforced. In Glasgow, for example, the proportion of the population living in one-room dwellings fell between 1871 and 1891 from over 30 per cent to 18 per cent and the proportion living in three-roomed dwellings correspondingly increased, at an accelerating rate after 1881.[125] It is worth adding that the much-lauded building schemes sponsored by the Peabody Trust, Octavia Hill and others by the mid-1870s were together housing only about 26,000 persons. Their stringent qualifications for tenants admitted only the 'well to do', the teetotal, the clean and the deferential. Visitors were struck by the 'peculiarly quiet and wistful — not to say depressed — air of some of the better class of lodgers'.[126]

In Aberdeen in 1892 the authorities 'registered' 6,169 'nuisances' and had owners 'abate' over 5,500 of them. They 'removed' almost 1,000 infectious patients to hospitals, 'supervised' another 6,700 at home and fumigated a similar number of dwellings; 1,052 sets of bedding were publicly fumigated and washed, and 28½ tons of meat, fish, jam, fruit and other items were seized as unfit for consumption. By 1898 Bradford was typical of many towns in having only the origi-nal insanitary core of 22,000 square yards, containing 7 streets, centred on Longlands Streets, still resisting improvement. The core contained 1,357 people, equalling 301 per acre, against an average of 21 for the whole city. The people were still grossly overcrowded and averaged 15 persons to every WC. The death rate for the city was 42.7 per 1,000; for Longlands Street, 69.9 per 1,000. The MOH called for the area to be levelled. He did not say where the displaced people were to go.[127]

In 1890, after a decade of rising death rates from scarlet fever and typhoid fever, the town council and colleges in Cambridge finally agreed to clean up the Cam and implement a water supply and sewer-age plan. But it was a near-run thing and skirmishes continued about their respective shares of the total costs. Gateshead, between 1882 and 1911, belatedly used its powers under the Common Lodging Houses Act of 1851 and other subsequent legislation to 'close' 362 tenement rooms and halve the number of lodgers.[128] The mechanism by which this was achieved needs further research but presumably 'closing' some rooms raised the rent of the remainder and thereby gradually closed the town to itinerants.

The water carriage of sewage was finally introduced throughout Leicester around 1890, after a decade of rising death rates and agitation by sanitarians. Some poorer towns still skimped on the engineering and construction costs. It seems that the authorities of Lowestoft built their main sewer outfall in 1896 so that it stopped short at high tide mark: the outfall was blocked by sand for 17 hours every day and the incidence of enteric fever and diphtheria had worsened. The poorer inhabitants used the failure as an excuse to retain their privy middens. By the mid-1890s, only the ten poorest wards of Middlesbrough remained dependent on the old polluted Tees water. Enteric fever, which had become rare elsewhere in the town, was still endemic in the ten wards. They were the unsewered and unscavenged parts of the town, but the MOH believed that an equally important cause was the defective nature of the sewers carrying the excreta of the sewered 10 per cent of the town. At times of high spring tide or heavy rainfall the sewage was dammed back from the sea and flowed into the cellars and yards of the ten wards. Almost 10 per cent of their houses recorded enteric fever cases in 1896, against 1.62 per cent in the sewered houses.[129] The process of paving, draining, sewering and bringing piped water to all the inhabitants, rich and poor, in Merthyr Tydfil took thirty years, beginning with the rich in 1855. Over the period the infant death rate fell by nearly half; typhoid mortality fell from 2.1 per 1,000 to 0.3 per 1,000, and the average age at death had risen from 17½ to 27½. The cottages of the labouring classes were still damp, the MOH admitted, but drainage had 'dried out' the place and made life much more comfortable, as it must have done elsewhere in Britain.

South Shields, which had long proved resistant to improvement schemes, acquiesced in the notification of infectious diseases in 1891, although the authorities still blocked the doctors' call to build an isolation hospital. Insanitary property was being levelled and a 'number of abominable midden privies abolished'. Between 1872 and 1889 West Bromwich had an average of 63 deaths from scarlet fever every year. In 1906 there were five. During the intervening period the town had acquired: a piped water supply, instead of half the population relying on polluted wells; deep drainage, instead of free run-offs into the Tame; a mortuary; notification of disease; an isolation hospital; inspection of food and milk. Next on the programme for improvement, the MOH announced in 1907, were the privy middens which persisted in the poorer parts of the town.[130]

In 1856 the parish of St Olave's, Southwark, had only one stand-pipe at which the people queued for hours, armed with dirty receptacles. Otherwise they depended upon open water butts in the yards of their dwellings. The privies were open pits, the drains were untrapped, the streets were unpaved, backyards were sodden and dirty, scavenging was irregular. After '30 years of effort' by the MOH and the local authorities, filtered water was piped to a covered cistern in every house, every closet had water connection and was trapped, 700 cesspools had been demolished, the drains to every house were trapped, the yards of the houses were paved, as were the streets, dustbins were 'general, and emptied regularly', and houses could be disinfected. The mortality from 'fever' had fallen from 4.3 per 1,000 in 1856-66, to 3.2 per 1,000 in 1867-76, to 2.0 per 1,000 in 1877-87. Dr Vinen, the MOH, was justifiably proud. Inner London had over 250 public drinking-fountains supplying filtered water by the 1890s, and in 1898 there were proposals to provide public lavatories for women, a boon males had enjoyed since the 1850s.

The worst overcrowding and abominations in water supplies and disposal of sewage probably continued longest in the rural parishes, powerless to raise the capital to improve things and beyond the reach of MOHs and Local Government Board Inspectors. Helmsley in 1909 still had dwellings constructed of thatch draped along the branches of trees.[131]

As this brief survey indicates, the domestic supply of water in Britain did not become safe, uninterrupted and near-universal until the later 1890s. In Liverpool between 1896 and 1905 over 100,000 more inhabitants, or one-sixth of the total, received mains water; in Manchester, over 400,000, or two-thirds of the population, between 1897 and 1908; in St Helen's the number supplied rose from 56,000 in 1880 to 85,000 in 1897 to 98,000 (almost 100 per cent) in 1908; in Sheffield, too, the whole town was effectively supplied by 1906. This decade also saw a prodigious increase in water consumption, over 100 per cent in Wallasey, for instance, and around 70 per cent in Manchester. As one informed commentator remarked: 'taps have become common in cottages . . . instead of stand-pipes'.[132]

At about this time commentators remarked among the labouring classes a change of attitude towards sanitary reform. Dr John Glaister reported in 1888 that householders had ceased to regard the sanitary department and 'sanitary police'

> on a footing with the school board officer with regard to their troublesomeness. The tendency then [until about 1880] was rather to thwart than assist the sanitary department. Now . . . the occupants of a tenement willingly inform the sanitary officials of the existence of an infectious disease.

The common people, he said, had become less 'careless' about disease, dirty wash-houses and WCs. Among these classes the greater accessibility of safe water and food had for the first time made the pursuit of health rationally possible. Moreover, Glaister believed that the spread of compulsory elementary education had increased the value parents put upon their children and encouraged parents to guard them from infection; 'Children are the wealth of a workingman in respect that when they have passed the Fifth Standard they become wage-earning.' If the children caught an infectious disease they might miss an examination and thereby lose a whole year.[133]

The doctors, the professional men, the middle-class ladies, the public-spirited aldermen, the radical artisans, the crusading clergymen and journalists who comprised the sanitary movement achieved the great clean-up against the odds. In 1803 the average local rate had been 4*s*. 5¼*d*., according to the Local Government Board. At the end of the Napoleonic Wars this had fallen to 3*s*. 10¾*d*. By 1868 the ratepayers had reduced it to 3*s*. 4*d*. and, by 1892, it was still only 3*s*. 8*d*. The total 'local government' debt of England in 1892 was £200 million, the largest single item of which was expenditure on water supply, at £38 million, with 'public improvements − mostly sanitary' next at £29 million, and then sewerage, at £20 million. It is reasonable to suggest that it could and should have been much larger. Britain is estimated to have spent £120 million on the American War of Independence and £600 million on the war against France. That £200 million in 1892, at about one-sixth of the national income, is a much smaller proportion of the national wealth than that which a less developed economy afforded for war a hundred years earlier. Sanitary improvement could also have been implemented less tardily and patchily: the sum annually borrowed for such works did not exceed £1 million until 1870.[134]

Cholera

Expenditure might well have been more prompt and lavish had the three great 'dirt' diseases among adults, Asiatic cholera, typhus and typhoid, been less specific to the lower orders and been seen by middle-class contemporaries to be so. Cholera appeared as a dramatic visitation upon the nation in 1831-2, 1848-9, 1853-4 and 1866. The first and the last epidemics, especially, coincided with times of economic depression and political disturbance. On each occasion, too, cholera arrived during seasons of increased general sickness and epidemics of scarlet fever and typhus.

In an age when many people believed in ascribing untoward events to the intervention of Providence, clergymen found a new opportunity to declare divine interest. In 1832 Bishop Blomfield warned his royal congregation on the national fast day that the cholera was a sign to the great in the land 'to increase the comforts and improve the moral character of the masses'. The Reverend Dr McNeale told his hearers in Gloucester in 1849 that cholera was a judgement on the country 'for favouring Popery'. At Leicester, the Reverend Mr Gutch 'attributed it to parliamentary electors voting for Dissenters and Jews, instead of Church of England men', while the Reverend Theophilus Toye of St Stephen's, Gateshead, assured his flock that cholera had been sent 'to deter people from marrying the sisters of their deceased wives'. The radical editor of *Reynolds's Political Instructor* took a more mundane and pertinent, if no less moralising view: 'We . . . fancy that cholera was a natural malady, terribly aggravated by the scandalous, cruel and heartless neglect, shown by the government, and the upper classes generally, towards the dwellings, wants, interests, and health of the poor.'[135]

Cholera killed quickly and nastily. It is a transient disease, affecting the sodium pump mechanism of the intestinal cell, and allowing the damaging loss of body fluid into the bowel. People die of sudden dehydration, shrivelled like raisins with blackened extremities, pale, staring, pouring watery fluid from their bowel on to the place where they lie. But if they survive, recovery is said to be rapid. When Asiatic cholera first spread in Great Britain in 1831-2, over 31,000 deaths were ascribed to 'cholera and diarrhoea', in 1848-9 about 62,000, in 1853-4 about 31,000, and in 1866 about 15,000. There are no well founded records of the numbers attacked. Cholera in recent outbreaks, when untreated, had a case-mortality rate of between 40 and 60 per cent and it seems reasonable to estimate the number seized during the nineteenth century on this basis. Excepting the fourth epidemic, cholera killed slightly more males than females and had its worst fatality rates among adults over 45. In 1866 deaths among females outnumbered those of males and the mortality among infants rose by 10 per cent.[136]

In each epidemic the working classes and poor were over-represented among the victims, by comparison with the middle and upper classes. In some places, such as Liverpool in 1866, the disease was virtually restricted to the poorer and topographically lower quarters of the town. Farr's table for London vividly illustrates the difference in life chances between the West and East Ends (see Table 4.3).

Table 4.3: Deaths by Cholera by 10,000 Living, London

	1849	1853-4	1866
All London average	62	46	18
Bermondsey	161	179	6
St George, Southwark	164	121	1
Newington	144	112	3
Rotherhithe	205	165	9
Kensington	24	38	4
St George, Hanover Square	18	33	2
St Martin-in-the-Fields	37	20	5
St James, Westminster	16	142	5

Source: William Farr, *Vital Statistics*, p. 384.

The West Enders were supplied with relatively safe water obtained upstream; the East Enders were drinking water fouled by their wealthy up-river fellow citizens as well as themselves. The East End suppliers, the Lambeth Company and Southwark Water-Works, until 1854 took their water from below Westminster Bridge and near London Bridge respectively.[137]

It is interesting that the over-representation of the poor parishes declined relatively faster with each outbreak than the rate of the West End. It would be a worthwhile research job to discover *who* contracted the disease in the West End.

At Hull, the town worst hit by the 1849 epidemic, with over 2,000 deaths among a population of 80,000, the topographically and socially lower Old Town and Myton had a mortality rate of 241 per 10,000, compared with Sculcoates, the wealthy suburb, with 152 per 10,000. One observer calculated that the 1,738 deaths among the 'labouring classes' comprised one in 38 among them, compared with the 122 deaths among the 'well off', or one in 106.[138]

Cholera is transmitted in drinking-water or food contaminated by the faeces of persons who have contracted the disease or who have very recently recovered from it. It is not normally a 'carrier' disease. It follows that it could only (before effective immunisation became widely available in the 1920s) be eradicated by adequate sanitation. The difficulty for doctors and administrators working to confine outbreaks was that until 1866, their ruling theories of the aetiology of disease prevented their proceeding effectively. Old-fashioned adherents of humoral-Brownian pathology believed in a muddled sort of way that the disease was generated on bodies which had been misused. 'Experience proves', the Edinburgh Board of Health reported, 'that notorious drunkards were numerous among the victims.' Dr Proudfoot, of Kendal, thought it 'remarkable' that cholera was nearly confined to the 'intemperate, the old and infirm, and poor . . . half-starved children . . . worn-out prostitutes'.[139] The bodies, especially the blood or, on other principles derived from Cullen, the nerves, of these wretched people had little resistance to the miasmata generated from stagnant water conveying the exhalations of putrefying animal or vegetable substances. In special climatic conditions, some miasmatists like Dr Southwood Smith believed the miasma could transform normally mild, infrequent fevers into epidemic killers. If these exciting substances were absorbed into the blood they were carried to the heart, brain and nerves and either poisoned these organs directly or induced further putrefaction and thence poisoning, or they affected the nerves to a degree that totally disturbed the mechanisms of the body and thereby induced vomiting, diarrhoea and the other symptoms. Moreover, contagionists believed in a more thoroughgoing way than the younger miasmatists that contagion, the communication of disease from the sick to the healthy by direct contact, was the chief means by which epidemics generated. The new men, Southwood Smith, Chadwick, Dr Neil Arnott and other Benthamite political economists, had by the late 1830s become thoroughgoing mechanists. They projected a closed circle of causation which avoided the moral questions of deprivation and redistribution. They argued that the 'source of high mortality incites' was '*not* due to want of food and greater misery . . . but in the generation of effluvial poisons'. This conveniently narrow doctrine was to be influential for the next hundred years, and beyond.[140]

Contagionists and miasmatists and those who accepted both theories were agreed that the indications for preventive action were to contain the probably noxious exhalations of the victim by his thorough isolation,

and removal of the stagnant water and decaying matter which furnished
the poisoned — or potentially poisonous — miasmata. Some local
authorities, like those in Exeter, sought to purge the exhalation by
burning barrels of tar in the streets, or as in Oxford, adding chloride of
lime to the sewers and the water supply. Several authorities, from
Exeter to Edinburgh, set about removing the putrefying vegetable and
animal matter. Others, like the Board of Health in Cheltenham in 1832,
stationed constables at the outskirts to turn away mangy-looking
itinerants. Private individuals could protect themselves against contagion
by being discriminate in their mingling in public, and preserving their
constitution by temperance and careful regimen, by avoiding vegetables,
for instance.[141]

The authorities resorted to these procedures for the first three epidemics and many people observed them still in 1866. But during this
last outbreak, isolation of patients, and careful disposal of their dejecta,
the boiling of the water and strict national quarantine came into their
own. Thereafter the Asian epidemics which spread through the European Continent in 1873, 1884-6 and 1892-3 were repulsed by a British
quarantine applied sufficiently reasonably as not to provoke evasion,
and never entered Britain.[142] Perhaps Britain was lucky, too. The advice
about prophylaxis issued to the public by the Royal College of Physicians during the cholera threat of 1892 was not essentially different
from that issued in 1831. It was a case of professional men talking to
their upper- and middle-class comrades, oblivious of the masses. The
house, the RCP declared, must be 'clean, light, thoroughly dry and well-
ventilated'. Its inhabitants must eat each day three or four 'nourishing
and ample meals', but avoiding soup and cheese, as 'indigestible'. Alcoholic beverages were permissible in moderation, but 'sparkling wines
were to be shunned, as well as over-fatigue, emotional excitement and
undue mental strain'. Regular exercise was also advised, 'early hours'
and the pursuit of 'an occupied and tranquil life'. This is sensible advice
for those who could afford to follow it, but it hardly bears on cholera.
Forty years after Dr John Snow had demonstrated that cholera was
conveyed by contaminated water and nine years after Koch had identified the micro-organism which caused it, the RCP still gave no special
warnings about care in handling the patient and his dejecta or about
boiling water intended for the household: the two procedures the masses
could best follow.[143]

Formal medical understanding of the aetiology of cholera was
blocked by two assumptions which had prevailed since classical times:
that 'fever' was a generalised form of disease and that it was static, even

spontaneously generated — in the putrefying matter, in the air, through-out the whole environment. Snow's marvellously elegant epidemiological demonstration of the specificity of cholera attacks and the dynamic nature of its transmission ran athwart these notions. Snow and his great contemporary, Dr William Budd, had grasped the central points about specificity but, working before Pasteur and germ culture, they were unable to prove their hypotheses. The *Lancet*, still intermittently radical, and the conservative RCP both condemned the new theories. The *Lancet* dismissed Budd's

> uncertain speculations, based upon the detection of the fungoid bodies . . . [as the] local cause of cholera . . . That in their growth they abstract the fluid parts of the blood to themselves, and thus cause the rice-water evacuations. Their special habitat he believes to be the human intestine, and water their chief mode of diffusion.

The *Lancet* editorialist used as a point against Budd's theory his inability to suggest a method of destroying the 'fungous growth' in patients' evacuations, other than the unconvincing proposal that the evacuation be doused in solutions of chloride of zinc. One 'ingenious Correspondent', the editorialist scoffed, 'indeed suggests that . . . it would be well to try the internal exhibition of fluid containing quantities of animalculae which . . . destroy minute fungi with the greatest rapidity'.[144]

The cholera subcommittee of the RCP, comprising William Gull and William Baly, both destined to be physicians to the Queen, reported in 1849 that they could not find Budd's bodies in water or in the air and concluded they were 'not the cause of cholera'. The 'whole theory . . . which has recently been propounded [was] erroneous'. Their report stopped there: they made no suggestions for future research.

Indeed, Snow's and Budd's emphasis on water as the transmitter reinforced the faith in miasmic propagation among otherwise radical-thinking potential allies. Dr Alison in Edinburgh argued that Budd's proof that the rice-water stools were 'poisonous' reinforced the need for control of water quality. Snow's explanation in 1855 that the 'specific morbid poison' had to be swallowed was rejected by the editors of the *Edinburgh Medical Journal*, because Snow and Budd had earlier 'supposed' that cholera had been spread among people after it had been 'extruded by the people using the same privy'. No one drank from the privy. Moreover, the act of individual swallowing of the poison appeared as a totally inadequate, even irrelevant, explanation of the survival unscathed of persons who had drunk contaminated water, and of the sudden rise and decline of epidemics. Snow's brilliant observation against the miasmic theory, that miners who shared water and did not wash their hands and nurses attending cholera victims caught cholera, while visitors to cholera patients, who drank nothing and washed their hands before they left, did not, passed unnoticed. Official opinion only accepted in 1866 after his death his view of the ingestion of a specific micro-organism.[145]

Even then, official understanding was right for the wrong reasons. The first generation of sanitarians had effectively captured radical medical opinion in 1838, when the *Lancet* embraced the formulations of Drs Neil Arnott and Southwood Smith that the higher mortality in cities resulted not from 'greater misery' but from 'effluvial poisons'. Their disciples, William Farr and Dr John Webster, between 1849 and 1855 calculated elaborate correlations between height above sea level and the incidence of cholera. During 1849 the mortality rate, in places under 20 feet above sea level, at 102 per 10,000 population, was one-third above the average mortality at 62 per 10,000. Taking the epidemics of 1849 and 1853-4 together, the mortality on the lower London ground was 15 per 1,000 population and 1 per 1,000 on the highest. Farr believed that his findings explained the two weaknesses in the Snow-Budd argument. First, that persons who ingested the poison but 'resisted its influence' must have absorbed poison of a lower 'concentration' than that which affected their neighbours who became sick. The 'concentration' was related to the amount of organic matter in the surrounding air, water and earth and this amount increased as the ground became lower. It followed then that 'although *elevation of habitation, with purity of air and purity of water, does not shut out the cause of cholera, it reduces its effect to insignificance*' (original italics). The fact that half the total deaths in 1849 occurred in seaport districts was now explicable; although Farr added that the mortality in lowland areas of Lincolnshire, Cambridgeshire and Northamptonshire was puzzlingly low.[146]

Farr's work inaugurated years of worthless speculation about the relation between the concentration of water in soil, water-tables and the incidence of cholera. There were several competing theories, the showiest of which was that promulgated by the Prussian Max von Pettenkofer, which was espoused in the 1860s by John Simon, the Medical Officer to the Privy Council, and George Rolleston, Linacre Professor of Anatomy and Physiology at Oxford. Pettenkofer renovated the miasmatic theory by asserting that the distribution of cholera mortality varied with the porosity of the subsoil and the height of the water-table. The higher the water-table, the worse the cholera. Pettenkofer and Rolleston based their argument on reports from India. But as Florence Nightingale robustly remarked, their theory hardly explained cholera outbreaks in villages in arid areas. Florence Nightingale and Edwin Chadwick have been mocked by historians for their hostility to 'scientific' research on cholera. But they were right in their estimate that in 1871 the urgent need was '*not to know but to do*' (original italics). In the short — or not so short — run it was the improvement of the water supply and domestic habits which mattered, not high laboratory investigations; or in von Pettenkofer's and Rolleston's cases, high theory based on false — and rather obviously false — information.[147]

There was no cure for cholera in the nineteenth century. Professional and lay treatment were much the same and varied little between 1831 and 1866. W. Price Evans, an obscure surgeon in Swansea, had suggested in 1849 that the injection of saline solution was of prime importance in repairing the loss of fluid and salts from the body, but his suggestion seems not to have received the attention it deserved, or even to have been properly tested.[148] The doctors' object was to clear the intestines of the morbid agent or action, activate the circulation and calm the febrile state. Thus the dosage comprised a purgative, aloes, castor oil with calomel and a sedative, opium. The procedure at the Glasgow Royal Infirmary in 1849 was representative: they 'tried calomel, alcohol, opium, castor oil, saline', yet two in every three patients died. Dr Buchanan's reminiscences of the Infirmary's procedures illustrate the incoherence of even the best medical opinion and indicate why surgeon Price Evans's suggestion could pass unremarked: 'What we did notice was, that after a few weeks, when the disease had killed off the more susceptible patients, it became less fatal.' The less susceptible subjects, he noted with some puzzlement, seemed to recover quickest 'under the simple treatment of keeping the patient clean, dry warmth, and sips of milk'. St Bartholomew's admitted 200 patients into special wards. They tried the saline plan, but it 'failed'. Their 'best results' came with an 'emetic of sulphate of zinc' 'repeated quickly'. St Thomas's administered enemas of turpentine and olive oil, and gave 'wine, brandy and tea ad libitum', with a 'mustard poultice, of course'. The authorities at Guy's refused to admit cholera patients in 1849, believing the disease to be contagious. The 'clerks' of the hospital worked among the out-patients giving 'opium . . . judiciously, but fearlessly'.[149]

The authors of popular herbal manuals were equally baffled. They recommended large doses of opium, rhubarb mixed with water and tincture of prickly ash berries, an aromatic shrub (*Aralia spinosa*, the 'tooth-ache tree'). 'Inject in ordinary quantity until the desired effect has been produced.' Private middle-class individuals were as eclectic as the professionals. In 1848 Samuel Palmer armed himself against the onset of the disease with home-made pills, each composed of Arabian specific (gum Arabic), 2 grains of opium, 2 grains of assafoetida, and 2 grains of black pepper. He intended to swallow each with a spoonful of brandy and water. He also got tapes ready, to apply as ligatures 'just above both knees and elbows – to keep [the] blood from rushing to the extremities'. He intended, too, to observe the official medical warning against perambulating near the Serpentine because of the 'noxious effluvia reeking from its lovely ripples'. Miners and iron-workers used brandy as a specific: bottles were taken to funerals of cholera victims and circulated.[150]

These illustrations of the defencelessness of the people almost lead us to expect that the ravages of cholera might have been greater than they were. But the manner of its transmission confined its attacks to localities, where it could be devastating. At Bilston, the place worst hit during the 1831-2 epidemic, there were 742 deaths among 3,568 cases in a population of 14,500. Four hundred and fifty children were left parentless. At Peahen Court, housing 150 people in 1849, there were seven deaths in one day, leaving seven orphans. After the epidemic in Bradford there were 27 new widows or widowers and 82 orphans, at Leeds, 35 widows or widowers and 73 orphans, at Lambeth, 81 widows or widowers and 234 orphans. Over 500 people who lived in an area only a few hundred yards square around the infamous Broad Street pump died within ten days. Old people living alone suffered during the epidemic and its aftermath. They had been relatively immune during the outbreak because their neighbours ceased to fetch water for them. After the outbreak there must have been few to fetch anything for them. In 1854 the disruption to the community in Soho resulting from deaths and from bereaved people moving away was sufficient to wreck Dr Joseph Rogers's medical practice. The plight of the orphans left by the 1866 outbreak impelled Dr Barnardo into his home mission crusade.[151]

Even so, cholera never ravaged Britain as severely as Continental countries, and it departed a generation earlier. French, Italian and Russian methods of combating the disease were much more desperate, barbaric and ineffective. In 1832 Paris had more deaths in one week in April (5,523) than London had in the whole year (5,275). It seems reasonable to speculate that this reflects an absolute difference in the general standards of well-being between the two populations, and the much fiercer purging and dirtier nursing to which the French sick were commonly subjected. In 1866 only the East End of London, at a death rate of 65 per 10,000, exceeded the reported rates of Paris, 39 per 10,000, Vienna, 51 per 10,000, Naples, 51 per 10,000, Rotterdam and The Hague, 107 per 10,000, and Brussels, 163 per 10,000. Even in 1892 the Russian and Italian authorities were still resorting to pleas to Heaven and to highly arbitrary and highly ineffective police quarantine, impregnating the clothes (of those who could not bribe at least) with hydrogen sulphide gas, and fumigating travellers with nitrous acid gas.[152]

Typhus and Relapsing Fevers

Typhus comprises a group of acute infections caused by species of the micro-organism *Rickettsia*. It is passed in the faecal dust of lice, which have earlier fed upon an infected human being. The dust can enter the human body through scratches on the skin, through the conjunctiva, or by inhalation. Consequently the new victim does not need to be lousy to catch the disease. Relapsing fever is also transmitted to man through lice. Some authorities hold that the organisms belonging to the genus *Borrelia*, causing the disease, remain in the louse and are trans-ferred to the host only when the structure of the louse is damaged by crushing or scratching, thereby allowing the louse's body fluid to exude on to the skin. The spirochaetes of relapsing fever distribute in the body of the louse but do not kill it and the organisms do not appear in the louse's faeces. It would follow that victims of relapsing fever were more likely to be infested with fleas. These possibly distinct modes of transmission bear on the differential class impact of the diseases. Now-adays louse-borne typhus is distinguished clinically from the other typhus fevers by its epidemic nature. Those who recover are generally immune. But in the nineteenth century the typhus fevers were endemic. This situation is especially important in the case of relapsing fever be-cause immunity after an attack lasts for only about two years and re-infection can be common.

Louse-borne (epidemic) typhus is the more fatal disease. After an incubation period of 6-15 days the symptoms begin to appear — head-ache, running nose, cough, nausea and chest pains. In a few days these symptoms are followed by high fever, chills, vomiting and bowel up-sets, muscular aching and perhaps delirium or stupor. A red rash may appear on the trunk and spread to the arms and legs. The symptoms subside after about two weeks. Fatal cases, seemingly overall about one in four in the nineteenth century, are often associated with pneumonia and heart disease. These latter two conditions help explain the higher than average case-mortality rate among the middle-aged and elderly.

Relapsing fever begins with a high fever, chills, headache, muscle aches, nausea and vomiting. The attack lasts about two to three days, after which the symptoms disappear during a crisis accompanied by severe sweating and a rapid fall in body temperature. This crisis often destroys elderly people, when the respiratory system and heart collapse. After three to four days the symptoms return. The cycle can continue for up to ten attacks. The disease is very debilitating.[153]

Typhus, 'fever' (including probably various forms of meningitis, etc.) and typhoid fever were not distinguished in the Registrar-General's returns until 1869. The traditional names for typhus, 'putrid fever', 'ship fever', 'gaol fever', all known from at least the mid-eighteenth century, suggest that epidemics were common from at least that time. In the early nineteenth century, there were major outbreaks in 1801, 1812, and most notably during the depression of 1816-19, an outbreak that was said to have begun among 'poor Irish' in Saffron Hill.[154] There were further visitations in the economically depressed, and sickly, years of 1837-8, 1847, 1855, 1862-3 and 1866. Nearly 19,000 people in England and Wales were reported to have died from typhus in 1837-8, and over 17,000 in 1847. In 1869 there were 4,281 deaths from typhus in England and Wales and 2,059 in Scotland. Thereafter a rapid decline set in until 1878, when the number of deaths fell below 1,000 in England and Wales and under 300 in Scotland. By 1886 there were under 250 deaths in England and Wales and fewer than 85 in Scotland. The disease lingered on to the First World War but, at home at least, was never a major killer again.[155]

In 1817 Dr C. Chisholm, the Senior Physician to the Clifton Dispensary, investigated the incidence of typhus deaths in Bristol. He was puzzled by the fact that the 'upper, more salubrious parts of Clifton' had 16 cases between 1813 and 1816 while the 'lower Hot Wells area' had none. He drew the inference that 'filth, etc., are not the causes of typhus, but that it proceeded from a specific virus introduced'. Chisholm confessed himself the more puzzled by this inference because he knew that typhus accompanied times of scarcity, as in 1795 and 1799. But again, it seemed it was not simple privation or the consumption of 'corrupted' food that brought infection, but 'the superinduction of infection, to which, under such distressful circumstances, the poor are more exposed'. And yet there still remained the bafflingly high incidence of typhus among the wealthy and in burgeoning manufacturing towns. Chisholm postulated that the 'unnatural' way of life which inhabitants led in manufacturing towns, disposed to the generation of 'that unknown virus, a poison, called typhus infection', whilst in commercial towns the bustling 'more natural' condition of life enabled the inhabitants to preserve a balance in their systems and throw off useless and potentially injurious bodily secretions. Sloth and 'despondency' among both the wealthy and the indigent might also induce typhus.[156]

The uneven incidence of typhus continued to worry doctors until its decline in the 1870s. Mr John Hiley, a surgeon of Elland, noticed in 1841 that during the fierce winter of 1840 typhus attacked rich and poor alike, but only killed the poor. He attributed the spread of the disease to the spread of railways: the badness of trade had forced otherwise healthy respectable men to become navvies and mix with the typhus-ridden Irish. By 1853 the Metropolitan Association for Improving the Dwellings of the Industrious Classes declared that typhus was 'pre-eminently the disease of the adult, the well-nourished, and the strong', and therefore could only result from '*filth*'. In six years the Association's tenants had not experienced typhus death.[157]

The concentration of relapsing fever among the poor could be more easily brought within the miasmic theory. Whether 'intermittent' fever developed into 'typhus' depended upon the degree of concentration of the poisonous miasma and the condition of the body at the time of the concentration. The concentrated effluvium was strongest in damp, crowded, ill-ventilated, dirty habitations. In these topographically low aggregations, the poor huddled; their 'dissipated habits' left their bodies weak and open to 'contagion'. Nurses, even respectable cleanly ones, were often carried off; presumably they suffered from the offensive odours of the patients' evacuations in close rooms. Unlike most other zymotic killers, typhus was a winter disease.[158]

In 1868 Dr R. Beveridge analysed the cost of an outbreak between 1863 and 1866 in Aberdeen. He noted that the incidence had risen during each winter, that women and, unusually, children suffered worse than males, and that the malady moved irregularly through the city, 'regulated more by the density of population than anything else'. He estimated, in a startling insight into the impact of a comparatively small epidemic on working-class families, that the immediate costs for support of widows and orphans occasioned by the death of heads of families was over £39,000. The total immediate charge to the Aberdeen community was over £55,000 or a tax of 15*s*. per head. His message was that preventive slum clearance and rehousing were kinder to rate-payers than the usual sequence of neglect and catastrophe.[159]

The reforms worked, if again for the wrong reasons. The diminution of overcrowding, provision of water for personal cleanliness, more strict control of common lodging-houses and a more regular food supply do seem to have reached a critical point during the early 1870s and to have overcome the lice which carried the diseases. Perhaps the post-famine recovery in Ireland helped, too, by lessening the flow into Britain of diseased itinerants; although it is significant in this respect that Liverpool was the last British redoubt of typhus and relapsing fever, until the close of the century.[160]

Fever Hospitals

The spread and increase in capacity of fever hospitals may also have helped diminish these zymotics, less by curing patients than by removing them, as continuing sources of infection, from their neighbourhoods. The provincial general hospitals did not admit typhoid sufferers before the twentieth century and the London hospitals only began to do so, as private paying patients, in the 1880s.[161] Yet even as isolation shelters the fever hospitals cannot have had a great impact. The actual numbers of cases they could handle remained very small throughout the century. The Manchester Fever Hospital was established in 1796 on the initiative of Dr John Ferriar after typhus epidemics in 1789-90 and 1794. Up to 1806 it handled around 440 patients a year, at an average death rate of one in nine. In 1818 the London House of Recovery had 69 beds and admitted almost 800 patients, with a death rate of one in 12.[162] The hospitals remained at around this size until the 1880s, when the new burst of building isolation hospitals began. Moreover, difficulties about diagnosis meant that the patient had to be into the sequence of symp-toms and well past the earlier lice-ridden infection stages before he was taken to hospital. The patients who really needed hospitalisation, the indigent and Poor Law patients, rarely got to the big fever hospitals because their Unions refused the fees the hospitals had to charge. The London Fever Hospital in the 1840s, for example, charged the Lambeth Union ten guineas a year, but if the Lambeth guardians sought to send more than ten patients a year they were charged an additional guinea per patient. The Lambeth Union ceased to send patients in 1844 and so thereafter the fever cases 'remained in their miserable abodes'. White-chapel was still refusing to send patients in 1864.[163]

Fever hospitals were unpromising objects for charitable support and until the 1860s, at least, ratepayers could easily block the spending of public moneys on what they regarded as essentially private charitable ventures on behalf of the lower orders. Even after the Sanitary Act of 1866 cleared the way for local borrowing to create such institutions there was never enough money for grandiose building projects. As Dr Perry lamented in 1844, funds for proper hospitals would never be forthcoming 'until some serious epidemic, such as typhus fever, has made such progress . . . as to commence its ravages among the upper classes'.[164] Typhus and relapsing fever remained too visibly specific to the lower classes for this ever to happen. Most hospitals even had trouble conveying their patients from their homes. There was a continued outcry against using public conveyances, but no hospital could afford to provide its own fever carriage until the early 1860s. The London Fever Hospital purchased such a vehicle in 1862, but had no funds for horses or a coachman. The hospital solved the problem some time in the late 1860s by employing paupers from the Westminster Union to pull the 'fever carriage' the three miles up the hill to the hospital at Hampstead. The paupers, who got 6*d.* a trip, arrived 'exhausted'. When questions were asked about the practice in the House of Commons, Goschen, President of the Poor Law Board, replied that the men liked the outing.[165]

Nearly all fever hospitals remained as wards of general hospitals set apart in sheds in the grounds, or as temporary structures and warehouses, erected or requisitioned during epidemics. Their very impermanence doubtless made them relatively safer places than the well endowed, solid, long-standing general hospitals their advocates envied. The poor hated being forced to enter the fever hospitals. Many institutions, like that at Reading (a small house with two beds) charged fees. The poor preferred to hide their fever cases and so evade possible eviction during fumigation and the loss of the breadwinners' jobs if the news went around that there was fever at home. The hospitals had a justified reputation as death-traps, the patients were cut off from their families and friends, the wards were cold (doctors believed that a 'free circulation of air,' lessened contagion) and the patients were peremptorily managed by underpaid, frightened and callous nurses. Such hospitals found it difficult to attract and hold staff and Sairey Gamp types persisted in fever hospitals after they had been cleared out of the big general institutions. The fever hospital at Ince Blundell, in Lancashire, was staffed solely by an infirm woman of 60 and her husband, aged 55. They were neglectful and could not cope with delirious patients: in 1887 a typhoid sufferer overlaid and smothered her child (who apparently was not in hospital as a patient) beside her in the bed. The Dover Fever Hospital still had no trained nurses in 1895. The medical officer was over 80 and lived miles away: he rarely visited. Patients died there unattended.[166]

In the larger, more efficient fever hospitals the patient was washed on admittance, often had her hair shaved off, and her clothes burned. If she had typhus, this treatment would not have saved her: further lice bites are harmless to the patient once infection has occurred; but the procedure probably saved sufferers from other diseases in the wards. At times of epidemic patients were crowded in three or four to a bed, despite the belief that the concentration of sufferers from the same disease intensified the virulence of the malady. Wealthy people who caught an infectious disease would not enter hospitals: their 'feelings were against it'[167] and they could be isolated at home.

The nurses were right to be afraid. The overcrowding and lack of effective antisepsis and fumigation in the wards meant that at the London Fever Hospital between 1861-70, for instance, there were 179 attacks and 42 deaths among the nurses and staff. In 1882 during a typhus outbreak in Newcastle-upon-Tyne, of 14 nurses engaged in tending cases at the infectious diseases hospital, nine contracted the disease and two died.[168]

Infectious diseases were not a popular study among doctors, until the 1880s at least. Doctors correctly regarded them as personally dangerous and socially degrading in that their incidence was highest among the lower orders. Their armoury did not equip them to fight the disease. They devoted much time to consulting about the initial diagnosis: pontificating upon technicalities and possibilities to the victim's friends preserved a doctor's standing and helped mask the real difficulties in diagnosis, especially in distinguishing typhus from typhoid and relapsing fever. Regardless of which fever it turned out to be, the regimen the doctor ordered was the same. Until the 1870s the fever had to be 'reduced' by bleeding, leeching and cupping, a low diet and '*strict confinement to bed*' in a darkened room, to lessen muscular exertion. The bowels had to be regulated with a mild purgative; mercury and chalk, followed by castor oil, was a common prescription. 'When the above precautions are observed', Dr Barlow remarked, 'the greater number of cases, in persons of sound constitution, will generally recover spontaneously.' Curiously, and perhaps not totally coincidentally, the death rate fell when treatment became more antiseptic, and less interventionist, through the 1870s. In 1864 the Metropolitan Association of Medical Officers of Health had noted that the death rate in the London Fever Hospital, the headquarters of intensive treatment, was 'much higher' than among patients 'outside'.[169]

In the early part of the century at least, some doctors, including Richard Bright, of Bright's Disease, recommended the traditional cobwebs as a styptic for the throat in intermittent fever cases. But by the 1820s radical young doctors, abetted by Wakley in the *Lancet*, were already turning to 'rational clinical procedures' like heavy depletion of blood, and they ridiculed cobwebs as fit only for 'country people' and 'lady doctors' among whom it was a favourite remedy. But the central point is that the dramatic decline in typhus and relapsing fever occurred before the building boom in fever hospitals set in after the Notification Acts and before the rise of medical interest in germ theory in the 1880s. The diminution also occurred independently of any advance in medical science. Short of some secular change in the virulence of the organisms which caused these fevers, and there appears to be no evidence of that, it does appear that the diminution of mortality and morbidity from typhus and relapsing fever, possibly occasioned most by increased washing of the body, was a triumph for the sanitary cause. By 1906 there were no deaths recorded in London. As Dr Rosen has pointed out, this was three years before Nicolle's discovery that typhus was transmitted by the body louse.[170]

Typhoid (Enteric) Fever

Typhoid fever is an infection transmitted by fouled water, milk or other foods. The causative organism is *Salmonella typhi*, harboured in human faeces. The bacillus enters the body through the intestinal tract and starts multiplying in the bloodstreams, causing fever and diarrhoea. The normal incubation period is about a week to a fortnight. A person who has had typhoid fever gains immunity from it, but may become a carrier. He might convey infection by the food he handles, or the vegetables he grows. The bacteria can also get into the water supply where sewage management is weak. Attacks last for up to a month and leave the patient severely debilitated.

Typhoid, although contemporaries gave it less attention than typhus, was reported to kill more people for a longer period. Historians have also remarked on the horrors of typhus, while overlooking its more formidable ally[171] (see Table 4.4).

In 1871 in Scotland there were 1,234 deaths reported from typhoid, in 1875 1,625, in 1881 1,004, and in 1885 889, down to 644 in 1892.

It was a disease associated with dirt rather than poverty. The average typhoid death rate for England and Wales from 1871 to 1880 was 0.32 per 1,000. London was only 0.24 per 1,000. But the mining areas, Durham, south Wales, the West and North Ridings and Nottinghamshire reported 0.56 per 1,000, 0.45 per 1,000, 0.45 per 1,000, 0.44 per 1,000 and 0.43 per 1,000 respectively. Stockton-on-Tees in County Durham recorded 1.09 per 1,000, and Pontypridd 0.71 per 1,000, and Middlesbrough in the North Riding 0.63 per 1,000.[172]

Table 4.4: England and Wales Deaths per 1,000 Persons Living

1847–50 (including typhus and 'pyrexia')	1.24
1851– 5 " " " "	0.98
1856–60 " " " "	0.84
1861– 5 " " " "	0.92
1866–70 " " " "	0.85
1881– 5 " " " "	0.21
1886–90 " " " "	0.17
1891– 5 " " " "	0.17
1896–1900 " " " "	0.11
1906–10 " " " "	0.07

Source: *PP*, 1916, vol. V, p. 60; *PP*, 1914-16, vol. XI, pp. cviii-cix.

Well before William Budd began his brilliant research into the aetiology of typhoid fever in 1839, the link between typhoid and bad drainage was recognised on general miasmatic principles. Dr Newell reported in 1832 that the incidence of typhoid in Cheltenham had declined since culverts had been constructed in the town, thereby 'furnishing an instructive example of the great importance of an efficient drainage to the public health'. Sanitary improvement worked dramatically: the rates for typhoid deaths before and after sewerage building and the extension of piped water are given in Table 4.5.

Table 4.5: Typhoid Deaths Before and After Sewerage Building (per 1,000 living)

Merthyr Tydfil	21.5	to	8.6
Croydon	15.0	to	5.5
Ely	10.4	to	4.5
Penrith	10.0	to	4.5
Stratford	12.5	to	4.0

Source: R. Thorne Thorne, *The Progress of Preventive Medicine during the Victorian Era* (1888), pp. 25-7; *Lancet*, 10 Nov. 1832, p. 211.

The importance of Eberth's discovery that the typhoid bacillus could live for up to 13 months in soil saturated with typhoid dejecta was demonstrated by the 500 cases in Stockport in the mid-1890s. Inhabitants of houses with a privy pit, who formed the bulk of the population (but far from exclusively comprising the poorer classes — over 1,500 of these dwellings were rated at £12 and upwards — or perhaps many poor families huddled into large, expensive houses?) were three times as likely to catch typhoid as those who inhabited houses with a WC.[173] (Incidentally, almost half the WC houses were rated at *under* £12. This is yet another reminder that future local studies may greatly modify the general picture presented here.)

The sanitarians' success in reducing the disease allowed medical authorities to continue their resistance to Budd's theory that typhoid was distinct from typhus and relapsing fever and was caused by a specific intestinal infection conveyed in water contaminated by 'excreted poison'; despite his having elegantly proved and reproved his case since the early 1840s.[174]

The objection that Budd's theory was 'too exclusive' was also sustained by the known vagaries in incidence of typhoid. The disease often went through wealthy families while it spared their servants and humbler neighbours. The hypothesis that typhoid was conveyed by milk had been published as early as 1858, but it was not followed up and demonstrated until 1870. After an outbreak involving 70 cases in Islington, Dr Ballard noticed that all were from families supplied from one dairy. The dairyman was among the victims. Ballard used the dairyman's list of customers to trace every family and then traced every member of the household who drank the milk. His inescapable conclusion was that the disease came with the milk. But Ballard clung to a miasmic theory of infection. The dairyman had not contaminated the milk: rather it was the water left in the cans after they were washed. The more milk people bought, the more likely they were to catch typhoid. This fact meant, of course, that they had ingested more of the water, and it explained why the comfortable, more cleanly households suffered worst.[175] Ballard's work was reinforced by the investigations of Dr Netten Radcliffe and Mr W.H. Power into the outbreaks in Marylebone in 1873-4. They traced 244 cases, 'mostly confined to the houses of the well-to-do and wealthy'. However, in a startling illustration of the ravages typhoid could effect among the working classes and poor, they found 26 families in these categories, among whom there had been 48 deaths. There is no report of the death rate among the wealthy or their indoor servants, partly because those families, if their servants contracted typhoid, 'went to the country', leaving the servants behind. If members of the family got the disease they 'stayed home', rather than enter the London Fever Hospital. The typhoid first arrived in special 'nursery milk' supplied from a farm near Chilton, in Buckinghamshire, where typhoid was endemic. Half the cases were among children under 15.[176]

Sudden explosive outbreaks, like those in Mountain Ash, Glamorganshire, in 1887, with 518 cases and 30 deaths between July and October, Lewes, Caius College, Cambridge, and the epidemic in Maidstone in August-October 1897, with over 1,800 cases and 132 deaths in a population of 34,000, were each attributed to contaminated water sources. Isolated deaths of celebrities, including the Duke of Grafton in 1882 and the Duke of Leinster in 1893, were attributed to the same cause. The extraordinary incidence among girls 14 to 24 during the Maidstone outbreak was explained by the assumption that women were 'more regular water-drinkers than men'.[177] The role of carriers, which Budd's work had originally pointed to, was not demonstrated until Koch did so in 1902.

Inoculation had been introduced by Sir Almroth Wright in 1896, but it did not become common among civilian populations until after the First World War. Thanks to inoculation and the lessons about strict hygiene learned during the second Anglo-Boer War and from the Japanese in the Russo-Japanese war, the British Army came through relatively free of typhoid. But the German, French and Russian armies continued to be decimated by typhoid, as armies had been decimated by it through the ages.[178]

Typhoid fever was treated until around the 1880s on the normal antiphlogistic plan, with depletion of blood and low diet. The special problem of the high body temperatures accompanying this kind of fever was tackled by 'pouring cold water over the whole surface' (of the body), and by shaving the scalp and applying cold embrocations.[179] By 1887 treatment was becoming less dramatic. Dr James Niven, MOH for Oldham, recommended 'quiet and good feeding'. The good feeding was to consist of 'restful, easily digested' items: 'milk, beef tea . . . fruit juices sugared, and raw egg'. Champagne was especially good. Niven had seen 'at least one case unquestionably saved' by it.[180] Herbalists treating the poor used hellebore root, usually in a tincture of alcohol: eight ounces of root to 16 ounces of alcohol macerated for a fortnight. Male adults could take eight drops of this brew every three hours, until nausea set in, and then resume the dose for up to a week after the symptoms had subsided. Female adults and persons aged between 14 and 18 could take six drops, and children one to three drops. People who doctored themselves used elm or holly bark decoctions. Infusions of pennyroyal also made cooling drinks and induced perspiration.[181]

Before the fashion of the quiet régime set in, ordinary people suffering from fever did themselves no harm by following their own treatments and keeping at bay the local surgeon, his techniques and the authority that accompanied them. Mr William Gourlay, a practitioner at Lenthrathen in Forfarshire, described the struggle for medical hegemony in 1819, during the outbreak of a fever that 'ran in families' and might well have been typhoid:

> The existing prejudices among the lower orders prove the greatest obstacle to the efficient practice of the country surgeon; and I found it no easy matter to persuade them to the necessity of losing blood [and swallowing heroic doses of calomel and opium] for the cure of fever, the old people declaring that they had had many fevers, and in their time no such thing was ever allowed, or thought of . . . 'they were *toasted sick for six weeks*, and often confined to bed for months'. Immediately after the doctor's visit, a consultation of the old women in the neighbourhood is held, each of whom has innumerable nostrums to propose, all equally infallible; and although they may dispute the superiority of their own individual plans, they invariably and unanimously agree on overruling the directions of the medical attendant, more particularly with regard to the use of cooling beverage, abstinence and the free admission of air . . . They [procure] the most dainty bits . . . for the sick because, forsooth, they cannot eat the common fare; and they are desired to force themselves to eat, in order to ward off ensuing weakness.
>
> [Gourlay remarked in parenthesis that this practice probably originated with the medical profession itself many of whose backward-looking members still ordered 'a nourishing diet']. This I found a very serious obstacle: as I could not make them sensible that the patients' weakness depended on causes quite the reverse of want of food. But finesse is sometimes very necessary, and I luckily hit upon a method to remove most objections, and at the same time save the credit of the old women's professional knowledge and thereby preserve their good opinion.

The women ascribed the epidemic 'to Providence'. Gourlay said that, while ultimately it might have been ordained by a higher power, the immediate cause was 'of foreign origin' and it had to be removed, to restore the body's natural balance. The women accepted the argument.

Gourlay then 'got busy': he took 32 ounces of blood and bled each patient to syncope; and then after the vomiting from the first bleeding ceased, dosed the patient with calomel, senna and digitalis and repeated the bleedings; he forbade fires in the rooms (it was autumn) and ordered all windows open; he prohibited visitors. Gourlay won his local war: every case recovered and rational medicine triumphed.[182]

2. HOSPITALS

The cholera crisis of 1831-2 inaugurated a change in function for British general hospitals. Their taking in a token number of sufferers began their slow transformation from private charitable recuperative asylums for the sick and injured into publicly funded curative, medical service stations.

The contribution of eighteenth- and nineteenth-century general hospitals to the well-being of the people has lately been much disputed. In 1926 G. Talbot Griffith and M.C. Buer asserted that general hospitals and the medical skills they nurtured played a fundamental part in the reduction of mortality and thereby furthered the increase of population that occurred during the early Industrial Revolution. This period also saw an increase in the number and size of hospitals, and Griffith and Buer implied that the coincidence was not fortuitous. These arguments reigned almost unchallenged until 1955 when Professor Thomas McKeown and Professor R.G. Brown published the first of their trenchant papers discounting hospital and medical practice as agents in the preservation and increase of the people. The scrutiny of records of patients and annual reports of individual hospitals by Professor Eric Sigsworth, Dr S. Cherry and Dr John Woodward has led them to argue that hospitals did rather better for their inmates than McKeown and his colleagues had alleged, but the debate is far from concluded, and I do not pretend that what I offer here will settle it.[183]

One fact not in dispute is that in 1800, at the centre of Griffith's and Buer's period of population growth, the general hospitals of England, with around 4,000 beds, could shelter only about 30,000 patients a year. They could cater for only a minute proportion of the population at risk and 30,000 lives among a young population of nine million could have made little impact on population trends. Talbot Griffith's and Buer's main contention founders on this point. The increase in the number of beds was gradual until the 1860s: in 1861 there were still only 12,000 beds catering for about 120,000 patients.[184]

There are questions bearing on the central one about the efficacy of hospitals as curative institutions which the present disputants have not explored very far. These include questions about the 'availability' of hospitals, their out-patient services, the costs and benefits of the money and effort invested in them, and their symbiosis with the rising medical profession.

The evidence about these matters is sketchy on essentials and profuse in ambiguities. Governors who had to raise funds and doctors whose reputations as teachers depended on their successes and professed acquaintance with unusual maladies had a shared interest in fudging the admission and discharge books and the annual reports. There was no independent audit. The hospital authorities did not begin to try to tell the truth or even in many cases to see the necessity for reliable statistics until Florence Nightingale and Dr W. Farr began to campaign publicly for them in the mid-1860s.

In 1840 Dr Davis described as 'supposititious' the number of inmates claimed in the annual report of the Birmingham General Hospital, and remarked that most hospital annual reports were 'delusive' and 'not exceeded as puffs by the advertisements of the vilest quacks'.[185] The average length of stay in hospital was around 40 days until the 1880s, when it shortened to around 35 days. Women tended to remain in hospital up to a week longer than men: the latter presumably were importunate for their discharge in order to get back to work; on the other hand, presumably they could also be more readily discharged to be nursed at home. The period was governed by the rules about subscribers' notes of admission. Patients whose condition required a stay beyond 40 days had to produce a fresh subscriber's note, obtained by their friends. Country patients sent and admitted as 'interesting cases' could stay as long as the doctors found them interesting, without a ticket. The important point, so far as the statistics are concerned, is that each of these patients was counted as a fresh admission after each set period. One country patient could often make six on the books. Governors liked the system; it caused less disturbance and made the bed occupancy and turnover rate look good. By 1860 the combined annual reports of the metropolitan hospitals claimed about 125 patients to every medical bed, which adds up to two occupants of each bed each week.[186]

Accurate numbers of out-patients are even more difficult to obtain. The *Lancet* alleged in 1858 that no British hospital kept proper records of out-patients. 'Full records, especially of accident cases' were not kept at the Leeds General Infirmary before 1870, at least. In 1887, the

Lancet remarked of the annual report from the Staffordshire General Infirmary that 'the books having been neglected, it was impossible to ascertain the number of patients who had been treated'. The North Staffordshire Infirmary was still not recording the names and illnesses of out-patients in 1891.[187] But even allowing for double and triple entries, the numbers of out-patients were enormous throughout the century. Guy's claimed over 50,000 a year in the 1830s. By 1869 the hospital reported nearly 80,000.[188] Bart's reported around 84,500 in 1859, 133,000 in 1865 and 128,000 in 1868. In 1900 the London hospitals combined were said to be treating 1.9 million out-patients annually.[189] Leeds General Infirmary claimed nearly 50,000 in 1909, and the Manchester Royal Infirmary 45,000. In that year, too, the Bristol Royal Infirmary and Bristol General Hospital claimed 90,000 between them, while the Glasgow Infirmary reported attendances of over 140,000, or about one-fifth of the population. Major Greenwood, the spokesman for the Poor Law Medical Officers' Association, remarked in 1909 that hospital out-patient wards still did not keep records of 'uninteresting' cases.[190]

In terms of proximity to their clients' dwellings and workplaces, those hospitals established in the eighteenth century or earlier in the old cores of the cities were well placed until the 1860s, when several began to move at least some parts of the institution to more salubrious environments on higher suburban ground. Depopulation of the core and a distorted growth of nearby working-class suburbs could push the clientele beyond reasonable walking distance and thereby isolate them from the hospital. This distortion was worst in London. By 1882 the enormous new population to the south of Guy's had no nearer hospital to serve them, and the new population to the north, apart from a small hospital at Dalston, remained dependent upon the London. Ten of the 15 large metropolitan hospitals, with three-quarters of the beds, were within 1½ miles of Charing Cross. Two, the London with 790 beds and the Metropolitan Free with 20, had to cope with the East End with a population of over one million. One, the Great Northern with 33 beds, had to serve north London with a population of over 900,000.[191]

The national proportion of beds to population in the 1880s, 1 to 980 in England, 1 to 2,340 in Wales, 1 to 930 in Scotland, reasonable by present standards (we now have four times as many beds) masked the geographical maldistribution of hospital assistance. When hospital authorities moved their institution they did so not to be closer to their clientele but for financial reasons and the doctors' convenience. When the Westminster Hospital Board discussed moving from Petty France to

Charing Cross in 1830 the reasons for the move were that Petty France dwellers were too poor to provide adequate subscribers and Charing Cross was in a 'wealthier district'. The doctors also found the old building 'repulsive'. But the local subscribers rallied and defeated the proposal. When the governors of the London Hospital discussed moving to 'a less congested, more salubrious site' in 1903, the discussions were blocked by the medical staff who had 'manifest objections' to having their commuting arrangements upset. The patients were not mentioned.[192]

This maldistribution was compounded by the admission policies of the hospitals. Outpatients comprised many of the categories of people precluded by the rules from becoming in-patients. Children under seven were normally excluded until the 1860s and children under two until after the First World War: in 1911 children under one year formed 25 per cent of all out-patients in Britain. Persons with contagious diseases were excluded from English hospitals, as were 'incurables' and 'chronic cases'; although incurable cancer victims and other curiosities were sometimes admitted as 'interesting cases'. Phthisis sufferers were classed as incurable. Pregnant women were barred by many institutions. The Scottish hospitals were less exclusive, especially after the 1850s. In particular, they were said to be much more likely to admit fever victims and paupers. By contrast, the medical men at the Exeter hospital, like many a struggling provincial group, instructed local GPs 'to select cases that [were] curable; cases that [would] do them credit; because they wished to have as few fatal cases as possible'. Obvious paupers were redirected to the workhouse, and dirty, disorderly or drunken persons were turned away by the porters. At many hospitals until the 1860s or later, the porters became effectively the admission officers.[193]

The suppliant sick, as objects of charity, were in no position to dispute the rules. 'Incurables' and chronics 'drifted about' from one out-patients' hospital room to the next, to dispensaries, and ultimately to the workhouse infirmary. As with fever victims, the small number of charitable long-stay and convalescent institutions (London had only one until the 1860s) could never house them. In 1875 a GP recommended a child with a paralysed arm and leg for admission to the Royal Surrey County Hospital at Guildford. The father carried the child and the GP's written recommendation several miles to the hospital. He was turned away: 'the case was hopeless.' He asked for some medicine, and was told to bring the child back in a week, on the out-patients' day. The father carried the child home. It had been a 'very cold day'. The patient seemed 'infirmed' by the cold journey, became 'drowsy' and died five days later. In 1914 a GP complained that a case with a contracted forearm resulting from a burn had been refused admission to a London hospital on the grounds of 'incurability'. The GP got him into another hospital 'by personal application to a member of staff, where the patient made a complete recovery'.[194]

In the first half of the century, the reigning conception of the hospital as a refuge ensured that if an in-patient developed into an incurable he could be quickly discharged. In 1834 a 'Pupil at the Westminster Hospital' sought help for 'an apothecary [named] . . . Cranwell . . . His disease is consumption; he appears to get daily worse, and is recommended by the physician to leave the hospital. This poor man has not a penny, nor a friend . . .'[195]

Porters and doctors found it hard to distinguish accident victims from drunks, who were not admitted. A 'man called Reed' was found insensible in the Strand in January 1853. He had a bruise on the right side of his head and his left hand was cut. He was carried first to Bond Street Police Station and thence to King's College Hospital, where he was given 'the stomach pump and the electrifying machine'. Then he was turned out as 'drunk' and therefore 'not for a hospital'. Reed collapsed in the street and never regained consciousness. His body was 'emaciated and covered with sores'. The bruise, cut and sores had not been treated at the hospital. The coroner found that Reed had not been drunk but 'merely insensible and unable to speak'. George Rockley, a cabman, suffered a similar fate in 1885. A chimney sweep was taken to the Middlesex Hospital in 1881, a day after he had fallen from a roof. The house surgeon said he was dirty, suggested that he had scabies, refused to deal with him, and directed the sweep's sister, who was apparently half-carrying him, to take him to a workhouse. There they waited two hours before he was admitted and treated for scabies. The sweep died a few days later. The post-mortem showed him to have had a fractured clavicle and two broken ribs.[196]

The subscriber's lines system of admission also curbed the number of would-be patients. In 1837 James Jewrey fell from the roof of a house and suffered 'severe injuries to his trunk'. He was carried, in agony, to the Westminster Hospital. There the porter ignored him 'for a considerable time'. A medical officer chanced to notice him and ordered 25 leeches 'immediately' to the affected parts. After 30 minutes a nurse arrived to announce that Jewrey should have no leeches and that he could not be admitted as an in-patient, 'being unprovided with a governor's ticket'.[197] He was taken home. Three weeks later he died in St George's Hospital. The post-mortem revealed that he had a ruptured urethra. The jury found 'accidental death'. This sequence was not as infrequent as its callousness might suggest. Even in the following month a bricklayer with a smashed leg was turned away from the St Marylebone Dispensary and the Western General Dispensary because he had no ticket. Even when the prospective patient had collected sufficient lines there was no guarantee that he could be admitted and treated. During the 1870s and 1880s 'a large number were turned away every day' from the Glasgow hospitals, for want of beds.[198]

The effort to obtain lines, as I remarked earlier with regard to expectant mothers, was demoralising, time-consuming and expensive. Chronics and incurables especially, 'pushing' for entry into the few convalescent or special retreats, found the going hard. A chronic sufferer could tramp from house to house for months acquiring lines against the next vacancy and then, like dozens of her competitors, find herself outscored by someone else, especially a subscriber's servant, who started with insider backing and the advantage that derived from the subscribers' practice of supporting each other's servants by way of mutual insurance. One lady with a large household in Portland Place, who possessed wide hospital interests, was issuing 1,500 letters a year to her friends' servants during the 1880s.[199]

At special hospitals, particularly, cases nominated by subscribers took absolute precedence for admission, as at the Liverpool Phthisical Hospital. These hospitals, too, often linked the number of nominations to the size of the subscription. At the Good Samaritan Hospital for Women in Glasgow ('for women of the poorer classes affected with serious diseases (not infectious) more particularly those peculiar to their sex, unsuitable for the wards of a general hospital') donors of £10 or more annually were entitled to recommend two patients yearly for every £10 subscribed; donors of £5 could recommend one patient annually, while donors of a guinea a year could recommend one patient a year for treatment, presumably as an out-patient.[200] In 1872 there were 298 candidates for 20 places at the Royal Hospital for Incurables: 8,640 subscribers had been canvassed for 24,000 votes; even the candidates who ran last had gathered over 1,000 votes.[201] The lines were good only for each particular month, year, or vacancy.

When defeated, the case had to begin again from scratch. Effectively the dirty and unrespectable, the very poor, women burdened with small children and the aged were excluded from the system because in the 1860s and 1870s at least, a competitor needed about £10 as a capital base from which to operate and considerable free time. Occasionally a benevolent subscriber would underwrite the seeker while she canvassed.

As hospital treasurers explained, when opposing moves to abolish lines, subscribers liked contests and such contests kept up the funds. Competition for lines also kept up a remunerative rivalry between church and chapel. In the mid-1850s a collier with five children, three of them mentally defective, used 48 guineas of his backer's money in gathering votes to get one child into a Nonconformist asylum. He ended up with insufficient votes. But for the unsubsidised majority, expenditure on canvassing was a desperate investment of their own narrow resources. An ailing widow on a pension of £20 a year sought to enter an old people's retreat in the 1850s. Her first try cost her £3.10s.0d. Her second canvass had necessarily to be larger than the first: 1,000 cards cost £2.5s.0d.; envelopes and paper, 10s.4d. stamps, £2.5s.0d.; journey expenses, £2.10s.0d.; a total of £7.10s.4d. She failed again. In 1858 she was embarking on her third attempt. With even more cards to dispatch she envisaged spending half her annual income.[202]

It is not surprising that the Reverend Arnold Pinchard of Birmingham should have declared in 1909 that 'the poor hate going' to the out-patients' wards. They were 'always harried' and had to 'sit for hours' waiting. The porters enjoyed their little authority and made the people 'feel that they [were] a nuisance'. The more sensitive, or less patient, simply went off to dispensaries, sixpenny doctors, or stayed away. 'The discomfort of waiting in close association with a set of dirty people', a *Lancet* observer explained, 'is, or ought to be, sufficient deterrent to those who can pay'.

The press of numbers ensured that the idealised subjects of the governors' and doctors' benevolence emerged as clinical objects. Guy's in the 1860s did not take the names or keep records of out-patients. Average waiting time at the London Hospital during the 1870s was seven hours. Hospitals with halls large enough provided benches, but others, never designed to cope with thousands of out-patients, provided a few seats packed around the entrance lobby. In 1869 a consumptive woman stood for five hours before finding a seat at the Victoria Park Hospital for Diseases of the Chest. The standing and waiting times were about normal. The wooden benches at St George's, as at most hospitals, it seems, were not supplied with backs until 1868.[203] Until mid-century and the explosion in the numbers of out-patients, even the great London hospitals only treated or admitted patients on two or three days in the week. This practice provoked very few patients' letters of complaint that got into print, so far as I have found. In 1835 H. Lee wrote to the *Lancet*:

Knowing your readiness to give publicity to anything which might benefit the lower classes . . . I take this opportunity of suggesting a trifling alteration in the management of hospitals . . . Having an ulcerated throat and violent pains in the head, I reported to *St Thomas's Hospital* on Thursday, in the hope that I might get advice and a little medicine, as I had not the means to pay for it, which is frequently the case with persons moving in the sphere of life in which I am. After waiting for . . . an hour, and actually fainting away . . . one of the students asked me the nature of my complaint and, upon satisfying him, he very coolly told me to call *on Monday at eleven*.

Lee replied that the physicians should attend out-patients for five hours every morning. But thereafter his temerity failed. He apparently chose to write to the *Lancet* rather than go back on the Monday.[204]

The procedure at St Bartholomew's in 1869 was representative of all the large hospitals. Bart's had one large hall which seated 600 on benches: males at one end, females at the other. On the north side were two small consulting rooms for 'medical' cases, and on the south side four for 'surgical' ones, and a room with a door for 'special examinations'. The doors of the examination rooms were never closed, as the doctors of the Westminster Hospital explained in 1879, 'because of the foul air admitted with each patient'. The Westminster waiting hall was heated by steam pipes from the kitchen. In winter the room was too cold, in summer the pipes were too hot to touch. Throughout the year the patients and porters insisted on keeping all external doors and windows closed, even those near the two WCs which served the hall. There was no effective registration of names or cases. The doors opened at 9 a.m. and shut at 10. Patients crowded about the hall, while the porters were busy all day sorting them into 'medicals' and 'surgicals' and in 'keeping order'. Eating and drinking were forbidden until the 1880s. Women were generally thought to be harder to keep quiet and in line than men. The dispensary stood in the centre of the hall. At the Great Northern one of the wall notices informed them that unless the women were obedient the surgeon would 'not see one of them'. On the other hand 'great strong men' regularly pushed ahead unhindered into the consulting rooms at Guy's. The 'really sick' had to wait till last.

Two of the house physicians, the most junior doctors in the hospital, arrived, on the unusual occasions when they were punctual, at 11.30 a.m. Customarily, they were one hour late. One worked among the males, one among the females. Patients were shuffled into the examination rooms 'several . . . at a time'. The rooms were too small to permit pupils or clinical clerks to attend to help with the examinations or keeping of records. Most examinations were in fact conducted by students in the hall. After the first hour, by which time the house physicians had done their normal 120 patients each, there was a speed-up, because the house physicians had soon to hurry off to attend the hospital physician on his ward round. Thereupon the students dealt with the patients, unsupervised. Occasionally, other house physicians or students attended and worked till 5 p.m., each seeing an average of 35 cases every hour. Patients left unseen had to come back on the morrow and try to push in earlier. The two morning house physicians were rostered weekly, so they rarely saw a case twice. If they did want to follow up an interesting patient they asked the porters to summon them when the person with those particular symptoms or dressings reappeared and came to examine the patient in the hall.

The four house surgeons controlled the admission of surgical cases. They retained the interesting cases for themselves, and quickly entered them as in-patients for examination and surgery later at their leisure. 'Uninteresting' patients they set aside, to wait for the hospital assistant surgeons and students, who might attend later in the day. Students complained about this discrimination throughout the middle decades of the century, as did the students at the Hospital for Chest Diseases who declared that their training was harmed because of the difficulty of examining cases while the patients were standing in a crush.

After each examination the doctors scribbled an order for the dispensary or hospital apothecary's shop. The patient carried the script back into the main hall and joined the crowd around the central dispensary, which contained six mixtures in jugs, and 'some gargles, lotions and pills of a simple character'. Bart's dispensed 900 gallons of cod-liver oil, 1,200 ounces of quinine and 3 hundredweight of ammonia in 1869. The mixtures at some hospitals, Guy's for instance, were concocted in a range of colours, black (mainly sarsparilla) to whitish (guaicacum) for ready dispensing. Even so, the dispensers were observed to give the patient whatever was in the nearest jug. The medicines in the jugs were dispensed by two female nurses, and were usually consumed on the spot. The dispensary handled between 250 and 300 cases every day. When the dispensers were presented with a more elaborate prescription they redirected the patient to the apothecary's shop across the quadrangle. Cursory though this procedure was, it fitted the patients' expectations. They wanted their dose of medicine, and no undue fuss. Mothers stopped doctors from pausing to take the temperatures of their children, or unbuttoning their shirts. They were not there to be experimented upon or investigated unnecessarily, particularly by students. But by 1909, Dr Lauriston Shaw said, patients who were turned away without a thorough examination felt themselves neglected.[205]

The 'surgicals' varied between victims with serious fractures, burns and bodily deformities and persons attending for vaccination, extraction of teeth (usually the largest single group), venesection and slight injuries such as cut fingers. The fracture and bodily deformity cases might be admitted as interesting in-patients, while the rest were treated by the students. Errors in the initial drafting by the porters were common, up to one-fifth of the total out-patients at the Birmingham General Hospital in the 1830s.[206] 'Medicals' (skin diseases, internal complaints, etc.) who turned up among the 'surgicals' were turned away untreated. Others were admitted and operated upon before the mistake was discovered. As Dr McVail remarked of the Glasgow Royal Infirmary in the 1880s, such eventualities were inevitable when five surgeons had to cope with over 300 cases. Most of the work devolved upon the students, for, after all, the hospitals were teaching institutions.[207]

Ellen Sheen went to the Westminster Hospital at 9 a.m. on a Friday in December 1850 to have an aching tooth drawn. She was, she wrote,

> in such great pain that I could scarcely live. I was told the tooth doctor [Clendon] was not within, and I was told to call again at one o'clock. I went again at that time, and then the tooth-doctor was there, with his two young gents, who had the tools in their hands, and the tooth-doctor nothing at all; and they handled me, he only looked on, and after a tug or two they got out my tooth, and the tooth-doctor . . . said it was a very bad one.

Ellen Sheen went on to ask whether it was 'right that at such a great place' the tooth-doctor did not do his job personally, at the advertised times. She hoped the 'tooth-doctor's master' would see her letter of complaint. Doubtless he did, but there is no evidence that he acted on it.[208]

John Cooper received burns on his arms while at work in Bermondsey in 1881. He was taken to Guy's on Thursday 7 July, when the burns were dressed (usual applications, until lanoline was found to be helpful in 1888, were turpentine, or vinegar, or most commonly treacle, applied on a dressing of calico), and he was told to return next day for a further dressing, which he did. He was dressed again on Monday 11 July. Cooper lived 3 miles from Guy's. The weather was exceptionally hot.

Cooper attended every day, until 20 July, when he complained of a sore ankle and found he could not walk. He became delirious. His employer called in a private doctor, who found Cooper's ankles to have abscesses and the burns to show signs of blood-poisoning. He died on 29 July. During his attendance at Guy's he had been seen twice by the house surgeon, who had not noted his name or address and had kept no case-notes. On the other visit he had been dressed by students or nurses, one among their regular 50 cases an hour. When Mabel Blanch, an infant, died 'very emaciated' in 1900 from marasmus and congestion of the left lung, she had been seen the previous day as an out-patient at Guy's by an unqualified student dresser, who told her mother there 'was nothing wrong with her' and to bring her back the next day. The hospital had no record of Blanch or her 'treatment'.[209]

There were three general stages in methods of handling in-patients during the century. During the first, until about the mid-1860s, the 'refuge' approach prevailed; then followed a period of about 30 years when the authorities gradually rearranged their aspirations for their hospital, widening its entry, tightening its nursing arrangements, towards making it a reparative, curative institution; the third stage began in the late 1880s when the hospital began to be transformed into an expensive scientific clinical, highly mechanised, research organisation the prototype of the hospital of the present. The two later stages coincide with, indeed partly result from, the decline of the power of the governors and the accretion of power to doctors within the hospital, especially in decisions about day-to-day management.

In-patient wards were harsh places, until the mid-1860s at least. They resembled a slovenly army barracks complete with submissive grubby soldiery, mean-spirited NCOs and negligent officers. Patients were admitted and discharged on set days, usually Thursdays, irrespective of the amount of preparation needed (in 1972 many British hospitals were still using this wasteful practice), and regardless of whether they had any money or anyone was waiting to receive them. Teaching surgeons, especially, required a quick turnover of cases. They were accommodated, as most poor patients still are, in dormitories. As hospitals were reconstituted from the old eighteenth-century homes in which they began, the wards became bigger and more dormitory-like. When the Westminster was partly rebuilt in the 1830s the *Lancet* especially commended the new airy wards, housing 15 patients each 'which experience shows to be most convenient for the enforcement of that regimental coercion which constitutes the principal advantage of hospital treatment'.[210]

On entering, patients' faces, hands and feet were washed. Most hospitals required them to bring their own bed attire and eating utensils. No hospital supplied cupboards for patients; so their belongings were stored under the beds. Petty theft and rows about alleged thefts and thieves were endemic. Hospital towels and sponges were shared. Patients were divided only by sex; cases of all ages and illnesses were mixed indiscriminately. Most hospitals had theoretically strict rules about visitors, but in practice, until the 1840s visitors came and went at all hours, together with food and porter vendors. Most patients had to supplement a hospital diet. The hospital supplied only a minimum of food and bed-ridden patients, dependent upon the nurses, got very little of it.[211]

The nurses were few and ill trained. It was an unhealthy job and few women of ability would undertake it. Governors were interested in keeping costs down and doctors had no desire to see nurses acquire skills or responsibility that might make them into rivals. In the 1830s sisters received 14s. to 16s. a week and nurses 7s., together with a food allowance that they had to supplement privately. They were subject to the matron, effectively the housekeeper, and the steward, a butler, and were hired and fired by them. Their day started at 6 a.m. and ended at 10 p.m. Nurses were expected to sit up on ward-watch every alternate night. Many nurses were unable to read or write and could be trusted only to perform the simplest tasks. The hospitals continually lost their best nurses, who joined ladies of diminished income as private nurses to the upper classes, at a going rate of 5 guineas a week in the 1850s.[212] Those who remained, with notable exceptions, were callous and unreliable. In 1845, at University College Hospital, Mrs Dean, head ward nurse, was discharged for drunkenness; in 1848 another head nurse was discharged for ill-treating patients; in 1850 a night nurse was discharged for pawning hospital sheets; in 1852 Nurse Rosaire was discharged for stealing two mattresses, a table and set of fire-irons; in 1854 Nurse Turner was discharged for selling morphine to patients.[213]

There had been calls since the 1830s for a Protestant sisterhood of trained lady nurses, but the calls had been rejected by hospital authorities, partly out of fears of Puseyism and 'popery' and mainly because of the expense and trouble. Florence Nightingale's work on the Crimea took fifteen years to have an impact in Britain itself. The nurses trained by the Nightingale Fund at St Thomas's Hospital were fewer than 15 a year during the 1860s, and only 20 a year in the 1880s, although this core provided many of the great late-Victorian hospital matrons and thereby had a much wider impact than might first appear.[214]

Guy's began to reform its nursing arrangements in 1871. The number of nurses was increased to 69, to give a ratio of one nurse to 12 patients on day shifts and 1 to 17 at night. Nurses were now differentiated from 'scrubbers'. The pay was also increased to £20 a year, plus board and costume, amounting to £37.5s.0d. a year, well above the going rate of £15-20 for provincial nurses. The hospital preferred 'a good class of domestic servant . . . and a better class of person for sister and superintendent'. No nurse could be promoted to sister.

Guy's had been compelled to move because of increasing pressure to admit Protestant sisterhoods to the hospital, as had happened at King's College and University College Hospitals. These 'most superior' sisters gave the authorities endless trouble from personal feuds, proselytising, refusals to do menial tasks or obey doctors' orders, and taking their directions from their outside mother-house. At University College Hospital 150 beds were serviced by the five sisters and 23 nurses and probationers from the All Saints Home, Margaret Street. They regularly complained about the smell from the students' urinal which pervaded one wing, but refused to help clean it. The nursing orders also demanded a level of comfort and support that Guy's refused to meet. Beds at University College Hospital each cost £77 a year, those at King's nearly £60, compared with Guy's £7.10s.0d. Effectively, the hospitals were sustaining the sisterhoods. But the sisterhoods were at least reliable at night. Charing Cross Hospital had wards on three floors and eight nurses (in most hospitals there was only one) on night duty. The wards, as in most hospitals, had no doors. This was to enable patients and the single nurse on duty, at night especially, to be heard when they shouted for help. The lady superintendent attempted, as was usual, to make 'surprise visits' but the nurses always saw or heard her coming. But the hospital, like most others, could not find 'a lady' to serve as night supervisor, and the nurses refused to accept supervision from 'one of our own class'.[215]

By the mid-1870s the sisterhoods had become the pattern of nursing among the public and their black merino habits (they would accept nothing less from the hospitals) became the known nursing uniform. By 1875, Miss Bertha Adams proudly reported, men were giving up their seats to them in the underground, 'even in the Third class'. By the late 1890s doctors were complaining vehemently about these officious, efficient females who increasingly were taking temperatures, dressing wounds and handling patients on their own responsibility. There was even a threat of the growth of male nursing, first launched in 1885.[216]

Nursing had entered its modern phase of being the most important and expensive, but still underpaid, component in hospital services.

In the earlier part of the century, the shortage of nursing help combined with prevailing domestic norms to make hospitals insalubrious. The sheets at St George's were changed every three weeks. Immobile cases were left longer, as a way of not harming the patient and lightening the work. John Hammond was admitted in 1825 with a cut on his leg. The wound was not washed, but stuck together with sticking plaster. As his leg mortified he was given increasing doses of aperients, to clear the poison. The bandage was changed every four days. After five weeks he died in a filthy bed, having lain unwashed throughout his sojourn. Nicholas Dawkins, a policeman, died in the same hospital also in 1825. He had a compound fracture of the leg and had been immobilised. After 12 weeks he and his bed were 'alive with maggots' and the bed was sprouting mushrooms. Dawkins had not complained, and his ward-mates had seen 'nothing particularly dirty about it'. In 1833 a coal-heaver with a broken jaw was carried to Guy's at 12 midday on a Saturday. He was left in the accident ward unattended until 11 a.m. on Sunday, when a passing surgeon noticed him and ordered that his jaw be set. There was no entry in the ward book, the dresser of the week had been absent the whole weekend and the nurse on duty had ignored the case. The Gloucester Infirmary had a case of maggots in an amputated leg stump in 1868.[217] In the following year Mr Richardson was admitted to Bart's as a medical patient. He was secretary to the London Dock Labourers' Association and a 'person considerably superior in character'. Richardson was in hospital for seven weeks. After that time he made a series of complaints to the hospital treasurer: the patients were cold from constant draughts from ill-fitting windows; the hospital did not supply flannel bed-jackets and most patients had only their own thin cotton nightshirts; the inmates had no slippers and the hospital supplied none; the inmates, having no dressing-gowns of their own, to cover themselves in making their way to the WC, used a dirty old bed quilt kept for the purpose; the hospital did not provide soap or towels and most patients had none; the only seats in the ward for patients were backless wooden benches, while the two armchairs in each ward were reserved for nurses; medicines were given only at 6 a.m., noon and 6 p.m. and they proved especially nauseous on empty stomachs; breakfast was at 6 a.m., then there was a gap of 6-7 hours till dinner, which was postponed if the doctor happened to enter the ward; the dinner usually arrived cold anyway; the patients often lay stripped and cold for hours during the morning while waiting examination by students, followed by the doctor and his retinue of 6-10 more students; the nurses did less than required, while many were so tired that they fell asleep in their chairs. The treasurer reported Richardson's complaints to Dr Farre, the senior physician. He dismissed them: Richardson had 'mistaken the purpose for which he was in hospital, and . . . [was] little better than a "firebrand" '.

Dr Farre's reaction was symptomatic of medical opinion through the century. Richardson was no more than an object of charity and a clinical subject. Doctors engaged in hospital practice as an interlude in their private practice. They benefited from the students' fees, which went to them rather than the hospital, and from the enhanced reputation among their private patients which a hospital teaching appointment brought. They had every motive for getting through their hospital rounds quickly, followed by as many pupils as possible. The great Brodie had an entourage of 60 at St George's in the 1820s, jostling around each bed and the operating table. Mr J.P. Vincent at Bart's in the 1830s did his rounds so quickly that there was *'a general run'*. He regularly 'knocked off' 70-80 patients in 75 minutes. Mr F.C. Skey, also at Bart's, 'visited' 30 patients in 20 minutes.[218]

Early nineteenth-century treatment, especially surgery, was a brutal business and students necessarily became callous. Those who did not, dropped out. It is also possible, reviewing the course of nineteenth-century medicine, that the fugitives included the more intelligent and sensitive aspirants. Erasmus, Charles Darwin's elder brother, in a family of doctors, could not endure the 'case-hardening', and never practised. Charles watched two 'bad operations' and abandoned his medical studies.[219] J.D. Hooker and T.H. Huxley also forsook medicine. The manners of the President of the College of Surgeons, William Blizard, at the operating table at the London Hospital in the 1830s were so gross that the 'jeers of the students . . . overpowered the complaints' of the patient. Ordinary people sought to avoid the London Hospital and Blizard, and walked further to other hospitals. Railings had to be placed around operating tables during the 1830s to prevent students and 'strangers' from crowding the operator and obscuring with their hats (which they wore — black beavers were the students' favourites — until the 1860s) in the theatre and the wards. Those who could not see would shout in unison — 'heads, heads'. As the patient was being fastened down, the students relieved their tension with 'hideous yells', which became louder as the patient began to writhe and 'get an itching in his heels'. There was a sudden silence as the first incision was made, and then a general hubbub ensued for the rest of the operation, interrupted by laughter as the students joked among themselves, or with the operator. The operating-room and wards were also full of cigar smoke, for students smoked incessantly, they said, to combat the 'very offensive' smells of the wards and the operating- and dissecting rooms.[220] Sir Anthony Carlisle, surgeon-extraordinary to the Prince Regent and Professor of Anatomy at the Royal Academy, was famous for his knockabout wit at the expense of patients. When one student asked, at the bed of a patient, whether wine would help the case, a junior surgeon retorted, to Carlisle's guffaws, that 'Nothing will do him any good.' Carlisle then capped the joke with a story about a patient with a red nose: 'he drank red wine, pissed it white and left the red in his nose.' In 1834 a man died in St Thomas's after two surgeons had failed in attempts lasting four hours to tie his subclavian artery. The surgeons could not agree over the site of the artery and fought over the operating table. There was no inquest. At the London Hospital in 1831 a boy lay on the operating table while the surgeons discussed whether the operation would kill him. He had been dismissed from three hospitals previously with an 'incurable' diseased knee. Finally the surgeons unstrapped him and decided upon a week's trial of another attempt to cure the 'chronic inflammation'. Other busy surgeons refused to wait to hear the patient explain his ailment.[221]

Medical students, as I shall argue in the next chapter, were regarded as cads for the first sixty years of the century. The riots that occurred about resurrection men (suppliers of bodies, sometimes recently buried ones, to anatomy schools) in the 1820s and early 1830s and again in Sheffield in 1862, were but one manifestation of popular mistrust of these brash, cigar-smoking, cold-hearted young men.[222] Once in hospital, the poor felt trapped. Instances of patients being dismissed for insolent and defiant behaviour are endless.[223] Doctors expected deference, not gratitude. As one London house physician explained in 1899, once a doctor showed sympathy with that 'class of patients' he found himself subject

to long-winded and totally unimportant details concerning the manner they received their injuries, accounts of their families and pecuniary condition, and often even requests for pecuniary assistance . . . A short and decisive manner is the only way to deal with people like this . . . The want of gratitude and civility shown by patients . . . is something appalling . . . gratitude is so rare . . . that it always calls forth a remark from the medical men to his assistants. Scarcely a day passes but a patient has to be ordered out . . .

or removed . . . for gross incivility.

As that cold genius, Joseph Lister, remarked of patients: 'who knows, it may be that whilst here they may have a chance of learning something of the meaning of the word Gratitude'; one of his house surgeons added that patients expressed gratitude astonishingly seldom, but shrewdly concluded, 'I think the poor are fatalists and take things as a matter of course.'[224]

A servant to a doctor was admitted to the Westminster Hospital in 1834 with a contused ankle and fractured humerus. A month passed before any surgeon touched him. Then Mr G.J. Guthrie, hurrying past, 'stopped for a moment to direct that splints be placed on the man's *arm*'. When James Chaplain was admitted to University College Hospital in 1837 with a bayonet wound in the abdomen the surgeons refused to see him; as Mr Edward Taylor remarked, 'the man was dying when he arrived and was not worth seeing.' Sir Anthony Carlisle regularly transferred his patients to junior surgeons when they showed signs of decline. It was still standard practice in the 1870s to herd all casualties, children included, together in the casualty room to await the surgeons. The rooms with block and tackle for reducing dislocations and the operating table was usually immediately adjacent. Patients with cuts were sewn up in the casualty room itself, 'midst the screams and blood'.[225] In the Magdalen wards, as one Magdalen complained of Bart's, the medical students 'tittered' when she showed 'her feelings' while she was examined. Their ward was always dark. The surgeon brought a candle on his rounds and

> without any ceremony whatever, he orders us to show our disorders with our own hands, and thrusting forward his light he makes his remarks upon our cases . . . We seek all sorts of excuses to avoid this . . . exposure, and some of us think that the better-looking are more leniently treated than the rest.

After the inspection, many of the women buried their faces under the bedclothes, trying to shut out the sound of the other patients who tittered and the students who tittered with them.[226]

Hospital Results

Sponsors of hospitals justified their institutions by their reported cure rates. There was controversy about these rates in the 1860s and a century later the argument has revived. On both occasions the debate has been inconclusive. I want to suggest some refinements to the old questions which might further the detailed research in these matters which remains to be done. The terms 'cured' and 'relieved' need definition. 'Cured' in the nineteenth century had a wider meaning than our notion of complete, or near-complete, permanent restoration of function. It retained part of the older connotation of 'caring for', as in a 'cure of souls', and could be extended to include a condition in which symptoms, grievous pain especially, had largely ceased. Here 'cured' merged into 'relieved', which apparently meant the mitigation of pain of malfunction without restoration to well-being or full capacity. Nineteenth-century writers avoided definitions of these terms. One of the few who tried was Dr J.C. Steele, in 1861:

> With reference to the class designated 'cured' or 'well', it is well known to those accustomed to hospital practice, that the meaning intended to be conveyed is not an absolute and permanent recovery from disease in all cases, but that it includes a very large number of cases where a restoration to temporary health is the utmost that can be expected . . . The same remark [applies] . . . to the division 'relieved' . . . Under this heading are included a large, perhaps the greater portion of the patients whose classification might, with equal propriety, have been inserted in the category of incurable, were it not the fact that they had received benefit from their temporary residence.

Steele went on to explain that the tiny category 'unrelieved' covered only those *discharged* from hospital as such. This small proportion 'would', he remarked disarmingly, '. . . be much increased . . . by the addition of the many cases . . . that have died in the hospital'. The lax keeping of records combined with the absence of any 'follow-up' also improved the hospitals' claims. Even when follow-ups did eventuate, doctors had no wish to discount their colleagues' achievements. In 1869 Mr Timothy Holmes reported the case of a man who had been discharged as 'healed entirely' from St George's Hospital after his arm had been amputated at the elbow. Next day he celebrated and got drunk. Rigors came on, and some days later he was readmitted with pyaemia. But this did not mean, Holmes implied, that the surgeons had not cured him, rather that the pyaemia 'was obviously induced by drunkenness, and could not be charged to hospital arrangements, since it did not come on till after his discharge'.[227]

Florence Nightingale argued that hospitals actually damaged their

patients' chances of being cured. Hospitals were insanitary and care-
lessly run, and bred infections which killed patients. Professor McKeown
and his colleagues have made similar criticisms in the present debate.[228]
Hospitals were indisputably insanitary, into the 1870s at least. Sanitary improvement only meant extra expense to governors, and irrelevant fuss to senior doctors. They did not live in the hospital, and deaths
in the hospitals did not come before the coroners' courts. In the 1850s
the ventilation shaft at the Manchester Royal Infirmary conducted
smells from the mortuary throughout the female surgical wards. The
WCs were ventilated directly into the wards, pervading them with a
'penetrating and sickly odour'. Patients were unused to flushing WCs
and the bad plumbing did not help: at Highgate Infirmary, the WCs
blocked before the building was occupied in 1870 because the discharge pipes were too narrow. The Manchester Royal Infirmary experimented in 1908 with WCs that flushed automatically when the patient
shut the door on leaving. They never worked.[229] Between 1862 and
1882 the trough closets in wards and lobbies of the Hull Infectious
Diseases Hospital were 'insufficiently flushed and their untapped soil
pipes . . . were blocked . . . and [the wards and lobbies] offensive'.
The drains under the scullery and kitchen of the Middlesex Hospital
were of the old brick square type; they contained nine feet of stagnant
sewage in them when the authorities finally moved to cleanse them in
1872. The drains under the Liverpool Lying-in Hospital, which had
finally to be abandoned in 1882 because of endemic erysipelas and
puerperal fever, were found to run uphill when they were lifted in
1884. Scarlet fever and smallpox had spread through the hospital. The
Westminster had two cesspools in the basement until 1895. One set of
ward WCs regularly leaked into the kitchen below and the hospital
was pervaded by a 'foul odour'. Occasionally the Tyburn stream, into
which the hospital chamber-pots were emptied every morning, flooded,
and the nurses' dining-room and the kitchen were awash with sewage.[230]

The wards were overcrowded, with the beds usually ranged along
blank windowless walls, and a second row against a partition, with
ventilating holes, separating a further two lines of beds in the other
half of the dormitory. During the 1870s authorities began to build
WCs into turrets on the external walls, but most hospitals economically
retained the privies, kitchens and nurses' rooms along a common corridor.[231] Operating-tables and rooms were not washed between operations: the wooden or linoleum-covered floor was simply sprinkled with
sawdust. Into the 1870s at least, the wooden table was covered with a
permanent, thick woollen red cloth, to absorb the blood. Some large

hospitals had two tables in the one room: operations proceeded simultaneously. It was usual, too, until into the 1870s, to re-use bandages and sponges after they had been 'washed'. They were not boiled.[232]

In 1882 Arthur Hill Hassall, the hero of the anti-adulteration campaigns of the 1860s and 1870s, suggested that the doctors' practice of carrying their clinical thermometers (and their favourite lancets) in their pockets and wiping them with their 'rarely washed' handkerchiefs was dangerous. Hassall proposed that the thermometers be left to stand in disinfecting fluid. Two notable country surgeons denounced the suggestion as impractical. Mr Arthur Flint of Westgate-on-Sea said that he always took temperatures in the armpit, or between the scrotum and thigh, or the rectum. He then unfailingly washed his thermometer in cold water and thus 'reduced the risk of conveying infection'. Mr George Jeaffreson of Framlingham was against unnecessary fuss. He washed the glass and rubbed it with a cloth 'till it slips in with perfect smoothness . . . [as] proof of sufficient cleaning'.[233] The doctors' education had helped make them unfastidious. Until the 1880s (and even up to the First World War from remarks I have heard from elderly surgeons) 'surgeons operated in old coats (or leather aprons), which, like England's flag, had braved the battle and the breeze of many a bloody operation'. The fashion for wearing cotton antiseptic gloves, masks and white ducks spread from Germany among younger surgeons between 1900 and 1908, but it then faded, as news arrived from Germany that the Germans were discarding their special dress. The fashion took on again after war was declared. In 1900 Wynter Blyth observed as a matter of humorous interest in his report on adulteration investigations that the mice in his St Marylebone laboratory ate only the butter samples, never the margarine.[234]

Dissection rooms stank and, because the nurses sensibly avoided them, they were rarely cleaned. Rats were numerous. They were said to be boldest at the Little Windmill Street medical school, where they took pieces off the dissecting tables during demonstrations. Grim though they were, British hospitals were better than French, Austrian or Italian ones. The British hospitals were much smaller, so that outbreaks of hospital gangrene wrought less destruction than, for example, among the 2,000 patients at the Krankenhaus in the 1860s.[235]

Patients may also have been treated more as individuals in British hospitals. Doctors were very overbearing grandees in Austrian hospitals and the students visited the wards in regiments of 200. (Incidentally, when the medical director entered a ward the nurses and patients had to kiss his hand — perhaps this was one main way in which infection was conveyed from the dissecting rooms to the wards and a reason why Semmelweiss's theory was so unpopular with his superiors.) In Continental hospitals patients were required to remain in bed; in British hospitals they were expected to get up and help themselves, at meal times, for example. In French hospitals all patients had their meals in bed. In French hospitals discarded bandages were left in baskets in the wards: in British hospitals they were removed 'immediately' to the wash-house. In British hospitals a bed was supposed to be 'aired' after a patient died in it; in France they simply refilled the bed. French hospitals did not give a full diet and alcohol after operations, as was common in Britain. French and Italian hospitals, with their 1,000-2,000 patients, were extremely crowded, yet each bed had curtains, which were rarely changed. Most British hospitals expected patients to do without curtains or screens: patients simply used the chamber-pot under the bedclothes. British doctors agreed that, though their hospitals might stink, they were less nauseating than Continental ones.[236]

Moreover, improvement did go forward. As hospitals gradually were rebuilt, hot and cold water was piped to each floor, steam heating replaced open fires, the walls were fire-proofed, skirtings cemented and non-porous floors laid. Kitchens were separated from the main hospital buildings in the late 1880s. Beds were placed further apart and patients' lockers were installed during the 1880s, although patients persisted in misusing them by placing their chamber pots in them, together with their food and eating utensils. Increasingly, as hospitals grew larger from the 1870s, 'fever' (but not diphtheria) patients were restricted to separate wards, although isolation wards were still rare in 1890. Flowers were introduced into wards in the mid-1870s and distinctive starched uniforms for all nurses were adopted through the 1880s and 1890s. Christmas parties for inmates began about 1869.[237] The new Addenbrooke's in Cambridge in 1866 was

> decorated with a very happy effect above the skirting, which is dark green, and up to the level of the . . . brackets to which cords are attached to enable the patient to raise himself, the dado is painted a cheerful red, which serves to relieve the blue and white of the bed furniture . . . [two lines at levels of the brackets contained] stencilled ornaments in blue, white and black, while the space between these bands is divided into styles and rails and panels in two shades of buff . . . [Above the brackets' line to the cornice] the walls are painted in a warm green, which gives a sort of subdued sunshining

effect; and the cornice itself has also stencilled ornaments in several bright and well-contrasted colours. The whole effect is that of . . . homeliness . . . It is not well to cherish in the hearts of the poor the ambition of luxury, but a life . . . destitute of luxury is . . . depressed . . . Taste is an expensive faculty if it be pampered into absoluteness; but a soul without it misses the . . . keenest relish of existence.[238]

During the 1870s nickel-plated and enamelled hospital instruments and utensils replaced the old iron ones which were prone to rust. The London Hospital introduced the first accident ambulance in 1882. Hitherto, public cabs or hand barrows had been used to convey incapacitated cases to and from hospital.[239] Above all, the ratio of nurses to beds fell. At the great charity hospitals by the mid-1870s there was about one nurse to every five beds, during the day at least.[240] Patients were cleaner and more regularly fed and dosed.

The best hospitals had by the 1870s become orderly barracks, and perhaps lost some of their earlier rough familiarity. The practice of making medical rounds early in the morning, which St Thomas's introduced from the Prussian practice in 1878, spread during the next decade.[241] Writing people did not often enter public wards as inmates and it is difficult to find evidence about the inmates' experience from the inmates' point of view. One inmate who did write was W.E. Henley, in Edinburgh Infirmary with tubercular arthritis between August 1873 and April 1875. He had been nominated by 'a lady in the South of England . . . of very considerable influence in London Society [Lady Churchill], and she has sent a pecuniary donation'. Incidentally he is an example of the deceitfulness of hospital statistics. His stay of 565 days presumably represented about 16 'patients' on the books.[242] His sequence of poems, *In Hospital*, provides vivid insights:

INTERIOR

The gaunt brown walls
Look infinite in their decent meanness.
There is nothing of home in the noisy kettle,
The fulsome fire.

The atmosphere
Suggests the trail of a ghostly druggist.
Dressings and lint on the long, lean table —
Whom are they for?

The patients yawn,
Or lie as in training for shroud and coffin.
A nurse in the corridor scolds and wrangles.
It's grim and strange.

Far footfalls clank.
The bad burn waits with his head unbandaged.
My neighbour chokes in the clutch of chloral . . .
O, a gruesome world!

STAFF-NURSE: NEW STYLE

Blue-eyed and bright of face but waning fast
Into the sere of virginal decay,
I view her as she enters, day by day,
As a sweet sunset almost overpast.
Kindly and calm, patrician to the last,
Superbly falls her gown of sober gray,
And on her chignon's elegant array
The plainest cap is somehow touched with caste.
She talks Beethoven; frowns disapprobation
At Balzac's name, sighs it at 'poor George Sand's';
Knows that she has exceeding pretty hands;
Speaks Latin with a right accentuation;
And gives at need (as one who understands)
Draught, counsel, diagnosis, exhortation.

Even allowing for the weaknesses in the statistics, it is reasonable to suggest that hospital mortality varied with the hospital's size and location — which partly shaped the kinds of patients admitted — and that it varied through time. In general, males were said to have higher mortality rates than females, the mortality rate among medical patients was higher than among surgical, and some hospitals, and Edinburgh Royal Infirmary and the Royal Infirmary, Glasgow, for example, had distinctly higher rates because they admitted elderly terminal patients.[243] The nineteenth-century debate centred on amputation statistics. Here the one certain thing is that the nineteenth-century figures are all to some extent delusory. The absence of follow-up information is crucial. Research in the 1950s suggested that over a third of patients released from hospital as cured after surgery died within two years and that half of all former surgical cases are 'dead or unimproved' within two years.[244] In general, until the advent of antisepsis in the 1860s, patients whose fingers or toes were amputated survived better than those who suffered amputation at the thigh, elbow or shoulder. These latter 'capital' operations were more common at the big metropolitan hospitals because they admitted those accident victims from the urban accident-prone occupations, building, stevedoring and transport. Bart's mortality ratios were said to be better than Guy's because Bart's received many lads injured in the nearby printing offices who quickly recovered, whereas Guy's had to deal with a large group of older men severely injured at the surrounding railways. Victims with compound fractures and internal injuries were operated on as terminal cases.[245]

The advent of antisepsis deserves much more detailed discussion than I can give here. It did expand the range of internal explorations, and conservative surgery for stone and uterine cysts, for instance, and thereby probably increased the death rate; and the death rate from generalised infection may well have increased. On the other hand, antisepsis probably diminished deaths from shock and it required slower, more considered procedures. Lister's antiseptic system, on his own careful figures, did reduce the death rate after the mid-1860s. At Glasgow the rate fell, for amputations, from 1 death in every 2.2 cases, in the pre-antiseptic period, to 1 in every 6.3.[246] The 70-90 per cent 'cure' rates claimed by surgeons before the 1860s are, as Professor McKeown and his colleagues point out, better than present rates, underpinned as they are by careful anaesthesia, antibiotics and chemotherapy, and are simply unbelievable. Lister's figures are impressive, even when qualified by the absence of follow-up information, because many more operations were being performed by the 1860s. At the Glasgow Infirmary in 1830, 81 amputations were performed for the whole year (70 were claimed as 'cures'). The surgeons were performing about 110 operations annually at the Manchester Infirmary about the same time. By contrast, Guy's in 1834 had announced a 'field day' with four operations, three of them 'capital' (ligature of femoral artery, lithotomy, amputation at shoulder joint, excision of tumour on on jaw — there is no report of how the patients fared).[247]

The advent of anaesthesia immediately increased the amount of surgery. In 1848 the Manchester hospital surgeons performed 169 operations, including 69 amputations a year. Patients were said to be readier to submit to the knife and 'promising young men' quickly found that they could 'carve their way into practice'.[248] Dangerous operations such as the excision of the head of the femur and 'explorations' for ovarian tumour by incision through the wall of the abdomen became fashionable. In 1854 alone the number of operations reported in London hospitals, 180, almost equalled the total reported for the five years 1837-42. In general, operations in voluntary hospitals appear to have increased about threefold between 1847 and 1857, while the overall amputation death rate declined from 33 per cent for 1837-41 to 28 per cent for 1854-6.[249] If we add the numbers for whom anaesthesia made conservative surgery possible these figures become even more telling. At King's College Hospital, before anaesthesia 73 per cent of patients admitted to surgical wards were 'judged unsuitable'. They remained untreated or were 'treated by other means' and had a death rate of 12 per cent, which slightly exceeded the mortality rate of those who underwent operations. By the 1860s only 16 per cent of surgical ward patients were judged unsuitable for surgery and treated by other means. Operative mortality was at 9 per cent, while the mortality rate of the remaining 16 per cent remained at 12 per cent.[250]

Antiseptic operating procedures became widely accepted in the charity hospitals by the mid-1880s, about fifteen years after Lister demonstrated their efficacy in saving lives. Dr Clarke noted that the new procedure had been first adopted as standard in 'private — uncounted — nursing homes for wealthy patients'.[251] But at present we know almost nothing about these institutions. They represent an important area of patient demand and medical innovation which deserves more research. The delay in acceptance within the profession resulted from the surgeons' fear that their traditional rapid cutting, sawing and sewing techniques were suddenly made obsolete. The change-over to the new deliberative procedures took half a generation. As with anaesthesia, the new technique wrought a dramatic increase in the number of operations. At the London Hospital the reported totals rose from 993 in 1843 to 1,317 (more serious) operations in 1883.[252] The West London Hospital went antiseptic in August 1881 after the younger medical staff won a battle with the administrators and their seniors. Before then the hospital had kept no records, it had been dirty, badly ventilated and ill drained. In the 12 months ending August 1881 there had been 69 operations with 11 deaths, mostly from sepsis. In the remaining four months there were 79 operations, with no deaths. In the next four years there were over 100 operations each year. At the Glasgow Royal Infirmary the totals rose from 397 in 1873, 542 in 1874, the antisepsis year, to over 2,000 a year by 1898.[253] Throughout the three decades, surgeons became increasingly venturesome. By the 1890s they were tackling 'in the last resort', intestine obstructions and pyloric (junction of stomach and duodenum) carcinomas.

The remarks about young surgeons 'carving their way' in the public hospitals and the earlier adoption of antisepsis provoke speculation about the patients' varying chances and influence on their treatment in public and private practice. Mr Timothy Holmes admitted in 1869 that

> the private practitioner would very rarely be permitted to perform such a grave operation as an amputation unless he could hold out much more confident hopes of success than any candid man could do in many of the amputations that we perform . . . [on the poor]. Then there is the dislike (and a very natural and proper feeling it is) of a private practitioner to perform an operation which is likely to prove fatal.[254]

Doctors could experiment and act on their prejudices in public practice. In general the results were bad for the poor, but not wholly so. In pre- and post-operative procedures on private patients, the surgeon probably exercised greater control over his patient's low (and debilitating) diet than he could in a public hospital. On the other hand, until the nursing reforms of the 1870s, at least, private patients probably got more opium, wine and spirits, while hospital patients were usually severely bled and purged before an operation and bled to syncope after it, especially if they were 'white and inclined to tetanus'.[255] Post-operative shock must have been more frequent in hospitals. Such results as we have suggest that private patients' chances of survival were much greater. Simpson obtained returns from nearly 400 private practices giving details of 2,000 operations in the late 1860s. These showed a 10.8 per cent death rate from amputations of upper and lower limbs, compared with 41 per cent in the large hospitals. Yet Simpson's figures probably overstate the difference. Holmes criticised his conclusions because private practitioners 'treasured up' records of success and happily forgot failures. They rarely touched the worst cases, but sent them to hospitals. When they could not escape operating, and death ensued, they 'would not bother to keep a record', or 'if they did, they ascribed the death to a 'previous disease or concomitant injury'.[256] The great advantage of private treatment was, of course, the relative safety from cross-infection and the patient's power to demand anaesthesia and antiseptic procedures.

Doctors could display their scientific scepticism in hospitals. Many older men resisted antisepsis because they recalled the exaggerated claims made for Gannal's antiseptic fluid as a preservative of cadavers. Pasteurism seemed to be only another fad out of France. Others preferred to experiment with Condy's crystals on burns, ulcers and amputation surfaces. Dr Wynn Williams preferred sulphurous acid, and Dr

George Ross chlorine. Both agreed in refusing to allow Lister's carbolic acid in their wards. Dr Nunnelly knew that antisepsis could not work and therefore never tried it, in public practice at least. Dr G.W. Callender, at Bart's, got good results with 'cleanliness alone'. Besides, he pointed out, Lister's carbolic sprays and the rest of the antiseptic method, especially the assiduous after-care, of regular draining and re-bandaging, was 'extremely complicated, expensive, irksome, and laborious', and hospital doctors were always short of time. Lawson Tait, the apostle of ovariotomy, still used only tap water as an aseptic agent in 1886 and insisted, in order to annoy the Listerites, that it be unboiled. He claimed not to have had a death among 139 cases in 1884-5. By contrast, two of Lister's disciples at Guy's, Henry Howse and Davies-Colley, set out to prove his techniques in 1871 by per-forming all their operations in the erysipelas wards, with what was reported as 'comparative safety'. Strict washing of patients and the part to be incised, together with the full hour-long boiling of the instru-ments did not become standard in Bart's until 1892.[257] Ultimately, asepsis was to triumph, with the maturing of hospitals as safe institu-tions based on exhaustive nursing and scrubbing.

When they were not under scrutiny, doctors evaded antiseptic pro-cedures in private practice too. This was especially true of midwifery. As late as 1898, doctors said that Lister's procedures were too elaborate and practically impossible to follow in the lying-in room. Moreover, as Dr J. Armstrong remarked, in 1883, in normal births there was no obvious need for it. He was content to wash his hands and smear the woman's labia with a solution of eucalyptus oil and boracic acid.[258]

Listerism opportunely saved the hospitals during a crisis of confi-dence about their effectiveness. Streptococcal infections had been endemic, but the increase of admissions and operations in the 1850s and early 1860s produced epidemics. James Simpson claimed in 1869 that many more patients suffered pyaemia or sloughing and phagedaena (rapidly spreading ulceration) than were admitted with it. And the larger the hospital, the worse the infection and mortality rates. Hospi-tals with 300-600 beds had rates of 1 death in every 7 amputations; those with under 25 beds, 1 in 21. Simpson's statistics were unreliable and his claims were exaggerated but none the less he was probably right in the general drift of his assertions. He, Florence Nightingale and William Farr argued from 1858 onwards for the dismantling of the big single-block hospitals and a change to pavilion-type wards or to cottage refuges. Only then could the causes of infection, over-crowding, deficient ventilation and careless nursing be overcome.

Their allegations and recommendations provoked a furious row about the worth of their statistics, and about the possible rebuilding and resiting of St Thomas's Hospital, or, as William Farr wanted, breaking up of the hospital into small units set among areas of patient need all over the metropolis. The St Thomas's story is well told elsewhere. The important point here is to see the row in its context of questioning the future of the mass clinical machine. As one of Simpson's supporters remarked: 'hospitals are necessary evils, good for paupers, good for medical instruction, and as fields of scientific observation, but worse than useless as hygienic resorts. Who would like to have a mortality of 11 per cent in one's private patients . . .' He went on to plead for more home treatment for the poor, as the rich enjoyed already, more cottage hospitals, and better workhouse infirmaries.[259]

Traditionalists joined with antisepsis missionaries to beat back the environmentalists. For the traditionalists, Mr T.P. Heslop of Birmingham disputed Simpson's figures. The county hospitals had a good record only because they uniformly excluded infectious diseases cases and, because they were still subject to lay governors, 90 per cent of their admissions were mild cases or chronics nominated by subscribers. Every patient had to be kept in for the full term of his letter, otherwise the subscriber would think he was not getting value for his donation. Chronic cases of rheumatism or consumption took turns for long-term stays, as at Colchester, of about two months each, or Gloucester and Ipswich, one month. In Oxford, 'lines' for the Radcliffe Infirmary were even called 'turns'. These 'sick club' institutions demeaned medical dignity.[260] For the missionaries, the great surgeon, James Syme of Edinburgh, Lister's father-in-law, was pressing in the late 1860s for a large single block for the new infirmary, in order that it could 'be kept clean with disinfectant'. Simpson declared that the large-scale antiseptic plan would never work. Syme spurned 'unscrupulous attempts to undermine confidence in large hospitals'. They had to be retained, and, if elaborate antisepsis had to become the means of keeping them, then antisepsis had to be 'doubled up'. Large hospitals aggregated medical skills and were the only economic way of dispensing those skills to the poor. And without the aggregation of such clinical material, medical advance would cease.[261]

Both sides won. The great hospitals remained, although some transformed themselves into pavilion systems or what were believed to be better-ventilated H shapes. Overcrowding, which Listerism and its prolonged after-care methods had recently intensified, and which had formed a basic cause of hospital mortality, was alleviated by rebuilding and rearrangement of wards. By provoking this improvement Simpson and Nightingale effected a major saving of life. Cottage hospitals also spread rapidly after the first at Cranleigh, in Surrey, in 1859. In 1865 there were 18; in 1889, 400, with about 4,000 beds. They were simple, homely places without elaborate equipment. The number of inmates was deliberately kept small, at between 4 and 20 patients. There was a charge, usually 2s. 6d. a week, for all patients. Personal payment usually received priority of entry over cases paid for out of charity funds or by the guardians. Independent patients also could occupy private rooms. Patrons who paid a guinea a year were entitled to nominate one patient for a three-week stay. Some hospitals ran insurance schemes whereby one penny per week insurers could gain admission without a patron's vote.[262] Most hospitals refused infectious and maternity cases and directed chronics and incurables to the county hospitals.

Cottage hospitals were open to all qualified GPs in the district, a provision that was crucial to their acceptance. Patients 'retained' the visiting practitioner: if they could not pay him, the charity officers or guardians did. Cottage hospitals effectively channelled to doctors a lot of local money that had been beyond their grasp. At Sudbury, for example, the local hospital board received £110 a year from an 'old lepers' charity'.[263]

Most patients, in East Anglia at least, were admitted for 'debility and anaemia', or as accident cases. As Dr Sinclair Holden of the Sudbury Hospital remarked in 1889, the Cottage Hospital movement coincided with the increased use of machinery in agriculture and a great increase in 'broken bones, cuts etc.'. At Mildenhall Hospital in 1868, J.T. aged 18, labourer, was admitted on 18 April with ascites of the left lung. He had been discharged from the County Hospital at Bury St Edmund's as incurable. He died, at home, in December. He had had two admissions 'for fluid to be drawn off'. W.S., a thatcher aged 18, was admitted in early September with 'tubercular peritonitis, with secondary effusion within the abdominal cavity'. In early November he was discharged, 'cured'. As Dr Sinclair Holden said, 'a few weeks' residence in the hospital, with nourishing food, pure air, cheerful companionship, and a spirit of briskness, work marvels of restoration.'

The boards of cottage hospitals claimed almost 100 per cent cure rates. But as J.T.'s case shows, the figuring must have helped by omitting the hopeless cases and in W.S.'s case, not following up. In 1871 the Bury Hospital had an outbreak of erysipelas after a woman with burns had been admitted. There were 6 cases and 2 deaths. All patients were sent home and the hospital closed for a week and those who still had erysipelas were not readmitted. Presumably the hospital's 'cure' record remained at 100 per cent.[264]

By the early twentieth century the cottage hospitals and nursing homes had shed much of their homeliness and become miniature general hospitals, embryos of what most of them are now. Bexley had almost as many out-patients as in-patients. Beckenham had 32 beds. Nearly all had operating-theatres and paupers were now almost completely excluded.[265]

The Hospital Crisis

The new fame of the great hospitals as reparative institutions induced increasing numbers to flock to them, quite apart from the ordinary increase of population and the lag, until the 1880s, in building additional big hospitals. By the mid-1860s doctors were saying that the solution of the hygienic and therapeutic crisis had issued in a new social and economic crisis for hospitals and the medical profession. Between 1859 and 1865, for instance, the annual number of out-patients at Bart's grew from 84,000 to 133,000. The notions that out-patients' departments had become 'unmanageable' and that their facilities were 'greatly abused' became increasingly attractive to doctors and hospital administrators.[266]

They sought to replace the charitable refuge conception of the hospital by an independent curative corporation. Hospital specialists claimed that their skills were being wasted on trivial ailments. Moreover, the race through the ward, dispensing nominal treatment, was now seen to be undignified for a senior hospital man. Private practitioners, especially GPs, alleged that hospitals were drawing off their natural clientele, patients with common ailments who could pay. Patrons' letters only compounded the abuse. The doctors launched a generally successful campaign in the late 1860s to limit or abolish 'lines'.[267]

Doctors agreed that out-patients comprised not the deserving poor but the classes above the labouring poor, 'the grades who follow sedentary occupations or those of no avocation at all', like many of the females. By 1879 the Charity Organization Society had defined them as the 'upper lower-classes'. In 1872 University College Hospital invited the COS to vet out-patients. The Royal Free Hospital followed in 1874. The COS investigated a sample of 641 applicants and decided that:

12 could have paid a doctor's bill;
231 could have subscribed to a provident dispensary;

169 were 'proper applicants';
57 were paupers and should have gone to the Poor Law officers;
103 gave false names and addresses;
69 no information.

The majority, they concluded, used the out-patients' wards as 'family doctor and chemist's shop'. The patients attended, not to save money, but because they believed they would receive 'superior advice'.[268]

The problem lingered on into the twentieth century. Times of distress, as in the mid-1880s, brought it into medical discussions while at other times doctors forgot about it. They could not solve it because they were divided. Some old-fashioned paternalists, like Dr Bristowe, believed that the close investigation of their out-patients' circumstances lowered the 'dignity of medicine'. 'Hospitals existed to bring to sufferers, without haggling as in petty shops, all the resources of surgery, physic and pharmacy.' Bristowe added that he mistrusted the existing definitions of poverty based only on income.[269] (The London COS seems never to have had a definition of 'deserving poverty'. Its Manchester equivalent in 1875 fixed a 'poverty scale' of 18*s*. maximum for a man and wife; 12*s*. for a single woman and an additional 1*s*. 6*d*. a week for every child. This scale eliminated 42 per cent of the Manchester out-patients.)[270]

There was also 'refined poverty' and sufferers 'whose means are hopelessly disproportionate to their necessities or their necessary appearance in society'. They simply could not afford specialist help and were, rightly, the doctors thought, too proud to beg from a private consultant. Against this view, younger doctors, like James Erskine in Glasgow, argued that hospitals had been much too free with their services. Not only did private GPs lose patients, but beginners who were accumulating capital by working for provident dispensaries also found their incomes cut, especially in bad times, when subscribers left the dispensary and joined the hospital out-patients' queues. Guy's, Bart's and the Scottish hospitals introduced small charges for medicines and bandages, but these angered the GPs, who claimed that this only legitimated the attendance of patients who otherwise could afford to go to them. Hospital specialists, on the other hand, argued that hospitals needed large flows of clinical material to maintain their reputations. Specialists with private opthalmic, orthopaedic or other hospitals to maintain were equally firm that GPs ought to direct such patients as could pay to them rather than to the hospitals. Yet the GPs did not dare send such patients to private specialists for fear of losing the patient: the specialist might 'take him over', or because cataract operations cost 100 guineas, for example, the patient might denounce the GP as a rogue in league with the specialist. Yet specialities were at the heart of the problem: they required long periods of treatment and even middle-class people could not afford private consultations.[271]

This difficulty is the real source of the hospital almoner system. They were not created to help the poor through the system but, as Miss Helen Nussey, the first almoner at the Westminster Hospital, put it, 'to check abuses' and to save doctors the unsavoury job of investigating the patient's social circumstances, and to find social reasons for continuing treatment of otherwise ineligible cases when the doctor, 'considering only the disease', deemed the case interesting. Miss Cummins, at St Thomas's, found her mission in fighting 'the want of backbone that is increasingly evident among the working classes'.[272] Finally, as the threat of Lloyd George's social insurance legislation loomed in 1909, hospital administrators, consultants, GPs, almoners and directors of friendly societies closed ranks to defend gratuitous hospital and dispensary treatment; questions about patient eligibility suddenly became unimportant.[273]

The growing sophistication of their services so increased hospital expenditure that by the 1860s most hospitals were near financial collapse. Indeed, disputes about provisions for patients were partly a symptom of this fundamental *malaise*. Even in the 1850s nine of the London hospitals were said to be 'crippled' for want of money. Whole wards had to be kept empty.[274] In 1857 Drs Farr and Guy estimated that £300,000 was spent annually on the institutional treatment of the sick poor in London. Dispensaries spent one-tenth of the sum upon one-third of the total patient population of 65,000 (who in turn amounted to 1 in 5 of the London population). Yet the entire income of 14 London hospitals was £155,000, half of which went to three Guy's, St Thomas's and Bart's. Guy's spent 18s. per patient, the Royal Free, 3s. 8d. Bart's received £34,000 a year, King's College Hospital, £6,000. St George's annual outlay exceeded its income by £6,000: it had been living on its £225,000 capital endowment since the 1830s. The Board had just spent £25,000 on a new building. The hospital now needed donations totalling £10,000 a year to save it from closure.[275] Such management, traditionally in the hands of a tiny self-perpetuating clique which met without proper minutes and reported without proper audit, had sufficed in the days of minor expenditures on asylum-type services. Now, in the days of anaesthesia, special wards and big buildings, the hospitals were overwhelmed. The voluntary hospitals' troubles worsened in 1866 with the decisions by the House of Lords in Jones *v*. Mersey Docks, which rendered them in England and Wales, at least, liable to local rates. St George's, for example, suddenly found itself levied for £600 annually for the poor and £300 for other parish rates. The Birmingham Infirmary was proposing to close wards capable of holding 123 patients, in order to find the £330 it needed for rates.[276]

Building costs soared, too, as the hospitals made sanitary improvements, and remodelled themselves on the standards set by the unprecedentedly expensive and luxurious new military hospital at Netley, which was built during the late 1860s at a cost of about £300,000. The new St Thomas's in the 1870s, constructed on the pavilion principle, cost £600,000. The largest suites were the Treasurer's house and the Board dining-room. The Manchester Royal Infirmary in 1881 had to spend £23,000 remedying sanitary defects, when their annual income was only £20,000, after having fallen consistently through the 1870s. In four years, the hospital had sold £60,000 worth of stocks.[277] Moreover, the fall in the value of land during the 1870s and 1880s must have hit the wealthier old hospitals, whilst there were difficulties for the newer hospitals in accepting gifts of landed property because of the law of mortmain. Subscriptions were stationary at the 1-, 2- or 10-guinea mark. Hospital treasurers avoided increasing them, for fear of losing the subscriber. Subscriptions were collected by fund-raisers such as Edgcumbe and Co., who kept half the proceeds as commission. Apart from Guy's, Bart's and St Thomas's, the subscriptions did not even cover the staff wages bill. This incidentally was the largest single item of recurrent expenditure and the second-fastest in its rate of increase. It would be worth trying to discover how much the Treasurer and other officials made out of their hospitals. Quite apart from their vaguely announced 'honoraria', their investment and share trading policies, which cumulatively must have been a significant part of the stock market, would be worth tracing. Meanwhile, medical staff continued to use much more expensive and showy instruments in hospitals than they did for their private patients. In hospitals they used yards of gauze, in their private practice, one layer of gauze and a calico bandage. 'Incidental expenses' were the fastest increasing item in London hospitals. They increased 310 per cent between 1871 and 1881. Voluntary income increased over the decade by 5 per cent.[278]

In the light of these calculations, it is difficult to explain how the hospitals survived. Given the evasions and exaggerations in their annual reports, the answer will only be found in their surviving accounts books.

There is some evidence that doctors decreased the average cost per patient by reducing the length of stay, especially in hospitals like the big Scottish ones, which abolished subscribers' lines. The poorer hospitals also allowed out-patients fewer treatments: 2.6 per patient at the Middlesex in 1908 against Guy's 3.3. They also apparently saved on nursing care, drugs and treatment per in-patient bed: Charing Cross spent £136 on each bed per year, Guy's, £529. Expenditure at St George's on bread and flour, tea, milk and alcohol per patient was cut over all by about one-third, while outlays on instruments and surgical appliances rose fourfold.[279]

The hospitals had three sources of new revenue: public begging, patients' charges and pay beds. Hospitals began to advertise for legacies and donations and sought, for instance, through a shady fund-raiser, Dr Benham, to cash in on the Queen's Jubilee. Benham let them down. Ladies' committees, fêtes, galas, medical students' and nurses' fund-raising stunts all became fashionable. Very occasionally someone would suggest, as Lord Derby did in 1870, that hospitals should be supported out of the rates, or that the allocation of hospital resources be centrally controlled by government, as Dr Sutherland proposed in 1888. But doctors and administrators always smothered the proposal with cries of 'charity' and 'liberty'.[280]

Hospital Sunday began in Birmingham in 1859. The practice spread through the provinces in the 1860s but did not start in London until 1874, because of the fierce opposition of the Bishop of London, who had his own hospital fund and did not want public money to go to Nonconformist dispensaries. The proceeds from Hospital Sunday in London were £26,600 in 1874, £32,000 in 1883, £40,000 in 1888, £60,000 in 1902, and up to £10,000 in the 1870s in Birmingham, Manchester and Liverpool. These could not have solved the hospitals' basic difficulties; but they probably enabled them to continue from year to year while waiting for legacies and other benefactions to turn up. In the share-out of the funds, hospitals took four-fifths, and dispensaries received the remainder. The Hospital Sunday Fund was not an unmixed blessing, so far as doctors and hospital administrators were concerned. Large regular subscribers fell away, to be replaced by working men contributing through the Sunday (in some places, Saturday) Fund, which was promoted as the small man's charity at 2s.-3s. per year. Working men began to join boards of governors, and to demand 'every attention' for working-class patients. At Leeds and Coventry working men had by 1889 gained an especially 'large say' and they proved 'intensely antagonistic to the medical men'. At the Newport,

Monmouthshire, Infirmary, the working-men 'directors' elected to the
Board by the Workingmen's Hospital Saturday Fund sacked Dr Henry
Ensor because he refused to treat two out-patients whom he believed
could afford to pay him privately.[281]

Working-men governors also fought the administrators and doctors
in their essays to develop patient charges and pay beds as new sources
of revenue. The big London hospitals, which managed to avoid working-
class governors, could, as Guy's did in 1884, smoothly introduce a 3*d*.
a week charge and 1*d*. per medicine bottle. But there was a row when
the Newcastle Infirmary followed suit in 1886. After a 3*d*. per visit
charge was introduced the number of casual out-patients fell by nearly
two-thirds, and there was a change in the class of patient: 'a superior
class . . . presented themselves, persons who would not accept of charitable assistance, but had no objection to be cured cheaply, while the
very necessitous "appear to be scared away" '. Yet hospital treasurers
found patient fees indispensable; the COS calculated that it formed 10
per cent of hospital income in the early 1880s. By 1897 at least 18
London hospitals were getting more from patients' fees than from
subscribers.[282]

Special hospitals, Moorfields Eye Hospital, for instance, had since
their inception been sought by wealthy patients, who were admitted
as private paying patients. Newly rebuilt hospitals with good reputations, such as Addenbrooke's, the London Fever Hospital and the
Edinburgh Infirmary, also met demands from middle-class cases for
admission by creating pay rooms at around three guineas a week;
thereby the hospital helped to amortise its building debt. When St
Thomas's experienced a sudden liquidity crisis in 1879, the authorities
set aside a whole block for paying patients. They also took the revo-
lutionary step of appointing a salaried resident doctor to treat them, in
conjunction with the hospital's consultants. The board hoped thereby
that 'the patients [would] be able to give somewhat larger fees to the
consultants'. Hitherto, pay patients had had their own doctors come in.
The St Thomas's 'Home Hospital' proved immediately remunerative
and was quickly copied by Guy's and other hospitals.[283] The Bradford
Fever Hospital, for instance, spent £3,000 adding a 'luxurious' wing, in
which the paying patients were to receive free attention from the hospital's consultants. A great row ensued. Local practitioners alleged that
the closed pay-bed system was robbing them. Norwich GPs declared
that a similar proposal before the Norwich Hospital board would turn
'the hospital into a hotel'. They combined with working-men governors
of the hospital to defeat the move. Over 200 GPs joined the protest

when the Great Northern Central Hospital started closed pay beds in 1894. It was the only hospital in the midst of a population of 400,000, yet during the 1880s and 1890s it increased the proportion of pay beds every year. Among the medical fraternity, only Dr C.R. Drysdale, the radical, opposed pay beds on the principle that the poor, because they were poor, had greater need of hospital beds than the middle classes, who could pay for care elsewhere. His colleagues appear to have ignored his argument.[284]

Pay beds brought a new class into the charity hospitals. While the dormitory wards continued to house the labouring poor and the 'upper lower-classes' in 1890, the pay-bed wings housed 'clerks, warehouse-men, clergymen and women of the middle classes with special diseases'. Treatment by the consultant in the hospital was still cheaper than the equivalent private treatment outside. In 1911 two investigations found that the 'surgical population' especially contained an 'admixture of the middle classes', due to 'the increased expense of medicinal surgical treatment'. Indeed, two years earlier a medical man in a pay bed sued Bart's for negligence during an operation on him. He lost. By 1956 social classes I, II and III were using the London teaching hospitals more than classes IV and V, although the two latter had higher death rates and probably higher morbidity rates.[285]

Entrepreneurs were quick to catch on to the pay-bed system. Fitzroy House opened in 1880. By 1882 it was paying 3 per cent profits to the six investors who put £6,000 into it. It had 14 beds at between 4 and 10 guineas a week, with 'specials' at 30 guineas. All medical fees were extra. Forty-nine leading London consultants had taken rooms in it. By 1903 Fitzroy House had handled over 5,000 patients. The board of directors had managed to have the clinic declared a charity. The re-building they completed in 1903 was paid for largely by donation. Copies of Fitzroy House opened in many provincial cities. The Medical and Surgical Home in Aberdeen, for instance, opened in 1890, as a 'strictly private and independent venture'. It too was willing to receive charitable help. The nominal proprietress was inappropriately named Sister Dorcas.[286]

3. REGULAR PRACTITIONERS AND QUACKS

Bone-Setters

Certain classes of patients remained beyond orthodox help and others held aloof from it. They included sufferers from dislocated bones, tuberculosis, cancer, and a range of internal complaints including venereal diseases and impotence. Here the traditional bone-setters and quacks held their own.

Bone-setters had existed for centuries in Britain. Their skills, which seem to have combined those of the modern physiotherapist, chiropractor and osteopath, were often handed down within families from father and mother to son and daughter, although most bone-setters were male. Many country bone-setters combined their practice with horse-doctoring. Some sufferers went to them always in preference to the local orthodox surgeon but most, like their present counterparts, resorted to a bone-setter after orthodox medicine had failed them. Bone-setters worked by feel, with only the vaguest knowledge of anatomy. Unlike orthodox practitioners, they used manipulation and brute strength to 'snap' things back into place (the patient always expected the 'snap', as a sign that the process was succeeding) rather than the agonising block and tackle at the hospitals. Some bone-setters also 'charmed' the joint after they set it. But this was extra: 3s. 6d. at Manchester in the 1880s. Bone-setters were of the people, and found their business at the local markets. Mason at Sleaford, 'old Roady', formerly a butcher, at Mareham, and Trolly, who worked mainly at Boston.[287]

Although they were of the people and there was great popular faith in them, bone-setters were not invariably dedicated and effective. The behaviour of some with large practices, Trolly, for instance, seems not too different from that of their orthodox brethren. In 1831 a lad was brought to Trolly with a dislocated shoulder. He did not inspect the injury but simply pronounced that the left shoulder was 'out'. He pulled that arm for 10 minutes and then put it in a sling. It was the wrong arm. In Morpeth in 1888 a woman went to a bone-setter with swollen rheumatic wrists, after her GP had said he could not help her. The bone-setter pronounced them 'out' and 'set' them for 2s. 6d. Soon after her fingers swelled 'like sausages' and after a fortnight the woman could not move her wrists. In 1898 a girl died in Gateshead from gangrene after a bone-setter had blistered her back and tightly bandaged her leg to 'ease down' the muscles. He was found not to have been negligent and thereby was acquitted of manslaughter.[288] Bone-setters also had frequent trouble with bad fracture cases. So also did orthodox practitioners. In 1849 at Allerby near Maryport in Cumberland Dr Pearson was called to a collier with a severe compound fracture of the leg. The bones had been set two days earlier by a local bone-setter, in a rough splint and a white bread poultice on the four inches of exposed bone. The muscles and flesh looked like 'half boiled beef', and no attempt had been made to bring the bones together. Talk in the village was that the wound was 'beginning to matter nicely'. The collier died from tetanus after 10 days. The coroner's jury found 'accidental death'. Pearson was shouted down when he tried to give evidence.[289]

Defections of patients to bone-setters made doctors wrathful, especially during the early and middle years of the century when they were slowly establishing their respectability. At Spalding in 1853 Henry Branton, a 'respectable yeoman', went to a bone-setter at Wisbeach after his damaged hip made no progress under the treatment of the local surgeon. The surgeon refused to act with the bone-setter, while Branton gradually sank and died. The coroner's jury rebuked the surgeon. In 1858 at Colneis in Suffolk a six-year-old son of an iron-worker broke his humerus at the elbow. The local GP refused to see the child, but sent his inexperienced assistant who bandaged the arm tightly with splints to the wrist. Five weeks later the wound suppurated and burst. The boy's mother then took him to a bone-setter who recommended 'warm formentations, cold water bandages, and whisky cloths'. Three months later she took the child to another bone-setter. He remarked: 'That's a lost arm; that hand is quite dead.' He told the mother to boil salt and nettles in water and apply the mixture to the arm. The wound healed, leaving the hand and wrist distorted. The mother sued the GP and his assistant, but failed to prove 'maltreatment'. At Nottingham the traditional bone-setter were the Maltbys, who were also innkeepers. In 1877 an old woman injured her thigh. Five days after the accident a surgeon visited her. He 'suspected' a fracture but did not pronounce positively. The old woman was ailing when her friends sent for Mrs Maltby. She declared that the hip was 'out' and proceeded to reduce the dislocation; whereupon the old woman died. By contrast, a solicitor went to a surgeon in Cockermouth in 1866 with an ankle injury. The surgeon said it was a 'sprain'. But the ankle became worse. The solicitor was helped to a bone-setter. He manipulated the ankle and brought 'almost instant relief'.[290]

This last case is doubtless more typical than the failures I have sketched. Bone-setters charged accordingly. After he successfully set a boy's fractured leg in 1850 Rhodes (son of 'old Roady'?) at Bishop Monkton in the West Riding charged £15.2s.0d. for the cure, and sued for it when it was not forthcoming. He won his case and Rhodes *v.* Atkinson became a crucial precedent for permitting other unqualified practitioners to claim fees. The going rate for a treatment for a poor patient seems to have been 2*s*. 6*d*., or rather more than many a six-penny doctor would have charged.[291]

By the 1870s, bone-setters had developed their own respectability. Richard Hutton, who had a notable practice among the upper classes, and over 1,000 patients a year, treated poor cases gratuitously. Professor Atkinson, a descendant of the Huttons, had his rooms in Park Lane and by 1904 was employing 12 assistants. H.A. Barker also had a fashionable clientele, headed by the Lord Mayor of London. By 1908 he was living in Park Lane, and dealing with up to 40 patients a day.[292]

From the 1870s, too, orthodox practitioners began to admit that bone-setters could succeed where they failed, to send patients to them, and to copy their methods. As one surgeon noted, doctors immobilised injured joints, whereas bone-setters moved them and got them working. The surgeon's smattering of morbid anatomy was less useful than the bone-setter's confident empirical skill. And in cases of severe fracture neither was able to achieve much, although desperate sufferers might have been readier to believe in the powers of the bone-setter than in those of the GP. By 1875 several orthodox doctors were using bone-setters' manipulative techniques. Many, unlike the bone-setters, applied anaesthesia during the manipulation. But the leaders of the medical profession remained supercilious and they finally forced the issue in 1911 when Frederick Axham was struck off for working with Barker. Barker did great work during the First World War and was knighted in 1922. Axham was never restored to the register.[293]

Tuberculosis

Tuberculosis is an infectious, communicable disease which commonly attacks the lungs, although it can manifest itself in various forms in almost any part of the body.

The tubercle bacillus (*Mycabacterium tuberculosis*) can enter the body in several ways. The source is normally the sputum of an infected person. The bacilli can spread by droplet infection, by carriage through the air, and on contaminated eating utensils. They can live for months in dried sputum. And they can also enter the body through the digestive tract carried in contaminated milk and dairy products. Persons in poor general health who live in crowded conditions for long periods with TB sufferers are at the greatest risk.

In the nineteenth century tubercular infection was often difficult to diagnose. The early listlessness and vague pains in the chest passed unnoticed as normal fatigue. The distinctive symptoms, the cough and spitting of purulent sputum, fever and light sweats, do not appear until the disease has a strong hold, possibly after a year. For this reason, and others, the mortality statistics are particularly suspect. Deaths and illness among infants and children ascribed to 'hydrocephalus', 'scrofula' and 'tabes mesenterica' undoubtedly included many deaths originating with tubercular infection. The Registrar-General recognised this in 1881 when he re-assigned deaths from 'hydrocephalus' and 'scrofula' respectively to 'tubercular meningitis' and 'other forms of tubercular scrofula'. Moreover, the prevailing belief that pulmonary tuberculosis-consumption was hereditary, and therefore a stigma on a family, led many kindly doctors to report the cause of death as 'pneumonia' or 'respiratory disease'. This stigma always blocked moves to make consumption a notifiable disease, until 1912, and even then notification remained patchy until after the Tuberculosis Act of 1921.[294] But the fact remains that it was a grievous killer throughout the century.

In 1838 there were 59,000 deaths reported in England and Wales from consumption. These formed two-thirds of all respiratory deaths and one-sixth of all deaths. By 1858 there were over 50,000 deaths reported from consumption, together with 8,000 more from 'scrofula' and 'tabes mesenterica'. Over all, reported consumption mortality halved from 380 per 100,000 in 1838 to 183 per 100,000 in 1894. This represents a saving of 75,000 lives a year by the 1880s.[295] We know very little about this process, achieved long before antibiotics, whether by region, social class, or age group. Tuberculosis, because it is related to overcrowding, seems to have been worse in the large cities, but was by no means confined to them. The distributions by age are also complicated, although the main point, that consumption mortality was highest among persons 25-45, is clear.[296] Dr Jones calculated that mortality reported among infants under five fell dramatically, as shown in Table 4.6.

Table 4.6: Mortality in Children under Five Years per 100,000 Living

	Consumption	Hydrocephalus	Other Tuberculoses
1851-60	130	253	192
1861-70	96	221	226
1871-80	76	190	255

Source: *JRSS*, vol. LVII (1894), p. 26.

The rise in 'other tuberculoses' might be accounted for by a better diagnosis over the period,[297] although even in 1912 school medical officers were still very uncertain in diagnosing tuberculosis.[298]

The fall in infant tubercular deaths was matched by a fall of about 33 per cent between 1851 and 1880 in the rates for 15- to 25-year-olds, which served to emphasise the concentration of the mortality among the 25-45 group at twice the infants' rate, and a slow but steady over-all decline of about 16 per cent. Until 1865, more females were reported as dying of tuberculosis than males; thereafter the rate among females decreased much faster than that of males. Possibly this change is con-nected with improving conditions of female employment. Within the adult age group TB was reported as the cause of one-quarter of all deaths.[299]

Tuberculosis was pre-eminently a disease of the poor (although it was always less common and less virulent in Ireland). In 1895 Hampstead had a reported rate of 93 per 100,000 while St Giles's, St Saviour's and St Olave's had 330 per 100,000. Dr C.R. Drysdale asserted that it was his experience that the poor had four times as much TB morbidity as the rich.[300]

Fifty years earlier in 1846, Benjamin Phillips, surgeon to the Westminster Hospital, and his colleagues had claimed to have examined nearly 134,000 children aged 5-15 in workhouses, schools and factories. They found 24 per cent with 'certain marks of scrofula', a high propor-tion of which must have been tubercular. The incidence was highest among those in workhouses. Convicts in Millbank Penitentiary had 'external scrofula' at the rate of 13.5 per 1,000 in 1844. Even so, Phillips remarked, the British rates among children compared favour-ably with those reported from orphanages, abroad: Lisbon 35 per cent; Amsterdam 42 per cent; Berlin 53 per cent; St Petersburg 41 per cent; and Calcutta 56 per cent.[301] As with other — most other — diseases, these are grounds, admittedly shaky because it is impossible to discover how the figures were derived, for suggesting that Britain had the lowest incidence in Europe — and, it might follow, the highest standard of living.

Doctors had long guessed that TB was associated with overcrowding and poverty. Before germ theory, they knew that the disease ran in families but they were puzzled about its manner of propagation. Dr Wynn Williams expressed the general medical opinion in 1867 in saying that he did not think TB 'contagious', that is, that it could not be 'communicated to a healthy person'. But

> if a person with any hereditary taint lurking in the system, were placed constantly in close contact with a person dying of consump-tion, such as nursing or sleeping with him, and breathing the exhala-tions from the expectoration, skin, etc., he would be certain to have

the disease, then dormant brought into activity . . . He had in this way seen sister after sister carried off.

He added that no reliance could be placed on the Registrar-General's statistics because 'there is great objection among the lower classes to have the disease registered as consumption'. And in Wales, where deaths could still be registered without a medical certificate, 'the disease was quite as likely to be registered wrongly as rightly'.[302]

Dr William Budd had suggested that consumption was a specific infection in 1867. But this hypothesis had been ignored. Koch's discovery of the bacillus in 1882 took about a decade to find general medical acceptance in Britain. Doctors and patients eagerly used his 'fluid' when he announced it in 1890; its failure set back acceptance of specific anti-germ treatments for years. Dr J. Andrew's writing on the aetiology of phthisis in 1884 still found it 'inexplicable' that married females should have a higher incidence than any other group. He guessed that they might be 'affected by a widely diffused exciting cause produced by the special duties and indoor nature of their occupations'. TB had long been known as the particular disease of seamstresses, tailors, bookmakers, indoor servants and unmarried daughters living at home.[303]

There was no cure. But with rest, quiet and good diet, the body may overcome attacks if they are found early enough. Before the 1860s wealthy sufferers had sought to avoid the dank British winter season by going to Torquay, the Isle of Wight, Cannes or Florence, or even emigrating to Australia. In 1868 Herman Weber publicised the notion that high, dry mountain air could arrest or even cure TB. He began the lucrative careers of places like Davos, where wealthy patients patiently 'freezed it out'. For those who could not thus escape, the treatment was much the same as that for other respiratory diseases and fevers;[304] until the 1850s venesection, with calomel, opium, Dover's powders and antimony; thereafter, to the 1880s, the treatment was 'eliminant and expectant'. The patient was dosed, if he could afford it, with bicarbonate of potash, ammonia acetate, nitric ether, combined with ipecacuanha and opium, and 'occasional doses of a mild mercurial'. When the patient's strength began to fail, stimulants — 'ammonia, brandy, or wine' — were given, and blisters or poultices were applied externally. By 1880 Dr Frederick Livy reported good results 'at the pre-tubercular stage of phthisis' with white of egg, 1 oz of brandy, and ammonia, and 4 oz of cod-liver oil.[305]

Tuberculosis both ravaged the existing poor and impoverished the families of victims. The period of 'decline', usually between 2½ and 5 years, was hopeless and nasty. Bread-winner victims had to cease working long before they died. Walter Rose, born in 1871 in Haddenham, Buckinghamshire, recalled that consumption was dreaded among the agricultural labouring families in country villages. His village 'was never free of it'. 'The symptoms were always the same, a delicate flush on an otherwise pale face, accompanied by a short hacking cough; this continued for about three years, the sick one becoming weaker, until the end.' The Rose family, like their neighbours, ate live snails as a preventive.[306]

There was virtually no hospital accommodation for poor TB sufferers. In 1897 there were an estimated 250,000 consumptives, of whom only 50,000 had the means to go abroad, rest at home, or enter a private sanatorium. Charity hospitals for consumptives had only 1,160 beds between them. The cure rate at the most notable hospital, the Brompton, was 4 per cent. The big general hospitals rejected them as 'incurables'. By 1900 only 3.4 per cent of their total admissions were TB cases.[307] The medical profession, like the government, had dismissed the problem as vast and hopeless. Most poor victims lingered on at home until they could no longer be nursed by their families, when they were removed to die in workhouse infirmaries.

Three case-histories collected for the Poor Law Royal Commission in 1909 provide insights into the disruption and anxiety that TB could produce in working-class families. 'M Mc M' was a male aged 44. He had phthisis but apparently had kept it quiet and was still working as a dock labourer. (Here the absence of compulsory notification was convenient.) He slept with his wife and two children in one room. He used pieces of paper to spit into, and then burned them. He had seen the district medical officer and the female sanitary visitor had called, seemingly infrequently. One of his children, aged 18 months, had acute pneumonia when the Royal Commission investigator called: the parents had not thought 'of troubling the district medical officer to attend the child'. GW was a male aged 35, with phthisis. He had a wife and four children. He had been a brass-founder, and first fell ill about three years before. Then he went to a charitable dispensary. His chest was not examined, because 'the doctor knew what was the matter by looking at him'. He continued at work for about two years, but then had to give up and go on outdoor poor relief. In 1909 he was attending the dispensary of a general hospital, where he received cod-liver oil and cough mixture.

He has a heavy spit. During the day he spits into the fire, and at

night into a chamber pot. No sanitary officer has called, and he has
had no instruction as to preventive measures. He and his wife and a
baby . . . all sleep in one bed.

'HB' was aged 41. He had phthisis and lived with his wife and two
children in one kitchen and two other rooms. He had been a book-
binder, but the family was now on outdoor poor relief. He was declining
and the local authorities had proposed that he enter the workhouse
infirmary. He had refused; not, he said, because he feared the stigma
of pauperism, but because he would be unable to get sufficient outdoor exercise under workhouse discipline. At home he 'walked about
continually'. For this man the workhouse infirmary loomed as the final
admission of defeat.[308]

The examples of the brass-founder and the book-binder bear out the
claim of Dr Nathan Raw that of 4,000 cases of TB in the Liverpool
Union infirmary, 60 per cent were 'paupers because they were consumptives, and not the other way round'.[309] The burden of supporting these
TB sufferers and their families fell on the local ratepayers. Had the
central government or rural taxpayers been more closely involved they
might have acted earlier. For there were ameliorations they and the
medical professions could have effected before the twentieth century.
Dr Jacob Hare of Pimlico had suggested as early as 1842 that phthisis
might be spread by milk from tuberculous cows and that the distribution of 'bad milk' be prohibited. His suggestion was ignored. Only in
1868 did Deléphine begin research into milk as a conveyor of TB and
his work was not finally accepted by medical and sanitary authorities
until the Royal Commission on TB in 1898. The Commissioners recommended that governments set standards for non-tubercular milk. In
1910 20 per cent of milk and 10 per cent of butter contained 'living
tubercle' but there was still no national legislation. This did not come
until the TB scare finally overcame the dairymen's lobby after the
war.[310]

The long-suspected association between TB and overcrowding was
demonstrated in 1904. Dr Chalmers, the MOH for Glasgow, told the
Physical Deterioration Committee that the death rate for phthisis varied
between 2.4 per 1,000 among families living in one room, 1.8 per 1,000
for families in two rooms, and 0.7 per 1,000 for 'all other houses'. In
Finsbury families living in one room had an overall death rate of 8.9
per 1,000, compared with 5.6 per 1,000 for families occupying four or
more rooms. This is but another index of relative poverty. In 1909-10
Chalmers calculated that at age 25-35 labourers' families had a phthisis

mortality rate of 7.1 per 1,000 compared with 1.9 per 1,000 for
'professional classes'; at 35-45 the gap was even wider: 8.6 per 1,000
against 0.7 per 1,000. Chalmers, Drysdale and other radical doctors
believed that the enormous social costs justified expensive-looking
rehousing schemes. But even they never carried their proposals into
detail.[311] The interference with private life and private property that it
entailed was unthinkable. It is fair to add that Drysdale and Chalmers
were also aware that the TB problem, though bad enough in Britain,
was better there, and improving faster, than on the Continent. In
Vienna in the 1890s, one-third of all deaths were ascribed to TB, in
Paris one-fifth, whereas London reported only one-twelfth (which still
represented 8,000 bereavements). France reported 160,000 TB deaths
annually, Germany 150,000, and Britain 65,000. Given that Drysdale
and Chalmers regarded TB as a precise indicator of poverty, their underlying complacency about Britain was not unfounded.[312]

Meanwhile anxious or desperate poor people persevered with their
live snails, maggots (soldiers still ate or smelled these during the First
World War), or breathed in the miasma of pigsties or foxes' lairs.
Suffolk people breathed in the breath of a stallion, as a preventive or
cure, Herefordshire people preferred the breath of a piebald. Scots put
their faith in cows. The practice seems to have rested on the notion of
a change, or exchange, of air, from the strong and unknowing brute to
the weak and human.[313]

Despairing sufferers turned to quacks. In 1848 Francis Pace took
his ailing daughter to the famous London Dutch Jewish quack, Meyer
Lotinga. He pronounced it 'no consumptions' and said he would cure
her after four days. He treated her for two months, until she died.
Lotinga's main medicine was brown sugar. His bill was £3.18s.0d. At
Oldham in 1850 John Liddell was 'in an advanced stage of consumption' and visited George Winterbottom, a former cotton-spinner who
had turned herbalist-hydropathist. He placed Liddell in a hot vapour
bath, then plunged him into a cold shower, and then gave him an
emetic. Liddell gained some relief at first, but after a few days of the
treatment 'he just lay down and died'. Winterbottom was acquitted of
manslaughter. He had acted in good faith and, as Judge Platt remarked,
there would be no improvement in medicine if practitioners were tied
to old notions. There were also various brands of 'anti-consumption
pills', the main constituent of which was cayenne pepper. A quack in
Hull in the 1860s and 1870s made a good living from selling butter as
the 'same kind of ointment as that with which Mary Magdalen anointed
the feet of Christ'. He got £60 from one farmer alone for a course of

treatment with this *Elixir of Life*. The farmer had been shown he had
consumption by being told to blow into a glass containing magic liquid.
It was citrate of magnesia which turns milky when blown into.[314]

4. VENEREAL DISEASES, CONTRACEPTION AND SEXUALITY

Orthodox medical men were evasive and ignorant about venereal
diseases and sexuality. They were proud of their skills in mending some
disorders of the urinary system, stone in the bladder, for instance, but
on other matters affecting the genital region they remained silent. Most
voluntary hospitals would not admit VD cases, for fear of losing subscribers. Guy's, Bart's and St Thomas's provided about 200 beds
between them in 1870. Hospitals in garrison towns, Winchester and
Colchester, for instance, also refused to open VD wards. Charitable
dispensaries would not supply medicines and workhouse infirmaries
would not admit venereally diseased paupers. There were numerous
small voluntary lock hospitals for diseased prostitutes, but these had
only 157 beds in the United Kingdom in 1883 and their wards were
half-empty. Lock hospitals still required 'lines'. Moreover, because few
respectable donors sponsored them, they were shabby, badly sited and
hopelessly short of funds.[315]

Yet VD was undoubtedly widespread. That self-appointed expert,
Dr William Acton, claimed in 1846 that one-half of Bart's out-patients
were VD sufferers.[316] Even allowing for Acton's habitual exaggeration,
they must have amounted to several thousands.

Doctors found VD hard to diagnose, especially in women. Syphilitic
chancres were often hidden inside the vagina and even in 1898 doctors
were not confident about distinguishing gonorrhoea from urethritis.[317]
Treatment consisted of applications of mercury salts, mostly calomel.
This did clear up small chancres, but repeated applications and internal
doses sometimes issued in salivation and mercury poisoning. Dr
Alexander Patterson, surgeon to the Glasgow Lock Hospital, believed
that syphilis became less virulent between the 1860s and the 1880s.
Cases of the mortification of the leg bones and destruction of the nasal
bones had become rare. Patterson speculated whether 'in many cases
of bone destruction, mercury, which in former times was administered
so lavishly [was] not the cause'. Cases of gangrenous destruction of the
prepuce and glans penis, common in the 1860s, had also virtually disappeared. Ulceration of the soft palate was still prevalent, but again
Patterson wondered if the standard treatment with nitric acid or caustic
gargles did not exacerbate the condition. Copper iodide salts and chalk

were other common ineffective remedies.[318]

The notion that syphilis was a specific infection caused by a microbe was pressed in the late 1880s by Jonathan Hutchinson, the great authority on syphilis, and by Charles Drysdale, honorary physician to the Rescue Society of London. But it made slow headway. Many doctors, like Alexander Patterson, continued to regard syphilis as an inflammatory poisonous disease, like hospital gangrene. There was also a lunatic fringe, and recognised as such by the *Lancet*, which probably included some silent lay opinion, represented by Samuel Solly, senior surgeon at St Thomas's. He opposed research into VD lest a cure was discovered: syphilis had been created as a punishment for fornication and if it could be cured, 'fornication would be universal'.[319]

The existence of this vociferous lunatic fringe obscures the evidence about medical opinion on sexuality. William Acton, much quoted by historians on prostitution, is another case in point. I have argued elsewhere that he cannot be trusted. His general approach is prurient, obsessive and authoritarian. Some of his claims, about the numbers of prostitutes in London for instance, are unbelievable when set against other contemporary estimates. As for his anecdotes about prostitutes, it is worth recalling that some come from the equally untrustworthy Mayhew narratives, and that Acton had an American medical-journalist collaborator, Horace Green. Some medical contemporaries recognised this dubious sensationalist point. The *London Journal of Medicine* dismissed the anecdotes in his *Practical Treatise on Diseases of the . . . Generative Organs* (1851) as 'mere fancy or gratuitous assertion'.[320]

There appears to have been no formal teaching in problems of sexuality in British medical schools. There are instances where opinions about sexuality were interspersed in lectures on diseases of the urinary organs and in each case they differ strikingly from the horrors threatened by Acton. 'Moderate use of sexual connection', or what another doctor called 'venereal combats', about twice a week, and the moral worth of sexual enjoyment in both males and females seem to have been accepted as the norm. Patients expected this as the norm and GPs counselled it.[321] Within the profession the prophets of doom were occasionally ridiculed, but more often ignored. When in 1826 Benjamin Brodie, the rising young surgeon at St George's Hospital, attributed one case of 'wasted testicles' and impotence to 'over indulgence in intercourse while a youth' (the patient, aged 31, had also had an injury to his testicles when he was 20), and another to 'onanism' (masturbation),

Wakley, the editor of the *Lancet*, dismissed Brodie's paper as 'trash' which would 'amuse his readers'. Brodie, incidentally, directed George P., the second case, to take sulphate of iron and tincture of cantharides internally, and apply blisters to the scrotum. There was 'no improvement'.[322] Later in the century a main reason for the profession's reluctance to adopt Lawson Tait's operation for ovariotomy was their fear that it might spoil women's sexual appetite and 'unsex' them.[323]

Similarly, when C.F. Lallemand, the French expert on the brain, revived the fear in the 1840s that 'spermatorrhoea', spontaneous ejaculation — 'wet dreams' — was a disease that ensued from masturbation, a few British doctors supported him, but it is significant, as Dr Thomas Chambers pointed out in 1861, that 'spermatorrhoea' was not recognised by the Registrar-General, and that this 'imaginary disease' was never reported in hospital case-books.[324] Writers in the *Lancet* continued sceptical about the more extreme statements of medical prudery, many of them emanating from the United States. (In this, nineteenth-century writers have been more critical than modern historians, who commonly underpin their allegations about British medical prudery with American examples, sometimes without admitting or even recognising that the example is American.) When the expatriate American T.L. Nichols published his *Human Physiology* . . . (1872), the *Lancet* reviewer noticed a 'curious vein of eccentricity' expressed throughout the book in a 'curious inequality in . . . knowledge and . . . common sense', especially when Nichols rode his hobby-horses of hydropathy, vegetarianism and spiritualism. In 1897, the *BMJ* dismissed as 'ignorant and untrue' the contention of another American writer, Dr Genevieve Tucker, that coition during pregnancy 'blights and blasts, if it does not destroy the life of the child'. Another of Dr Tucker's warnings, that the daughter of a father who smoked would have 'poisoned nerve centres, laying the foundation for hysteria', was also nonsense, the *BMJ* declared.[325]

None the less, the growing respectability and distinctive professionalism of the doctors during the 1860s did make them more censorious and open to doom theories. Dr Edward Smith, the dietitian, announced in 1862 a study of 600 male phthisis sufferers proving that their conditions derived from 'Smoking and immoral conduct': 48 per cent smoked, 24 per cent drank, 29 per cent had indulged in 'a bad life for a period', 14 per cent had had syphilis once. Overall, 11.8 per cent had been given to 'sexual abuse in early life', 18.2 per cent to masturbation, and 22 per cent to 'seminal emission'; 70 per cent, Smith remarked in an aside, had had 'hard occupations, with especially long hours and exposure'. Smith's paper exhilarated Acton. For the first time 'professional observation' proved what had been 'vague notions' before. Acton added that 'marital excess was productive of ill-effects not generally supposed' and the proof that masturbation helped cause phthisis would confound the sceptics. Two notable spokesmen in the field of medical trade unionism, Drs Greenhow and Sutro, publicly supported Smith's thesis.[326]

By 1863 country GPs were finding spermatorrhoea to be widespread and in 1870 the *Lancet* was offering advice on how to gain the confidence of boys and young men so that they would confess to masturbation. Fig leaves first appear on anatomical illustrations in the *Lancet*, so far as my casual observation goes, in November 1872. The *BMJ* denounced Chapman's frank discussion of prostitution in the *Westminster Review* in 1869. Evasion was now the best professional policy:

> If a physician were . . . to explain to a lady-patient the doctrines of syphilis, under any circumstances excepting those of the most urgent necessity, he would be guilty . . . of a gross departure from his duty . . . we deny that any possible good could come of enlightening . . . 'a trusting maiden' . . . before marriage as to her risks . . . If suspicions have arisen, they are for her father, or her brothers to deal with, not herself . . . delicacy . . . that beautiful quality of mind . . . interfered with by obtruded information.[327]

The *BMJ* also endorsed the views of such reforming headmasters as the Rev. J.M. Wilson of Clifton that exercise and cold baths lessened the proclivity to masturbation. Exercise was better than telling boys about the dangers, because too much detail could only lead to 'unsavoury suggestiveness'. The remedy for boys who did indulge in 'low talk' was a whipping.[328] But other opinions persisted, somewhat timorously. 'A Doctor and a Father' pointed out to his colleagues in 1886 that the young were legitimately curious about sex, for they read about it in the Bible and watched animals. He wanted 'a very elementary but explicit . . . treatment . . . with special reference . . . to the human species, and with appropriate scriptural references'. Copies were to be given to girls on their 13th birthdays. Mr C.G. Wheelhouse replied that he had written such a work, *The Special Temptation of Early Life*, commissioned by the social purity committee of the Ripon Diocesan Conference. I have been unable to find a copy, but it sounds indistinguishable from the dozens of horror primers about masturbation which appeared during the 1880s and 1890s. 'FGV' urged that girls be left in '*innocence*'. Boys had to be instructed before they left for school, but girls possessed an 'instinct of delicacy' which could be nurtured to overcome their natural curiosity and help them 'to shut [their] eyes to things that married life will reveal'. 'Heaven forbid', exclaimed 'Another Doctor and a Father', 'that such a treatise, however elementary, should ever reach . . . my children'. Children already lost their 'charming innocence' too early in 'this wicked world'. Besides, such knowledge would place 'parents and offspring too much on a footing': awkward situations might ensue and cause ' "un embarrass mutuel" '.[329]

During this narrowing of opinion after 1870 many ideas which had last appeared in the 1840s surfaced again. The *BMJ*'s faith in cold water as an antidote to sexual arousal echoed the advice of Dr Ramsay, published in 1814. Dr Thomas Graham in 1834 attributed many female genital disorders to the excessive nervous excitability of females as compared with males and their 'more capillary' circulation of the blood. They became over-amorous and damaged themselves. Forty-five years later Edward Tibbits, physician to the Bradford Infirmary, explained that the essence of the difference between the mind of man and woman sprang largely

> from peculiar bodily conformation. In a normal woman the sensations connected with the organs of generation (especially if we include the mammary glands) are . . . more voluminous, if not more intense, than in [males] . . . The woman has less control over her . . . sexual . . . feelings than a man.

Similarly, Francis Eagle declared in 1835 that 'the most fruitful' source of epilepsy was '*indulgence in venery*' exacerbated by onanism. In 1883 Mr Teale won acceptance for an almost identical hypothesis from the Royal Medical and Chirurgical Society.[330]

Antisepsis and the enhanced authority of the profession also made some new procedures possible after 1870. Doctors advocated universal male circumcision. The foreskin was a 'harbour for filth and . . . a constant source of irritation', Jonathan Hutchinson said in 1890. 'It conduces to masturbation and adds to the difficulties of sexual continence. It increases the risk of syphilis in early life, and of cancer in the aged.'[331] Little girls of 9 or so who masturbated might have their vaginas caged. Younger children needed different treatment. Dr Heywood Smith was proud of his invention. An anxious mother had brought him a child aged 2. She was fretful and 'its expression bordered on imbecility'. Heywood Smith first of all ringed the clitoris, passing a silver wire through it and twisting it over a penholder. This had the desired effect for a time, as it prevented the child touching itself for a fortnight. At the end of that time . . . she began the old habit again, when I removed the ring and gave bromide of ammonia and tincture of Indian hemp, with the result that [she] . . . got quite well, the expression becoming quite rational.

Dr Alex Leadman of Pocklington in the East Riding agreed with Heywood Smith, but remarked that he preferred cocaine to Indian hemp. Circumcision does not appear to have been part of the usual childbirth and infant care services provided by the charity hospitals. One might speculate that male circumcision and the nasty things done to little girls were peculiar to private practice among the middle classes. In 1899 Dr H.S. Webb, self-described as 'country doctor' of Welwyn, Hertfordshire, remarked that 'of late years most parents' of his private practice asked him to circumcise their new-born boys.[332] It is possible, too, according to medical hearsay, that nowadays circumcision is rarely sought among the British professional classes, but is still popular among the working classes. At some time – the 1930s? – it seems to have filtered downwards. During the mid-1860s there had been a brief vogue for extirpation of the adult clitoris as a cure for self-abuse and epilepsy, but after the expulsion from the Obstetrical Society of the main – obviously insane – proponent, Isaac Baker Brown, surgeons abandoned it.[333]

Lesbianism appears to have passed unnoticed by doctors, and male homosexuality only came into medical discussions after Oscar Wilde's conviction in 1895. The *BMJ* deplored the growth of 'perverted tendencies' which threatened the 'basic animal instincts upon which the survival of the race and the Empire depended'. In part, the advance of civilisation had rightly reduced these instincts, but a point had been reached when in the interests of civilisation itself these tendencies had to be prevented from being transmitted. Mere gaoling and release soon afterwards did no good: 'it simply lowers the social stratum on which the pernicious influence is exerted.' The *BMJ*'s recommendations were obscure, but they seem to have begun with castration. The *Lancet*, commenting in 1898 on the prosecution of the bookseller who sold copies of Havelock Ellis's *Sexual Inversion*, was more confident than the *BMJ* about the aetiology of the disease: 'homo-sexuality is [nothing] . . . else than an acquired and depraved manifestation of the sexual passion . . . Such matters should not be discussed by the man in the street, not to mention the boys and girls in the street.'[334]

Contraception did not emerge in public medical discussion until 1870, when the *Lancet* published a letter from Charles Drysdale advocating it. His elder brother George's anonymous *Elements of Social Science* commending various methods of mechanical contraception had been a best-seller since its appearance in 1854. Drysdale argued that family limitation was the only sure means of reducing the mortality and hardship of the poor. At present they were poor and vulnerable because their numbers made them press too heavily upon the supply of food and employment. Family limitation was cheap and depended on their own self-discipline (Drysdale meant careful mechanical contraception, not coitus interruptus). It could only advance the poor and improve society. The differential rates of mortality between rich and poor suburbs showed that the prodigious expenditure on sanitary reform and coercion by MOHs and health visitors had not succeeded.

The *Lancet* inserted Drysdale's letter only to condemn it. 'The expedients recommended for preventing conception are as injurious to morals and to health as they are physically loathsome and repulsive.' The *Lancet* opposed to Drysdale's argument a tautological Spencerism:

Disease and overcrowding are not the result of large families or surplus population; but of that neglect of natural laws, which has allowed the population to herd together in insanitary conditions . . . There are matters of taste or opinion in which the rulers may be guided by the will of the people; and there are matters of science, in which it is the duty of the rulers to teach the people to be guided by the laws of nature . . . [these] . . . natural laws . . . [include] this, that a nation fruitful in healthy organisms must, in the struggle for existence, displace and swallow up a nation that is abandoned to conjugal onanism.[335]

Drysdale and the Malthusian League battled on through the 1870s and finally the Medical Society of London allocated a meeting to the subject in 1879. Together (the Bradlaugh Besant trial of 1877 passed unmentioned in the *Lancet*) with the discussion at the BMA gathering at Worcester in 1882, these constituted the only formal medical meetings on the topic in the nineteenth century. Drysdale rehearsed his arguments, but he encountered only hostility, at least from those who are recorded as having spoken. Dr Routh 'accepted' Drysdale's figures on the disparity between the death rates of the rich and the poor. But the poor's death rate was not due to poverty, 'but rather to their ignorance, intemperance and improvidence, as well as their unhealthy surroundings'. He rejected any proposal to diminish poverty by limiting children, because an increasing number of births indicated increasing national prosperity. Dr Paramore agreed. 'Intemperance was the case of the misery among the poor.' Limitation of births among them 'should not be entertained'. Dr Crisp settled for intemperance, too. So did Dr Rogers. Mr Gould did not think poverty had anything to do with the high mortality rate. Rather, it was the 'want of good clothing, healthy dwellings, and care'. No one, except Drysdale, discussed the clinical aspects of various forms of contraception.[336] After this, Drysdale appears to have given up trying to convert his colleagues. Thereafter contraception was rarely mentioned in the medical press. Dr W. Ewart summed up the likely mainstream of opinion in 1898: 'Malthusianism . . . is probably opposed by the conscience of the profession as a false notion politically, socially, and morally, its attitude has been . . . one of reserve . . . Love of offspring is the healthiest sign of a race, and the natural strength which is its reward stands revealed in connexion with armaments and now more than ever in connexion with colonising power.' He added that the state ought in future to take more advice from the profession about how best to manage breeding.[337] The doctors' public advice presumably would have differed from their personal practice: as I noted above, medical practitioners limited their families earlier and more strictly then any other group in the nineteenth century.

'Medico-Chirurgis' complained wistfully in 1843 that because of *opprobria medicorum* the 'lucrative form of practice' covering impotence, VD and other sexual disorders was almost wholly in the hands of quacks.[338]

Quacks, like the abortifacient sellers I mentioned earlier — indeed, they were often the same persons — advertised VD and impotence cures and doom warnings about masturbation extensively from the late 1830s. Undergraduates in the 1860s received 'obscene' letters up to three times a term. Another quack posted 'certain circulars' to every barmaid who advertised for a job in the *Morning Advertiser* during the mid-1870s. 'Obscene hand bills' were handed out to passers-by in the streets. The trade must have been big and lucrative. The Society for the Discouragement of Vicious Advertisements calculated in 1850 that as few as three advertisements in nine daily papers cost £3,780 a year, and in 220 provincial weeklies, £15,400. One of the first of the sex quack magnates, Dr Samuel Solomon, lived in a large house in Liverpool, amidst large grounds adorned with statues. He underwrote Lord Sefton's candidature in the election of 1818. The election flags alone cost Solomon £1,000.[339]

Anxieties about sexuality provided the minatory class of quacks with an open field. Kahn was the unqualified proprietor, under the protection of his qualified brother, of an anatomical museum which displayed models showing the effects of VD and 'weakness'. He charged a commercial clerk £51 for treatment in 1857. The clerk sought to stop the treatment and further payments. Kahn threatened to reveal his name and the fact that he masturbated. Kahn told the clerk that his 'brains were passing into his water'. The clerk was treated with antimony and told to stay in his room for 28 days and keep off pork. He lost his job. The clerk sued and got back his £51.[340]

The doctors' antipathy to sex quacks was the deeper because they shared so many beliefs and practices. Fox, in the *Working Man's Guide*, warned that the emission of this 'subtle, vital . . . fluid enfeebles the constitution', debilitated the nervous system, and, echoing Drs Smith and Acton, asserted that it induced consumption. He advised cold water and cayenne pepper and a vegetarian diet. Mr Jordan, MRCS, informed a reverend patient in 1863 that he had spermatorrhoea. Jordan placed some of the reverend gentleman's urine under a microscope and showed him a multitude of lively paste-eels twisting about (paste-eels are nematode worms which develop in sour pastry). He then gave the patient some medicine which blackened his teeth (mercury), made him walk around the room, and then pass some more urine. In the second specimen only one animacule was observed. The power of the medicine was proved. Jordan then demanded £100 for a box of it. The patient did not have £100. Jordan settled for a bill at four months for £80. Acton used opium and bleeding for orchitis (swollen testicle) in his public dispensary practice. But he told the Medical Society of London that opium was useless and in his 'private practice and in good institutions' he used tight strapping with adhesive plaster (which cannot have been useful either).[341]

In 1837 a footman went to Mr S. of Regent Street, fearing he had the pox. Mr S. suggested mercury, which would cost two guineas. But the 'safest way was without mercury, and would be four guineas . . . The weather was bad for taking mercury; the mercury would work up and down, and [the footman] . . . would be like a weather-glass'. The footman agreed, and paid up the four guineas. Then he found he had not had VD. His penis had been cold for ten days after he had lain with a woman who had been cold and he thought he had caught something.

After his visit to Mr S. his penis warmed up and he did not return.[342]

These fundamental notions about the functional relation of opposites in health and disease, cleanliness and dirt, hot and cold, purity and pollution, sympathetic colours and shapes, engrained in orthodox and unorthodox practitioners alike, also permeated the thinking of the common people. The madonna lily was traditionally associated with female purity. Wise women sold the bulb as a remedy for suppressed or purulent menstruation. The gradual conquest of orthodox medicine is illustrated by the grandmother in Keyworth, near Nottingham, who, in 1892, finally brought to the doctor her grandson who was suffering from incontinence of urine. She had fed him on the traditional cure 'moleywhaup' (mole pie) and it had failed.[343] The doctor would not have been able to help either.

The theme of purity and pollution runs through seven representative cases of rape in 1859, 1884 and 1887. They all occurred in Liverpool, where the belief was said to be strongest. Men believed that intercourse with a virgin child would cure VD. In 1884 a man with 'bad syphilitic ulcers' raped a girl of 14. His defence was that he had not intended to harm her, but only to cure himself. Amos Greenwood was tried for a similar offence upon a girl of 9. She was the daughter of illiterate costermongers. When sores suddenly appeared on her genitals they believed that it was the result of her having swallowed sixpence and were loath to give evidence against Greenwood. 'Quack doctoresses' had kept special brothels in Liverpool, since 1827 at least, to provide this cure. The children used were often imbeciles. Three who had become infected and were placed in the Liverpool Lock Hospital were 9, 7 and 5½ respectively. These doctoresses had never been prosecuted, even by 1887, two years after the law had been tightened by the Criminal Law Amendment Act. Folk medicine could be as damaging, expensive and ineffective as its orthodox rivals. Historians, including the present author, have lately tended to scepticism about W.T. Stead's child-saving histrionics in 1885.[344] Histrionic Stead certainly was, but our scepticism was partly the result of our ignorance of what he was up against.

Notes

1. Sheila Ryan Johansson, 'Sex and Death in Victorian England: An Examination of Age- and Sex-Specific Death Rates, 1840-1910' in Martha Vicinus (ed.), *A Widening Sphere* (Bloomington, 1977), pp. 163-81.

2. *JSS*, vol. XLVI (1883), pp. 189-213; see also a second article by Humphreys, *JRSS*, vol. LII (1890), pp. 225-45; *L*, 9 Jan. 1897, p. 115.

3. *BMJ*, 27 Jan. 1894, p. 205; Chadwick in *JSS*, vol. VII (1844), pp. 4-16.

4. *L*, 13 May 1848, p. 525.

5. J.H. Houghton (MOH), *Journal of Public Health and Sanitary Review*, vol. II (1856), pp. 67-73; T.J. Raybould, *The Economic Emergence Of the Black Country* (Newton Abbot, 1973), p. 24.

6. F.W.D. Manders, *A History of Gateshead* (Gateshead, 1973), pp. 172-84.

7. *L*, 7 Oct. 1871, p. 527.

8. John Billing, 'The Sanitary Condition of . . . Reading', *JSS*, Vol. X (1847), pp. 259-60; *L*, 28 Nov. 1874, p. 769.

9. M.W. Flinn, 'Introduction' to Chadwick's *Report on The Sanitary Condition of the Labouring Population . . .* , pp. 1-73; Royston Lambert. *Sir John Simon 1816-1904* (London, 1963); Oliver MacDonagh, *Early Victorian Government* (London. 1977).

10. *Nonconformist*, 15 Mar. 1848, quoting *Leeds Mercury*.

11. *L*, 2 July 1831, p. 433.

12. *Nonconformist*. 26 Apr. 1848.

13. *The Times*, 9 May 1848.

14. *L*, 15 Oct. 1853, p. 383; *PP*, 1854, vol. XXXV, Report of General Board of Health . . . 1848-54, pp. 35, 43.

15. Benjamin Scott, *A Statistical Vindication of the City of London*, third ed. (London, 1877), pp. 154-7.

16. Alexander P. Stewart and Edward Jenkins, *The Medical and Legal Aspects of Sanitary Reform* (1867, reprinted Leicester, 1969), p. 24.

17. *Examiner*, 8 Oct. 1853, p. 652.

18. *Examiner*, 16 Sept. 1854, p. 593.

19. John Whitmore and Dr Tripe, in *St Andrews Medical Graduates' Transactions* (1870), pp. 40-63; *L*, 8 Dec. 1894, p. 1365.

20. *L*, 12 June 1858, p. 597; 12 Feb. 1848, pp. 187-8.

21. *BMJ*, 19 Oct. 1889, p. 887; *L*, 5 July 1890, p. 34 (Stratford Local Board of Health *v*. Malton Farmers' Manure and Trading Co.).

22. E.g. Anon., 'An affectionate Address to the Inhabitants of Newcastle and Gateshead' – a Temperance tract of 1832, in Louis James, *Print and the People 1819-1851* (London, 1976), p. 174.

23. *BMJ*, 23 July 1881, p. 128; cf. 30 and 31 Vict. ch. 101 (Scotland).

24. John F. Sykes, *Public Health Problems* (London, 1892), pp. 226-40.

25. *L*, 22 June 1895, p. 1601.

26. C.R. Drysdale in *BMJ*, 13 Aug. 1887, p. 351.

27. *JSS*, vol. XXVIII (1865), p. 197.

28. *L*, 4 Mar. 1843, p. 841; *Once a Week*, 10 Sept. 1864, p. 317.

29. *BMJ*, 2 Sept. 1899, p. 584; D. Oddy and D. Miller, *The Making of the Modern British Diet* (London. 1976), p. 96.

30. *L*, 29 June 1895, p. 1631; Oddy and Miller, *The Making of the Modern British Diet*, pp. 323-4.

31. *L*, 17 Dec. 1836, p. 443; *Medical Chronicle*, vol. V (1896), pp. 264-6; see also J. Drabble, *Textbook of Meat Inspection* (Sydney, 1960), p. 327, and A. Wilson, *Practical Meat Inspection* (Oxford, 1975), p. 103.

32. *Once a Week*, 10 Oct. 1863, p. 425.

33. *L*, 1 Nov. 1902, p. 1213.

34. *L*, 27 June 1868, p. 825; J.S. Gamgee in *L*, 21 Mar. 1857, pp. 303-4.

35. *Once a Week*, 10 Oct. 1863, p. 425.

36. *L*, 18 July 1857, p. 65, 26 Jan. 1861, p. 94, 2 Dec. 1865, p. 635.

37. *Annual Register* (1861), p. 356; Richard Perrin, 'The Meat and Livestock Trade in Britain, 1850-70', *Economic History Review*, vol. XXVIII (1975), p. 396.

38. Anthony Trollope, *The Last Chronicle of Barset* (1866-7), ch. IV.

39. Oddy and Miller, *Modern British Diet*, p. 216.

40. *L*, 9 Feb. 1861, p. 144. Cf. Pye Henry Chavasse, *Council To A Mother* (London, 1869), p. 159.

41. *L*, 13 Apr. 1861, p. 378.

42. *L*, 15 Nov. 1862, p. 542, 2 Dec. 1865, p. 635. Scott, *Statistical Vindication*, p. 162.

43. *BMJ*, 14 Mar. 1908, p. 652.

44. *L*, 16 Jan. 1858, p. 76.

45. *L*, 3 Nov. 1860, p. 448, 14 Sept. 1861, p. 254; *Sanitary Review*, vol. II (1857), pp. 128-9.

46. *Truth*, 11 June 1885, p. 920; *L*, 3 May 1884, p. 814.

47. *L*, 12 Jan. 1861, p. 49, 16 Apr. 1870, p. 571.

48. *Truth*, 19 Mar. 1885, p. 444; *L*, 29 Oct. 1898, p. 1148, 17 Feb. 1866, p. 184.

49. *L*, 16 Aug. 1879, p. 252.

50. *L*, 18 Nov. 1871, p. 736; *BMJ*, 2 Dec. 1871, p. 648; *The Times*, 4 June 1872, p. 9.

51. *Second Report of the Association for the relief of the ... Poor, relative ... to the ... Supply of Fish* (London, 1815), pp. 554-7.

52. *L*, 22 Aug. 1846, p. 201; *Journal of Public Health and Sanitary Review*, vol. I (1855), p. 179; Oddy and Miller, *Modern British Diet*, pp. 130-8; S.D. Chapman, *Jesse Boot the Chemist* (London, 1974), p. 58.

53. *L*, 19 Feb. 1825, p. 214, 12 Mar. 1825, p. 317.

54. Palmer to George Richmond, 14 Oct. 1834, in *The Letters of Samuel Palmer*, Raymond Lister (ed.) (Oxford, 2 vols., 1974), vol. I, p. 62.

55. *Medical Gazette*, 14 May 1831, p. 201; *L*, 20 Feb. 1836, p. 824; W.B. Pringle of Master Bakers' Protection Society to SC on Adulteration Act, *PP*, 1874, vol. VI, Q. 3862.

56. R.D. Thomson, Professor of Chemistry at St Thomas's Hospital to SC on Adulteration ..., *PP*, 1854-5, vol. VIII, Q.1212; John Snow in *L*, 4 July 1857, pp. 4-5.

57. *L*, 22 June 1872, p. 882, 6 July 1872, p. 21.

58. *L*, 17 Aug. 1861, p. 166, 15 Feb. 1862, p. 183, 6 Jan. 1872, p. 26; Ernst W. Stieb, *Drug Adulteration: Detection and Control in Nineteenth-Century Britain* (Madison, 1966), p. 192; Report of the SC on Food Products Adulteration, *PP*, 1896, vol. IX, p. iii; Margaret Hewitt, *Wives and Mothers in Victorian Industry* (London, 1958), p. 77.

59. *Once a Week*, 10 Mar. 1860, p. 236.

60. Harriet Martineau, 'The Baker', *Once a Week*, 10 Nov. 1860, pp. 540-1.

61. *L*, 21 Sept. 1872, p. 427.

62. *L*, 4 Apr. 1863, p. 391, 7 Apr. 1866, p. 375, 22 Apr. 1882, p. 661, 5 Jan. 1884, p. 25; *Medical Chronicle* (1895-6), pp. 15-20; *Birmingham Trades Council. Enquiry into the Conditions of Labour in Bakehouses* (Birmingham, 1910), pp. 3-14.

63. *Once a Week*, 9 May 1863, pp. 551-2.

64. *L*, 15 Nov. 1902, pp. 13, 37; *Once a Week*, 10 Mar. 1863, pp. 236-7.

65. *Bell's Weekly Magazine*, 22 Feb. 1834, p. 92; *L*, 11 May 1844, p. 225; *Edinburgh Medical and Surgical Journal*, vol. LXXIX (1853), pp. 373-4; *Punch*, 4 Aug. 1855, p. 47.

66. *L*, 10 Aug. 1861, p. 145; SC on Food Products Adulteration, *PP*, 1896, vol. IX, p. ix.

67. *L*, 30 Nov. 1861, p. 532, 16 Nov. 1872, p. 718; SC on Food Products Adulteration, *PP*, 1896, vol. IX, p. xl.

68. A.H. Hassall to SC on Adulterations of Food ..., *PP*, 1854-5, vol. VIII, Q.73; *Once a Week*, 12 Mar. 1864, p. 321; *BMJ*, 27 Mar. 1880, p. 479.

69. *L*, 13 Feb. 1830, p. 673, 15 Feb. 1845, p. 197; *Edinburgh Medical and Surgical Journal*, vol. LIX (1843), p. 477; Alexander Morrice, *A Treatise on Brewing*, fifth ed. (London, 1825); Samuel Child, *Every Man his own Brewer*, sixth ed. (London, 1798).

70. *L*, 2 Mar. 1867, p. 281, 29 Jan. 1870, p. 169; *BMJ*, 10 Apr. 1869, p. 336.

71. A.H. Hassall to SC on Adulteration Act, *PP*, 1874. vol. VI, Qs. 6407-9; *L*, 19 Sept. 1868, p. 388.

72. *L*, 2 Mar. 1867, p. 281; SC on Habitual Drunkards, *PP*, 1872, vol. IX, Qs. 492-5; SC on Prevalence of Habits of Intemperance, *PP*, 1877, vol. XI, Joseph Chamberlain, Q.2448, 1878-9, vol. X, Qs. 2086-90; Brian Harrison, *Drink and the Victorians* (London. 1971), p. 315; SC on Food Products Adulteration, *PP*, 1896, vol. IX, p. xxxix

73. Albert J. Bernays, 'On the Working of the Adulteration Act', *Saint Thomas's Hospital Reports*, vol. VII (1876), pp. 95-7; *PP*, 1878-9, vol. X, Qs. 4-10; *PP*, 1896, vol. IX, p. xxxix.

74. *L*, 24 Aug. 1850, p. 239, 4 July 1857, p. 16, 8 Nov. 1862, p. 508; *Medical Chronicle*, vol. VII (1897), p. 104.

75. *Sanitary Review*, vol. IV (1858), p. 91; *L*, 16 Oct. 1869, p. 553; *Medical Chronicle*, vol. VII (1897), p. 97; *GMJ*. vol. LXIII (1905), p. 212; Oddy and Miller, *Modern British Diet*, p. 146.

76. *Truth*, 9 Apr. 1885, p. 564; *Medical Times & Gazette*, 22 Nov. 1856, p. 533; *L*, 15 June 1856, p. 674.

77. *L*, 14 June 1860, p. 43, 30 Aug. 1862, p. 244.

78. SC on Food Products Adulteration, *PP*, 1895, vol. IX, pp. iv-v, vol. X, Qs. 7562, 7604, 7785-7; *L*, 9 Aug. 1890, p. 293; *Truth*, 9 Apr. 1885, p. 567; *BMJ*, 14 Jan. 1888, p. 90, 8 Nov. 1890, p. 1099.

79. *L*, 17 Nov. 1894, p. 1186; *PP*, 1896, vol. IX, p. vi.

80. E.H. Whetham, 'The London Milk Trade 1860-1900', *Economic History Review*, vol. XVII (1964), p. 377; *PP*, vol. XXXII, p. 53; *Medical Chronicle*, vol. LII (1910), p. 75; Oddy and Miller, *Modern British Diet*, pp. 272-3.

81. J.C. Kearley, Butter importer, to SC on Food Adulteration, *PP*. 1895, vol. IX, pp. xxvi, 1, vol. X, Qs. 33-40, 281, 563; J.C. Forster, another butter importer, Qs. 6261-2.

82. David Taylor, 'The English Dairy Industry, 1860-1930', *Economic History Review*, vol. XXIX (1976), p. 590.

83. Oddy and Miller, *Modern British Diet*, pp. 211-22; Dorothy E. Lindsay, 'Diet of the Labouring Classes in Glasgow', *GMJ*, vol. LXXIX (1913), pp. 285-8; *BMJ*, 21 June 1913, p. 1343. For a typical 'full' diet for the early part of the century see *L*, 25 Nov. 1826, p. 242 which gives the dietaries for St Bartholomew's Hospital, which are basically bread, beer, porridge and potatoes.

84. A.E. Dingle, 'Drink and Working-Class Living Standards in Britain, 1870-1914', *Economic History Review*, vol. XXV (1972), pp. 608-22.

85. *BMJ*, 15 Oct. 1887, p. 842; Oddy and Miller, *Modern British Diet*, pp. 211, 247-52.

86. R.A. Lewis, *Edwin Chadwick and the Public Health Movement 1832-1854* (London, 1952); MacDonagh, *Early Victorian Government*.

87. *Edinburgh Medical and Surgical Journal*, vol. LXVI (1847), pp. 36-9; *JSS*, vol. XXII (1859), p. 244.

88. John Simpson, 'A Public Health Petition', *Medical History*, vol. V (1961), p. 389.

89. Robertson, *Yorkhill Story*, p. 13.

90. *JSS*, vol. XXVII (1864), p. 545.

91. *L*, 18 Oct. 1879, p. 560. See also E.C. Midwinter, *Social Administration in Lancashire 1830-1860* (Manchester, 1969), p. 102.

92. *Chambers Encyclopaedia* (1860s ed.), 'Sanitary Science', p. 717; *L*, 28 Sept. 1872, p. 455.

93. *Examiner*, 15 Jan. 1853, p. 40.

94. *JSS*. vol. XXII (1859), pp. 233-45.

95. Michael G. Mulhall. *The Dictionary of Statistics* (London, 1892), p. 542; Charles Wilson, *History of Unilever* (London, 1954), vol. I, pp. 9-20.

96. J. Liddle, Surgeon, Whitechapel, in *Medical Gazette*, 25 Nov. 1842, p. 292.

97. *Speeches of the Earl of Shaftesbury*, K.G. (1868, new ed. Shannon, 1971), pp. 218-19 (1848); *Examiner*, 8 Oct. 1853, p. 651, 4 Nov. 1854, p. 705; G. Kitson Clark, *Churchmen and the Condition of England 1832-1885* (London, 1973), pp. 196-224.

98. *L*, 30 July 1859, p. 126, 4 May 1861, p. 450, 31 May 1862, p. 578.

99. Mr Rendle to SC on Medical Poor Relief, *PP*, 1844, vol. IX, Qs. 2389-97; *L*, 27 Apr. 1844, p. 165, 26 Nov. 1870, p. 753; Royal Institute of Public Health, Aberdeen Congress 1900. pp. 549-50; Edward H. Gibson III, 'Baths and Wash-houses in the English Public Health Agitation, 1839-48', *Journal of the History of Medicine*. vol. IX (1954), pp. 392-404.

100. *L*, 10 Oct. 1868, p. 495.

101. *Sanitary Review* (Apr. 1857), pp. 17-18. *L*, 17 Oct. 1868, p. 515 (Birmingham), 26 Nov. 1859, p. 547, 10 Dec. 1859, p. 600 (Maidstone), 28 June 1884. p. 1175 (Manchester); Royal Sanitary Commission, *PP*, 1868-9, vol. XXXII, Qs. 6937-7005 (Basingstoke).

102. *L*, 12 Feb. 1887, p. 315.

103. *L*, 24 Nov. 1883, p. 917; *Pall Mall Gazette*, 8 Aug. 1885.

104. John Simpson, 'A Public Health Petition', p. 388; Lord Shaftesbury, *Speeches*, quoting Dr Neil Arnott, p. 221; *Blackwoods Magazine*, vol. LXXXV (1859), p. 229, quoting *Journal of Agriculture*; *L*, 13 Oct. 1860, p. 368, 19 Oct. 1861, p. 382, 29 Mar. 1862, p. 332, 18 Oct. 1862, p. 429, 25 Apr. 1863, pp. 471-2 (reporting Lawes' experiments at Rugby).

105. *Truth*. 14 May 1885, p. 760; *L*, 27 Nov. 1886, p. 1055.

106. *L*, 16 July 1898, p. 168, 11 Aug. 1883, p. 253, 27 Aug. 1898, p. 565 (Bradford); *Medical Times & Gazette*, 22 Apr. 1876, p. 441.

107. H.J. Dyos, *Victorian Suburb* (Leicester, 1961); J.R. Kellett, *The Impact of Railways on Victorian Cities* (London, 1969); Gareth Stedman Jones, *Outcast London* (Oxford, 1971), p. 213.

108. *Sanitary Review*, vol. II (1858), p. 392 (Cardiff); *L*, 12 June 1875, p. 838 (Keighley), 13 May 1882, p. 800 (Quarry Bank).

109. *L*, 19 Oct. 1901, p. 1072, 29 Nov. 1902, p. 1489 (Nottingham); 28 Mar. 1891, p. 738 (Wirksworth), 9 Oct. 1909, p. 1097 (Gravesend).

110. *BMJ*, 18 Dec. 1897, p. 1808 (Reigate, Maidstone and King's Lynn), 10 Mar. 1888, p. 556; *GMJ*, vol. LXXII (1909), pp. 116-17 (Liverpool).

111. *L*, 31 May 1862, p. 587.

112. *BMJ*, 12 Mar. 1887, p. 584.

113. *Chambers Encyclopaedia* (1860s ed.), 'Sanitary Science', p. 728.

114. *BMJ*, 10 Apr. 1886, p. 695, 8 July 1893, p. 99; *L*, 14 Mar. 1885, p. 487, 5 June 1897, p. 1557.

115. 'Report of Special Commission on Plumbers' Work', *L*, 4 July 1896, p. 73, 22 Nov. 1890, p.1105, 6 May 1893, p. 1090 (Folkestone); *BMJ*, 1 Jan. 1887, pp. 27-8, 22 July 1899, p. 258; *Truth*, 2 Apr. 1885, p. 526.

116. Horace Mann, '. . . Church Lane, St Giles's', *JSS*, vol. XI (1848), pp. 19-24.

117. J.S. Storr, 'The Anarchy of London', *Fortnightly Review*, vol. XIII (1873), pp. 757-8.

118. *Medical Times & Gazette*, 22 Apr. 1876, p. 441.

119. *Charity Organization Reporter*, 26 Mar. 1873, p. 53; J.M. Macintosh, *Trends of Opinion About the Public Health* (Oxford, 1953), p. 40.

120. Kellett, *Impact of Railways*, pp. 324-36.

121. *Charity Organization Reporter*, 18 Feb. 1874, p. 210 (Westminster); *L*, 11 Mar. 1876, p. 410 (Derby), 10 Jan. 1891, p. 113 (Newcastle).

122. *Truth*, 21 Aug. 1885, p. 802.

123. Helen Bosanquet, *Social Work in London 1869-1912* (1914, reprinted Brighton, 1973), pp. 174-5.

124. *Truth*, 14, 28 May 1885, pp. 761-2, p. 843 (Chelsea), 12 Nov. 1885, p. 754 (Oxford), 16 May 1895, p. 1192 (Castle Combe); R.C.K. Ensor, *England 1870-1914* (Oxford, 1936), p. 295.

125. John F.J. Sykes, 'The Results of State, Municipal, and Organized Private Action on the Housing of the Working Classes . . .', *JRSS*, vol. LXIV (1901), pp. 213-14.

126. Thomas Archer, *The Terrible Sights of London and Labours of Love in the Midst of Them* (n.d. [1870?]), pp. 441-8; Storr in *Fortnightly Review* (1873), p. 758; *Charity Organization Reporter*, 16 Dec. 1874, p. 344; Stedman Jones, *Outcast London*, pp. 179-96, has an excellent discussion of this matter.

127. *L*, 21 Jan. 1893, p. 170 (Aberdeen).

128. *BMJ*, 15 Nov. 1884, p. 975; *L*, 8 Nov. 1890, p. 988 (Cambridge); Manders, *Gateshead*, p. 172.

129. *L*, 20 June 1891, p. 1401 (Leicester), 15 May 1897, p. 1363, 8 June 1897, p. 1457 (Lowestoft), 23 Jan. 1897, p. 271 (Middlesbrough).

130. *L*, 14 Aug. 1886, p. 309 (Merthyr Tydfil), 6 Aug. 1892, pp. 340-1 (South Shields); *BMJ*, 27 July 1907, p. 241 (West Bromwich).

131. *BMJ*, 8 May 1886, p. 896; *L*, 6 Aug. 1898, p. 333; *Truth*, 26 Dec. 1895, p. 1588 (Helmsley).

132. W.R. Baldwin-Wiseman, 'The Increase in the National Consumption of Water', *JRSS*, vol. LXXII (1909), pp. 272-88.

133. *GMJ*, vol. XXIX (1888), pp. 254-6.

134. *BMJ*, 30 Sept. 1893, p. 752; *L*, 18 May 1872, p. 686.

135. R.J. Morris, *Cholera 1832* (London, 1976), p. 148; *Reynolds Political Instructor*, 29 Dec. 1849, p. 54.

136. William Farr, *PP*, 1867-8, vol. XXXIII, pp. 9-20; R. Thorne Thorne, *The Progress of Preventive Medicine during the Victorian Era* (1888), p. 59; Morris, *Cholera*, p. 83.

137. *L*, 12 Jan. 1867, p. 55; Farr, *Vital Statistics*, pp. 348.

138. Henry Cooper in *JSS*, vol. XVI (1853), pp. 247-50.

139. *Edinburgh Medical and Surgical Journal*, vol. XXXVII (1832), pp. 219-20, vol. XXXIX (1833), pp. 82-3.

140. [Robert Gooch], *Quarterly Review*, vol. XXXIII (1825), pp. 219-20; *L*, Dr Tweedie on Contagion, 22 Sept. 1827, p. 776, 28 July 1838, p. 632 (Southwood Smith), 6 Feb. 1841, p. 687 (reporting Liebig's views), 17 Aug. 1844 (Dr Robertson on miasmata); *Edinburgh Medical and Surgical Journal*, vol. LXXI (1849) (on relation between atmospheric pressure and spread of cholera in 1832), p. 311.

141. Morris, *Cholera*, p. 173; *L*, 10 Nov. 1832, p. 211.

142. *L*, 5 Jan. 1867, p. 18, 4 Sept. 1886, p. 454, 23 July 1892, p. 205; Charles Creighton, *A History of Epidemics in Britain* (London [1891-4]), vol. II, pp. 859-60.

143. Herbert Preston-Thomas, *The Work and Play of a Government Inspector* (London, 1909), pp. 218-20.

144. John Snow in *Edinburgh Medical Journal*, vol. I (1855-6), p. 669; *Snow On Cholera, with a Biographical Memoir by B.W. Richardson* (New York, 1936); *L*, 13 Oct. 1849, pp. 406-7, 3 Nov. 1849, p. 493, 7 July 1855, pp. 10-12.

145. *Edinburgh Medical Journal*, vol. I (1855-6), pp. 481-3, 670, 944; *L*, 5 Jan. 1867, p. 18.

146. Farr, 'Influence of Elevation on the Fatality of Cholera', *JSS*, vol. XV (1852), pp. 155-7; *Vital Statistics*, p. 351; John Webster in *London Journal of Medicine* vol. 2 (1849) pp. 994-7; Charles Kidd, *Dublin Quarterly Journal of*

Medical Science, vol. XVIII (1854), p. 349.

147. *L*, 3 June 1868, p. 752, 8 Aug. 1868, p. 183, 2 Sept. 1868, p. 339; Lambert, *Simon*, pp. 52, 380, 522.

148. *L*, 6 Jan. 1849, p. 19.

149. George Hilaro Barlow, *A Manual of the Practice of Medicine* (1861), p. 700; *GMJ*, vol. XLII (1894), pp. 443-6; *L*, 11 Aug. 1849, pp. 154-9.

150. D. Phelps Brown, *The Complete Herbalist or the People Their Own Physicians* (1867), p. 204; *Letters of Samuel Palmer*, vol. I, p. 463; Creighton, *Epidemics*, vol. II, p. 825.

151. Creighton, *Epidemics*, vol. II, p. 823; Shaftesbury, *Speeches* (1851), p. 279; Joseph Rogers, *Reminiscences of a Workhouse Medical Officer* (1888), pp. 1-2; S.P.W. Chave, 'Henry Whitehead and Cholera in Broad Street', *Medical History*, vol. II (1958), p. 97.

152. Scott, *Statistical Vindication*, p. 159; Preston-Thomas, *Work and Play*, pp. 213-14; J.C. McDonald, 'The History of Quarantine in Britain During the 19th Century', *Bulletin of the History of Medicine*, vol. XXV (1951), pp. 22-43.

153. R. Dudley Edwards and T. Desmond Williams (eds.), *The Great Famine* (New York, 1957), pp. 263-89.

154. *Medical and Physical Journal*, vol. VI (1801), pp. 196-7; Skinner, *Journal* (28 June 1812), p. 74.

155. Creighton, *Epidemics*, vol. II, p. 212; George Rosen in G. McLachlan and T. McKeown (eds.), *Medical History and Medical Care* (London, 1971), pp. 63-4.

156. *London Medical and Physical Journal*, vol. XXXVIII (1817), pp. 133-9.

157. *L*, 15 May 1841, p. 260; *Examiner*, 9 July 1853, p. 435.

158. John Armstrong, 'Some Observations On The Origin . . . Of Typhus Fever', *Medical Intelligencer* (May 1822), pp. 159-60.

159. *L*, 16 May 1868, pp. 630-1.

160. Creighton, *Epidemics*, vol. II, pp. 214-15; *L*, 10 June 1899, p. 1583; *Medical Chronicle*, vol. XXXVI (1902), pp. 1-4.

161. Steele, *JRSS*, vol. L (1891), p. 289.

162. *Medical and Physical Journal*, vol. XVI (1806), pp. 340-1; E.M. Brockbank, '. . . Fever Hospitals in Manchester', *Medical Chronicle*, vol. XXXVII (1902-3), pp. 400-4; SC on Contagious Fever, *PP*, 1818, vol. VII, pp. 6-10; *L*, 30 Sept. 1871, pp. 483-4.

163. SC on Medical Poor Relief, *PP*, 1844, vol. IX, Qs. 2611-14, 2859; *L*, 14 May 1864, p. 548.

164. *Edinburgh Medical and Surgical Journal*, vol. LXII (1844), pp. 90-1.

165. *L*, 22 Feb. 1862, p. 208, 19 Mar. 1870, p. 427; *Parl. Debs.*, vol. XCIX, col. 1736.

166. *Truth*, 28 Nov. 1895, p. 1319 (Reading), 5 Dec. 1895, p. 1381 (Dover); *L*, 21 May 1887, p. 1051 (Ince Blundell).

167. W.T. Gairdner to Royal Sanitary Commission, *PP*, 1868-9, vol. XXXII, Q. 8246.

168. Thorne Thorne, *Progress*, p. 11.

169. Barlow, *Practice of Medicine*, pp. 650-2; *L*, 14 May 1864, p. 548.

170. *Medical and Physical Journal*, vol. XXII (1809), pp. 94-5; *L*, 'On the Medicinal Properties of Spiders', 15 Apr. 1826, p. 85; J.B. Russell in *GMJ*, vol. XXX (1888), pp. 20-9.

171. *PP*, 1916, vol. V, p. 60; *PP*, 1914-16, vol. XI, pp. cviii-cix;

172. Creighton, *Epidemics*, vol. II, p. 288.

173. Charles Porter, *L*, 29 Oct. 1898, p. 1121.

174. *L*, 6 Dec. 1856, pp. 617-18, 27 Dec. 1856, pp. 694-5, 2 July 1859, pp. 4-5, 30 Nov. 1860, p. 534; see also E.W. Goodall, *William Budd, M.D.* (Bristol, 1936), pp. 46-53.

175. *L*, 30 Nov. 1861, p. 534, 26 Nov. 1870, p. 752. Dr Michael Taylor of Penrith claimed to have published the theory that infectious diseases were conveyed in milk in the *Edinburgh Monthly Medical Journal* for May 1858, but I have been unable to trace this issue (*L*, 10 Dec. 1870, p. 835).

176. *PP*, 1874, vol. XXXI, pp. 103-21.

177. *L*, 25 Aug. 1888, p. 381, 27 May 1882, p. 883 (Grafton); *St Bartholomew's Hospital Reports*, vol. XXXIII (1898), pp. 93-4; *Sanitation in the West* (Mar. 1894), p. 4 (Leinster).

178. A.G. Butler (ed.), *Official History of the Australian Army Medical Services 1914-18*, vol. II, pp. 539-40.

179. Barlow, *Practice of Medicine*, p. 648.

180. *Medical Chronicle*, vol. VI (1887), pp. 208-10.

181. Phelps Brown, *Complete Herbalist*, p. 85; *L*, 20 Jan. 1838, p. 577; William Fox, *The Working Man's Model Family Botanic Guide; or, Every Man His Own Doctor*, 19th ed. (Sheffield, 1909), p. 43.

182. *Edinburgh Medical and Surgical Journal*, vol. XV (1819), pp. 332-6.

183. T. McKeown and R.G. Brown, 'Medical Evidence related to English population changes in the eighteenth century', *Population Studies*, vol. 9 (1955-6); E.M. Sigsworth, 'A provincial hospital in the eighteenth and early nineteenth centuries', *The College of General Practitioners*, *Yorkshire Faculty Journal* (1966); S. Cherry, 'The role of a provincial hospital: the Norfolk and Norwich Hospital, 1771-1880', *Population Studies*, vol. 26 (1972); John Woodward, *To Do the Sick no Harm* (London, 1974). Dr Woodward's bibliography provides an excellent guide to this debate.

184. Woodward, *The Do the Sick no Harm*, pp. 36, 144; *L*, 27 Feb. 1864, pp. 248-9.

185. *L*, 13 June 1840, p. 426.

186. John Clenndinning, *JSS*, vol. VII (1844), p. 300; *L*, 11 Jan. 1851, p. 55, 28 Jan. 1860, p. 98, 9 Apr. 1870, p. 496, 29 Oct. 1870, p. 615; *Charity Organization Reporter*, 18 May 1882, p. 151; *GMJ*, vol. XXI (1889), p. 191; *Westminster Hospital Reports*, vol. XXII (1929-33), pp. 238-9, 'Average stay should not exceed 19 days'; Robert Kohn and Kerr L. White, *Health Care: An International Study* (London, 1976), p. 206. (In the early 1970s 25 per cent less than one day – 47 per cent less than 14 days.)

187. *L*, 3 July 1858, p. 14, 29 Jan. 1870, p. 150, 12 Feb. 1887, p. 303, 10 Jan. 1891, p. 102.

188. *Guy's Hospital Reports*, vol. I (1836), p. x; *L*, 30 Oct. 1869, p. 613.

189. *L*, 23 Oct. 1869, p. 577, 5 May 1900, p. 1305.

190. *L*, 28 Aug. 1909, p. 619 (Manchester), p. 620 (Leeds), p. 622 (Bristol), p. 640 (Glasgow), p. 735 (Greenwood). Dr. Steele Muir, *GMJ*, vol. LXV (1906), p. 57.

191. *Charity Organization Reporter*, 28 June 1883, p. 211; *L*, 6 Sept. 1890, p. 515 (distribution map).

192. Sutherland, 'The Breakdown of the Hospital System', *GMJ*, vol. XXX (1888), p. 349; *L*, 17 July 1830, p. 611, 20 Nov. 1830, p.276, 7 Mar. 1903, p. 676, 14 Mar. 1903, pp. 750-1.

193. *GMJ*, vol. LXXV (1911), p. 162; *L*, 22 July 1826, p. 531, 23 Jan. 1846, p. 109, 20 June 1914, p. 1784; John Fox to SC on Medical Poor Relief, *PP*, 1844, vol. IX, Qs. 5842-5 (Exeter).

194. *L*, 16 Jan. 1875, p. 103, 23 Jan. 1875, p. 130, 20 June 1914, p. 1784.

195. *L*, 25 Jan. 1834, p. 696.

196. *Examiner*, 15 Jan. 1853, p. 43; *Truth*, 3 Sept. 1885, p. 362; *L*, 6 Aug. 1882, p. 250.

197. *L*, 4 Nov. 1837, p. 203, 11 Nov. 1837, p. 238.

198. *GMJ*, vol. XXX (1888), p. 396.

199. A.P. Stewart, *L*, 10 Oct. 1868, p. 494.

200. *GMJ*, vol. XXX (1888), pp. 102-3, 444.

201. *Charity Organization Reporter*, 1 May 1872, pp. 78-9.

202. *BMJ*, 23 Jan. 1858, p. 76; Bosanquet, *Social Work*, pp. 371-2; RC on Poor Laws, *PP*, 1909, vol. XLI, p. 781; *L*, 23 Oct. 1869, p. 579.

203. *JSS*, vol. XXIV (1861), p. 389; *Charity Organization Reporter*, 27 Mar. 1879, p. 87; *L*, 29 Feb. 1868, p. 295, 14 Aug. 1869, p. 240, 2 Oct. 1869, p. 482.

204. *L*, 19 Sept. 1835, pp. 822-3.

205. *L*, 14 Aug. 1869, p. 240, 2 Oct. 1869, p. 482, 3 Oct. 1869, p. 577, 13 Nov. 1869, p. 678, 5 July 1879, p. 20, 4 Sept. 1909, p. 735; RC on Poor Laws, *PP*, 1909, vol. XI, Q. 33370.

206. *L*, 13 June 1840, p. 426.

207. *GMJ*, vol. XXIX (1888), p. 167.

208. *L*, 21 Dec. 1850, p. 696.

209. *L*, 13 Aug. 1881, pp. 293-4, 24 Mar. 1900, p. 871, 31 Mar. 1900, p. 975. For other similar cases see *Medical Gazette*, 3 Nov. 1838, p. 192, and *BMJ*, 19 May 1888, p. 1072.

210. *L*, 18 Aug. 1832, p. 671; Report of discussion at National Association for the Promotion of Social Science, *L*, 10 Oct. 1868, p. 494; Michael H. Cooper, *Rationing Health Care* (London, 1975), p. 72.

211. *L*, 20 Nov. 1824, p. 252; *Medical Gazette*, 31 Jan. 1835, pp. 633-4.

212. *Medical Gazette*, 12 Dec. 1835, p. 398; Mrs Gaskell to Emily Shaen, 27 Oct. 1854, in J.A.V. Chapple and Arthur Pollard (eds.), *The Letters of Mrs Gaskell* (Manchester, 1966), p. 319.

213. S.W.F. Holloway, 'The All Saints' Sisterhood at University College Hospital 1862-99', *Medical History*, vol. III (1959), p. 148; Henry E. Clark, 'Changes', in *GMJ*, vol. LII (1899), p. 306.

214. *L*, 13 Jan. 1855, p. 53, 16 June 1860, p. 606, 14 July 1884, p. 81.

215. *L*, 1 Apr. 1871, p. 452, 11 Nov. 1871, pp. 680-1, 30 Dec. 1871, p. 929; Florence Nash (ed.), *Florence Nightingale to her Nurses* (London, 1914), p. 10 (May 1872).

216. *L*, 2 Oct. 1875, p. 499, 23 Oct. 1875, p. 615, 6 Feb. 1897, p. 409; *BMJ*, 8 July 1899, p. 121.

217. *L*, 6 Aug. 1825, pp. 134-8, 12 Nov. 1825, pp. 261-3, 21 Dec. 1833, p. 499, 10 Oct. 1868, pp. 488-9.

218. *L*, 12 July 1828, p. 643, 28 Sept. 1839, p. 26, 18 Dec. 1869, p. 845.

219. Ralph Colp, Jr., *To Be an Invalid* (Chicago, 1977), p. 4.

220. *L*, 17 Apr. 1830, p. 95, 28 Aug. 1830, p. 380, 20 Nov. 1830, p. 286, 27 Nov. 1830, p. 318, 6 May 1837, p. 234, 20 July 1844, p. 541, 12 Feb. 1859, p. 179.

221. *L*, 12 Oct. 1839, p. 26, 5 Apr. 1834, p. 57, 21 May 1831, pp. 252-3, 7 Jan. 1882, p. 27.

222. *Medical Times & Gazette*, 14 June 1862, pp. 617-18; *L*, 24 Nov. 1832, pp. 274-5, 6 Dec. 1834, pp. 382-3, 16 Jan. 1858, p. 69; *Once a Week*, 27 Feb. 1864, p. 266.

223. E.g. *L*, 20 Oct. 1877, p. 584.

224. *BMJ*, 23 Sept. 1899, p. 797; Richard B. Fisher, *Joseph Lister 1827-1912* (London, 1977), p. 106.

225. *L*, 6 Sept. 1834, pp. 855-6, 4 Nov. 1837, p. 206, 11 Nov. 1837, p. 236, 2 Nov. 1872, p. 654.

226. *L*, 6 Nov. 1869, p. 660.

227. *JSS*, vol. XXIV (1861), p. 376; *L*, 14 Aug. 1869, p. 229.

228. Florence Nightingale, *Notes on Hospitals*, third ed. (London, 1863); McKeown and Brown, 'Medical Evidence', *Population Studies*, vol. IX (1955).

229. *Charity Organization Reporter*, 4 Aug. 1881, p. 179, 13 Oct. 1881, p. 190; Brockbank, *Portrait of A Hospital 1752-1942 . . . the Royal Infirmary Manchester* (Toronto, 1952), pp. 97, 154; *L*, 15 Jan. 1870, p. 95.

230. *PP*, 1892, vol. XXI, p. 196; *Transactions of Clinical Society of London*, 19 Oct. 1872, p. 587; *Medical Times*, 31 May 1884, p. 735; *Westminster Hospital Reports*, vol. XIX (1924), pp. 39-53.

231. *L*, 30 July 1859, pp. 117-18.

232. *L*, 18 Apr. 1863, p. 455, 8 May 1875, p. 667; Creighton, *Epidemics*, vol. II, pp. 733-4.

233. *L*, 14 Jan. 1882, p. 83.

234. F. de Havilland Hall, *Westminster Hospital Reports*, vol. XI (1899), pp. 32-3; *BMJ*, 10 July 1897, p. 114, 11 Sept. 1897, p. 692, 20 June 1908, p. 1479; Curt Proskauer, 'Development and Use of the Rubber Glove . . .', *Journal of the History of Medicine*, vol. XXII (1958), pp. 374-80; *L*, 26 May 1900, p. 1538. There is a vivid description of the operating-theatre at St Thomas's in the 1890s - sawdust on the floor, oak table, lead sink - in N.R. Barrett, 'The Contribution of Australians to Medical Knowledge', Medical *History*, vol. XI (1967), p. 321.

235. *L*, 9 June 1832, p. 320; T.G. Wilson, *Victorian Doctor: Being the Life of Sir William Wilde* [1942] (reprinted Wakefield, 1974), pp. 98-100.

236. *L*, 8 Feb. 1862, p. 152.

237. *L*, 24 Apr. 1858, p. 426 (Bristol General Hospital), 23 July 1881, p. 137 (Guy's), 25 May 1872, p. 737, 19 June 1875, p. 872 (flowers), 15 Jan. 1870, p. 96 (Christmas parties); *GMJ*, vol. XXX (1888), pp. 18-19 (Victoria Infirmary, Glasgow)

238. *L*, 28 Apr. 1866, p. 464.

239. *L*, 14 Oct. 1871, p. 568, 31 Oct. 1846, p. 491; T.C. Hunt, *The Medical Society of London 1773-1973* (London, 1972), p. 58.

240. Holloway, 'All Saints Sisterhood', *Medical History*, vol. III (1959), p. 150; *PP*, 1909, vol. XLII, pp. 48-9.

241. *L*, 2 Oct. 1858, p. 355.

242. Fisher, *Lister*, p. 207.

243. G. W. Callender, *L*, 20 Feb. 1864, p. 211, Guy, 20 Apr. 1867, p. 498, Simpson, 16 Oct. 1869, pp. 535-7, Lamond, 29 Jan. 1870, p. 175.

244. Cooper, *Rationing Health Care*, quoting Ferguson and MacPhail (1954), p. 96.

245. Spencer Wells and Callender, *L*, 20 Feb. 1864, p. 211.

246. *L*, 8 Jan. 1870, p. 40.

247. *GMJ*, vol. III (1830), p. 111; Brockbank, *Portrait*, pp. 61-2, 92; *L*, 31 May 1834, p. 367; Thomas McKeown, R.G. Brown and R.G. Record, 'An Interpretation of the Modern Rise of Population . . .', *Population Studies*, vol. 26 (1972), p. 346.

248. *L*, 11 Jan. 1851, p. 54.

249. A.E. Sansom, *L*, 30 Apr. 1859, p. 442.

250. F.F. Cartwright in F.N.L. Poynter (ed.), *Medicine and Science in the 1860s* (London, 1966), pp. 81-2.

251. *GMJ*, vol. LII (1899), p. 308.

252. *JRSS*, vol. LXXIV (1911), pp. 367-8.

253. *Proceedings of the West London Medico-Chirurgical Society*, vol. II (1887), pp. 86-8; *GMJ*, vol. LII (1899), pp. 308-9.

254. *L*, 14 Aug. 1869, p. 229 - for a similar earlier opinion see 18 Aug. 1832, p. 530.

255. Bransby B. Cooper, *Guy's Hospital Reports*, vol. IV (1839), p. 324; James Wardrop, *L*, 3 Aug. 1833, pp. 596-7.

256. *L*, 7 Aug. 1869, pp. 194-5, 14 Aug. 1869, p. 230, 28 Aug. 1869, p. 296.

257. *Medical Gazette*, 19 Jan. 1889, p. 621; *L*, 1 Jan. 1859, p. 8, 16 Oct. 1875 (Callender), 24 Jan. 1914 (Howse and Davies); *St Andrews Medical Graduates' Association Transactions* (1870), pp. 64-6 (Wynn Williams and Ross); 'Address in Surgery at 37th Annual Meeting of BMA', *BMJ*, 7 Aug. 1869, p. 156 (Nunnelly), 15 May 1886, pp. 921-3 (Lawson Tait); Henry Butlin, *St Bartholomew's Hospital Reports*, vol. XXX (1894), pp. 277-83.

258. Simpson, 'The Obstetrician's Toilet', *London Journal of Medicine*, vol. II (1851), p. 747; John Patrick, *GMJ*, vol. XLIX (1898), p. 447; Armstrong, *Liverpool Medico-Chirurgical Journal*, vol. IV (1883), pp. 127-9.

259. Lambert, *Simon*, pp. 344-5, 478-83; *Sanitary Review*, vol. IV (1858), p. 119; Florence Nightingale, 'Notes on the Health of Hospitals', *BMJ*, 23 Oct. 1858, p. 892; Percy Leslie in *BMJ*, 4 Sept. 1869, p. 282; *L*, 5 July 1862, p. 21; B.W. Richardson, *Vita Medica: Chapters of Medical Life and Work* (London, 1897), p. 264.

260. *BMJ*, 24 July 1869, pp. 82-3.

261. *L*, 25 Sept. 1869, p. 451; *BMJ*, 2 Oct. 1869, p. 377.

262. R.M.S. McConaghey, 'The Evolution of the Cottage Hospital', *Medical History*, vol. XI (1967), pp. 132-3.

263. J. Sinclair Holden, *BMJ*, 3 Aug. 1889, pp. 231-2.

264. H.G. St M. Rees, 'A Note on the Mildenhall Cottage Hospital', *Medical History*, vol. VI (1968), pp. 185-7.

265. *PP*, 1909, vol. XL, p. 645, Qs. 33312, 33375.

266. Charles West, *L*, 19 Feb. 1887, pp. 394-5; T. Holmes and A.P. Stewart, *L*, 2 Apr. 1870, p. 497.

267. Hugh Thomson, 'Breakdown of the . . . Hospital System', *GMJ*, vol. XXXI (1889), pp. 97-8; *L*, 23 Oct. 1869, p. 577.

268. Steele, *JSS*, vol. XXIV (1861), pp. 389-90; Bosanquet, *Social Work*, p. 209; *L*, 10 Feb. 1872, p. 197; *Charity Organization Reporter*, 27 Mar. 1879, p. 87.

269. *L*, 28 Mar. 1885, p. 572.

270. *GMJ*, vol. XXXII (1889), p. 361.

271. *GMJ*, vol. XXVI (1886), pp. 334-5; Steele, *JRSS*, vol. LIV (1891), pp. 268-72; *L*, 22 Apr. 1882, p. 663, 26 Jan. 1884, p. 171, 2 Jan. 1897, p. 71.

272. *Westminster Hospital Reports*, vol. XIII (1903), pp. 191-4; *L*, 17 July 1909, 160-1.

273. *GMJ*, vol. LXXII (1909), p. 46.

274. *L*, 1 Sept. 1855, p. 203; John Langdon-Davies, *Westminster Hospital: Two Centuries of Voluntary Service, 1719-1948* (London, 1952), p. 67.

275. *L*, 19 Dec. 1857, p. 634, 28 July 1860, p. 88, 9 May 1868, p. 600.

276. *L*, 30 June 1866, p. 716, 25 May 1867, p. 637.

277. *L*, 23 June 1860, p. 625, 12 Feb. 1870, p. 246, 22 Oct. 1881, p. 727.

278. Steele, *JRSS*, vol. LIV (1891), p. 290; *Truth*, 4 Apr. 1895, pp. 840-1, 13 June 1895, p. 1452; *L*, 19 Feb. 1887, p. 395, 22 Dec. 1888, p. 1241, 18 Feb. 1893, p. 378; *Charity Organization Reporter*, 9 Aug. 1883, p. 255.

279. A.W. Russell, 'Glasgow Western Infirmary', *GMJ*, vol. XXXI (1889), pp. 4-5; *L*, 18 Sept. 1909, p. 886; *Daily News*, 8 July 1881.

280. *Truth*, 7 Feb. 1895, pp. 338-9; *L*, 27 Aug. 1870, p. 312, 11 Oct. 1902, p. 1006; Sutherland and Hugh Thomson in *GMJ*, vol. XXX (1888), pp. 348-51, vol. XXXI (1889), p. 99.

281. *L*, 6 Nov. 1869, p. 651, 11 Jan. 1873, p. 62, 4 July 1874, p. 22, 22 June 1889, p. 1261, 17 Apr. 1897, p. 1118, 16 June 1900, p. 1777, 9 Aug. 1902, p. 397; E. Montefiore to RC Poor Laws, *PP*, 1909, vol. XI, Q. 35026; *BMJ*, 18 Dec. 1897, p. 1808 (Ensor).

282. *L*, 12 Feb. 1887. p. 342; *Charity Organization Reporter*, 12 July 1883, p. 236.

283. *L*, 11 Jan. 1873, p. 68 (Moorfields), 6 Jan. 1866, p. 5 (Addenbrooke's), 23 Dec. 1871, p. 893, 21 Nov. 1874, p. 745 (London Fever Hospital), 15 Oct. 1870, p. 552 (Edinburgh), 9 Aug. 1879, p. 217, 26 June 1880, p. 1009; *BMJ*, 8 Jan. 1881, p. 61 (St Thomas's).

284. *L*, 16 July 1881, p. 121 (Bradford), 13 May 1882, p. 794, 3 Jan. 1885, p. 32 (Norwich), 27 Oct. 1894, pp. 993-4, 2 Mar. 1895, p. 561 (Great Northern Central), 24 Dec. 1870, p. 895, 31 Jan. 1885, p. 214 (protests from GPs); *BMJ*, 27 Mar. 1869, p. 293 (Drysdale).

285. Steele in *JRSS*, vol. LIV (1891), p. 273; Greenwood and Candy, *JRSS*, vol. LXXIV (1911), p. 366; *L*, 31 July 1909, pp. 317-18; Frank Field, *Unequal Britain* (London, 1974), p. 44.

286. *L*, 17 June 1882, p. 997, 17 Jan. 1903, p. 185 (Fitzroy House); *BMJ*, 22 Nov. 1890, p. 1207 (Aberdeen). For earlier examples of 'private sanatoria', usually operated or proposed by leading radical sanitary reformers, see *Medical Gazette*, 6 Dec. 1839, p. 406 (Southwood Smith's proposed 'Sanatorium' in London) and 22 July 1842, p. 643 (B. Phillips's sanatorium in Wimpole Street).

287. *L*, 22 Jan. 1831, p. 572, 20 Oct. 1883, p. 710.

288. *L*, 19 Feb. 1831, p. 702, 15 Dec. 1888, p. 1215, 27 Aug. 1898, p. 587.

289. *L*, 5 May 1849, p. 475.

290. *L*, 10 Sept. 1853, p. 257, 3 Apr. 1858, p. 355, 8 Dec. 1877, p. 867, 9 Oct. 1886, p. 689.

291. *L*, 29 Aug. 1840, p. 831.

292. *L*, 15 Apr. 1871, p. 50, 10 Dec. 1910, p. 1739; *BMJ*, 25 June 1904, p. 1505, 18 Jan. 1908, p. 165; Leonard Le Marchant Minty, *The Legal and Ethical Aspects of Medical Quackery* (London, 1932), pp. 81-3.

293. *L*, 1 Apr. 1871, p. 451, 24 Apr. 1875, p. 597, 17 Apr. 1880, pp. 606-7; *BMJ*, 10 July 1880, p. 591; Brian Inglis, *Fringe Medicine* (London, 1964), pp. 96-7.

294. *PP*, 1883, vol. XX, p. 141; Reginald Dudfield, 'Note on the Mortality from Tuberculosis', *JRSS*, vol. LXX (1907), p. 454; *L*, 7 Jan. 1899, p. 41; Macintosh, *Trends of Opinion*, pp. 80-1.

295. *Edinburgh Medical and Surgical Journal*, vol. LXXIX (1853), p. 383; Arthur Ransome in *Medical Chronicle*, vol. VIII (1897-8), p. 163; Byrom Bramwell, *L*, 5 July 1902, p. 6.

296. John Tatham, Registrar-General's Office, *L*, 27 July 1901, p. 233.

297. *L*, 17 Dec. 1898, p. 1609.

298. Jane Walker, *Child-Study*, vol. V (1912), pp. 127-9.

299. Thorne Thorne, *Progress*, pp. 47-51.

300. T.C. Speer in *Dublin Hospital Reports*, vol. III (1822), pp. 177-9; *L*, 8 Aug. 1896, p. 427.

301. *JSS*, vol. IX (1846), pp. 152-3.

302. *St Andrews Medical Graduates' Association Transactions* (1867), p. 143.

303. *L*, 2 Feb. 1895, p. 298, 13 Dec. 1890, p. 1303 (Koch's fluid), 3 and 10 May 1884, pp. 786 and 836 (Andrew).

304. *BMJ*, 30 Sept. 1882, p. 628; Preston-Thomas, *Work and Play*, p. 308.

305. Thomas B. Peacock, *St Thomas's Hospital Reports*, vol. V (1874), pp. 2-21; *BMJ*, 31 Jan. 1880, p. 167.

306. Pamela Horn, *The Victorian Country Child* (Kineton, 1974), p. 178.

307. J.A. Lindsay in *BMJ*, 11 Dec. 1897, p. 1727; W.B. Thorne in *L*, 12 Jan. 1895, p. 119.

308. *PP*, 1909, vol. XLII, pp. 98-100.

309. *PP*, 1909, vol. XXXVII, p. 289; Macintosh, *Trends of Opinion*, p. 81.

310. *L*, 29 Oct. 1842, p. 160; *Royal Institute of Public Health Transactions 1900*, p. 221; *Medical Chronicle*, vol. LII (1910), p. 75.

311. *PP*, 1904, vol. XXXII, Qs. 6020-2, 12952; *L*, 16 July 1910, p. 168; Alexander Scott, *GMJ*, vol. V (1873), pp. 301-5; C.R. Drysdale, *Sheffield Medical Journal*, vol. I (1892-3), p. 115.

312. *L*, 8 Aug. 1896, p. 429.

313. Wayland D. Hand, 'Folk Medical Inhalants in Respiratory Disorders', *Medical History*, vol. XII (1968), p. 157.

314. *L*, 17 June 1848, p. 665, 30 Mar. 1850, p. 390, 5 and 12 Feb. 1848, pp. 158 and 185, 4 Jan. 1873, pp. 25-60, 1 Feb. 1873, p. 70.

315. Cavendish Bentinck, *Parl. Debs.,* vol. CCLXXVIII, col. 826; C.F. Pollock, *GMJ*, vol. XXX (1888), pp. 48-9; [John Chapman], 'Prostitution . . .', *Westminster Review*, vol. XXXVII (1870), pp. 121-2.

316. *L*, 7 Nov. 1846, p. 511.

317. *BMJ*, 4 June 1898, p. 1499.

318. *GMJ*, vol. XVIII (1882), pp. 414-15.

319. *BMJ*, 7 Apr. 1888, p. 768; *L*, 3 Mar. 1860, p. 226.

320. F.B. Smith, 'Sexuality in Britain, 1800-1900' in Vicinus (ed.), *A Widening Sphere*, pp. 182-98; *London Journal of Medicine*, vol. II (1851), p. 644; *Medical Times & Gazette*, 31 Oct. 1857, p. 458; *Sanitary Review*, vol. II (1858), pp. 329-30.

321. G.H. Bull, *L*, 9 Dec. 1843, p. 328, 30 Dec. 1843, p. 437; Lawson Tait, *BMJ*, 30 June 1888, p. 1387.

322. *L*, 21 Oct. 1826, pp. 78-9.

323. *BMJ*, 30 June 1888, p. 1387.

324. *L*, 13 July 1861, p. 48.

325. *L*, 25 Jan. 1873, p. 134 (Nichols came to Britain around 1861, when he was about 46); *BMJ*, 13 Nov. 1897, p. 1431.

326. *L*, 5 Apr. 1862, p. 356; *Dublin Quarterly Journal of Medical Science* vol. XXXV (1863), pp. 35-6.

327. *L*, 2 May 1863, p. 512, 30 July 1870, p. 159, 16 Nov. 1872, p. 702; *BMJ*, 23 Oct. 1869, p. 442, 26 Mar. 1881, p. 489.

328. [Ernest Hart?] 'A Grave Social Problem', *BMJ*, 3 Dec. 1881, p. 904.

329. *BMJ*, 30 Jan. 1886, p. 236, 13 Feb. 1886, p. 331.

330. *Medical and Physical Journal*, vol. XXI (1814), p. 212; Graham, *Females*, pp. 1-3; *L*, 20 Sept. 1879, p. 423 (Tibbits), 4 Apr. 1835, p. 13 (Eagle); *BMJ*, 14 Apr. 1883, p. 720.

331. *BMJ*, 27 Sept. 1890, p. 769.

332. *BMJ*, 26 Jan. 1895, p. 325; *St Bartholomew's Hospital Reports*, vol. XXXIV (1899), pp. 327-9.

333. *L*, 16 June 1866, p. 663, 12 Jan. 1867, p. 67; Hunt (ed.), *Medical Society of London*, p. 76.

334. *BMJ*, 1 June 1895, p. 1226; *L*, 19 Nov. 1898, p. 1344, 26 Nov. 1898, p. 1431.

335. *L*, 5 Nov. 1870, p. 658.

336. *L*, 8 Nov. 1879, pp. 693-703; *BMJ*, 16 Sept. 1882, pp. 515-16.

337. *L*, 17 Dec. 1898, p. 1611.

338. *L*, 14 Oct. 1843, p. 68.

339. *L*, 30 July 1842, p. 623, 5 May 1866, pp. 493-4, 30 Oct. 1875, p. 650, 14 June 1884, p. 1102, 29 May 1897, p. 1492 (Solomon).

340. *L*, 8 Aug. 1857, p. 150.

341. Fox, *Working Man's . . . Guide*, pp. 207-8; *L*, 2 May 1863, p. 505 (Jordan), 10 Dec. 1853, p. 559 (Acton).

342. W. Farr in *British Annals of Medicine*, 10 Mar. 1837, p. 315.

343. *L*, 12 Apr. 1851, p. 416; *BMJ*, 19 Mar. 1892, p. 639.

344. *Dublin Quarterly Journal of Medicine and Science*, vol. XXVII (1859), p. 134; *L*, 24 May 1884, p. 963, 22 Jan. 1887, p. 169; Ann Stafford, *The Age of Consent* (London, 1964); F.B. Smith, 'Labouchere's amendment to the Criminal Law Amendment Bill', *Historical Studies*, No. 67 (Oct. 1976), pp. 170-2.

5 OLD AGE

1. MALADIES

Middle age settled into old age at about 45 years during the nineteenth century. Although the proportion of the old in the demographic pyramid was held stable by the reduced death rate of under-45s, their absolute numbers increased dramatically.[1]

The class distribution of longevity is difficult to fix. The few calculations we have at present of expectation of life after 45 are sketchy, ill matched and partly contradictory. But there are some conclusions which look plausible. The first is that 'gentlemen', as Chadwick classed them in 1844, and those whom Charles Ansell junior, the actuary, called 'the richer classes' in 1874, had higher life expectancies than other classes, except 'paupers'. Chadwick, using figures for 1839, claimed that 'gentlemen' who survived 21 had an average age at death of 60 in London and 65 in Hereford. The gentry's better chances of longevity were also demonstrated by the proportions of deaths by age and class for over 25,000 deaths, mostly in 1840, from Manchester, Liverpool, Bath, the Strand and Kendal Unions, Wiltshire and Rutlandshire.[2]

Dr William Guy calculated from the London mortality records for 1839 and ascribed class by reported place of residence. He found that 'gentry' had an average age at death of 58.6 years.[3] Ansell estimated a mean age at death of 55 for the 'richer classes of England and Wales'.[4] Guy's and Ansell's totals are lower than Chadwick's because they averaged all deaths in the class, including infants. 'Paupers' equalled gentlemen at 60 in Chadwick's London calculations and surpassed them, at 71, in Hereforc. This is an unexpected conclusion and I shall return to it later. 'Tradesmen' and Labourers', in every calculation, had must the lowest life expectancy. London tradesmen surviving 21, in Chadwick's tables, had a mean age at death of 51, and labourers, 49. In Hereford, the 'Labourers' average was 58. Dr Guy put 'Tradesmen' at 48.8 and 'the labouring class' at 48.1. Ansell, calculating life expectancy from birth in Lambeth, a place with a high infant mortality, asserted that the 'wage receiving class' there had a mean average age at death of 29½. Another actuary, F.G.P. Neison, calculating from two burial societies operating among 'the lowest class' (presumably unskilled but fairly

316

Table 5.1: Total Population, England and Wales, Aged Over 45 and Over 65 (thousands)*

	1841	1851	1861	1871	1881	1891	1901	1911
				Both Sexes				
45+	2,811.1	3,346.2	3,839.4	4,413.5	4,896.3	5,526.5	6,363.2	7,705.2
65+	706.5	830.8	931.8	1,074.9	1,188.6	1,372.5	1,517.8	1,878.6
				Males				
45+	1,344.4	1,597.3	1,833.0	2,093.8	2,291.4	2,568.5	2,965.3	3,588.9
65+	324.8	376.2	423.0	490.5	535.5	606.5	661.1	809.4
				Females				
45+	1,466.7	1,748.9	2,006.4	2,319.7	2,604.9	2,958.0	3,397.9	4,116.3
65+	381.7	454.6	508.8	584.4	653.1	766.0	856.7	1,069.2

* The figures are rounded.
Source: Calculated from B.R. Mitchell and Phyllis Deane, *Abstract of British Historical Statistics* (Cambridge, 1962), pp. 12-13.

Table 5.2: Total Population, Scotland, Aged Over 45 and Over 65 (thousands)*

	1841	1851	1861	1871	1881	1891	1901	1911
				Both Sexes				
45+	456.0	537.5	597.0	659.4	714.2	785.9	870.2	1,000.0
65+	116.8	137.9	149.1	173.9	186.0	203.1	216.5	257.4
				Males				
45+	203.6	237.7	263.8	291.3	313.6	346.7	393.6	457.6
65+	50.5	57.7	61.4	72.6	77.1	82.8	88.2	105.2
				Females				
45+	252.2	299.6	332.9	368.2	400.6	439.2	476.6	542.4
65+	66.1	80.0	87.3	101.5	108.9	120.2	128.3	152.3

* The figures are rounded.
Source: ibid.

Table 5.3: Persons Aged Over 45 as Percentage of Persons Aged Over 5

	Persons Over 45 as Percentage of Total Over 5 Years	Males Over 45 as Percentage of Those Over 5 Years	Females Over 45 as Percentage of Those Over 5 Years
	England and Wales		
1841	20.3	19.9	20.7
1851	21.4	21.0	21.9
1861	22.1	21.7	22.4
1871	22.4	21.9	22.9
1881	21.8	21.0	22.5
1891	21.7	20.9	22.4
1901	22.0	21.3	22.7
1911	23.9	23.1	24.6
	Scotland		
1841	20.0	19.1	20.8
1851	21.3	20.0	22.5
1861	22.6	21.3	23.6
1871	22.3	21.2	24.0
1881	22.1	20.3	23.7
1891	22.3	20.5	23.9
1901	22.0	20.6	23.4
1911	23.6	22.4	24.8

Source: ibid.

Table 5.4: Persons Aged Over 65 as Percentage of Persons Aged Over 5

	Persons Over 65 as Percentage of Total Over 5 Years	Males Over 65 as Percentage of Those Over 5 Years	Females Over 65 as Percentage of Those Over 5 Years
	England and Wales		
1841	5.1	4.8	5.3
1851	5.3	4.9	5.7
1861	5.3	5.0	5.6
1871	5.4	5.1	5.7
1881	5.2	4.9	5.6
1891	5.3	4.9	5.8
1901	5.2	4.7	5.7
1911	5.8	5.2	6.3
	Scotland		
1841	5.1	4.7	5.4
1851	5.4	4.8	6.0
1861	5.6	4.9	6.2
1871	5.9	5.2	6.6
1881	5.7	5.0	6.4
1891	5.7	4.9	6.5
1901	5.4	4.6	6.3
1911	6.0	5.1	6.9

Source: ibid.

Table 5.5: Proportion of Deaths by Age and Class

Age	Gentry and Professional Persons	Farmers, Tradesmen and Persons Similarly Circumstanced	Agricultural and Other Labourers, Artisans and Servants
40-50	1 in 16	1 in 13	1 in 18
50-60	1 in 12	1 in 14	1 in 20
60-70	1 in 6	1 in 12	1 in 18
70-80	1 in 6	1 in 14	1 in 23
80-90	1 in 10	1 in 29	1 in 43
90+	1 in 115	1 in 122	1 in 338

Source: Edwin Chadwick, 'On the best Modes of representing Accurately . . . the Duration of Life . . . amongst different Classes of the Community', *Journal of the Statistical Society*, vol. VII (1844), pp. 4-16.

continuously employed labourers) in Liverpool who paid a 'few pence a week' found among those surviving 15 an average age at death of 38. By contrast, the English friendly society life tables, which relate principally to the better-paid working-men, show an average age at death — calculated from birth — of 45.7 years.[5] Finally, in 1888 Chadwick claimed that the mean age at death of 'well to do' people in Brighton was 63, compared with 28.8 among the 'not well to do'.[6]

Morbidity Rates

At about 45 the morbidity rates showed a sharp increase. It follows that the absolute increase in the numbers of persons surviving beyond 45 occasioned an enormous increase in the amount of morbidity. Virtually the only published figures we have come from the affiliated orders of friendly societies. Although these and other provident societies nominally covered about one-quarter of the population by the 1890s, the bulk of their membership was in the 20-37 age-band and it was largely upper-working class.[7] The lowest subscription to the Manchester Unity in the 1890s was 1s. 2d. per week. This rate tended to exclude agricultural labourers. To gain entitlement to a benefit of 10s. a week which might better sustain a family, a contributor had to pay 1s. 6d. or more a week.[8] The affiliated orders of friendly societies, especially, did not admit the chronically ill, the elderly, those with consumption, gout or hernia, or those employed in dangerous trades. The Royal Standard Benefit Society, for instance, refused all police officers, sailors, glaziers, colour-grinders, journeymen bakers, brass-casters, draymen and coalporters.[9] Moreover, the societies' figures cover only those who kept up their payments and we know there was a high drop-out rate: up to 50 per cent of the Manchester Unity of Oddfellows in the 1890s. The societies probably could not have survived without filtering out the worst risks. Contributors lapsed, most of them totally, when they became unable to work, because of prolonged sickness in their family, or old age. They also dropped out when a slump in employment occurred, as in Burnley in 1879, just when the concomitant deprivation raised the illness rate. Men on piece-work dropped out as their earning power declined with age: thus contributors who had paid for years without claiming suddenly found themselves unprotected as they entered their fifties.[10] The friendly societies, except perhaps the colliers' sick clubs, had little capacity for developing family affectiveness or local cohesion. Members who moved to live near their children or a hospital or into a workhouse commonly lost their benefit because it was not transferable between branches.[11] In 1881 the Local Government Board reported over 11,000 former members of friendly societies in English and Welsh workhouses: 7,400 had dropped out — 'non-payment, withdrawal or dismissal'; 4,000 had been left unprotected after their society had failed; over 2,000 had been members for ten years, some for more than thirty years.[12] Among the callous stupidities perpetrated by Chadwick's 1834 Poor Law Report was a recommendation that friendly societies be encouraged without any provision for securing their funds or preserving their actuarial safety.[13] Finally, the friendly societies and sick clubs excluded or catered less well for women.

For all these reasons the reported morbidity rates must be grossly understated. But even these conservative figures show a doubling of morbidity between 50 and 60 (see Table 5.6).[14]

Table 5.6: Sickness in Friendly Societies 1836-40 According to Various Returns and Actuaries' Calculations (average number 'constantly sick' per 100 living at each age)

Age	Scotland (the Highland Benefit Society)	England (Ansell's calculation)	Scotland (Neison's calculation)	England (Neison's calculation)	East India Company Labourer's Benefit Society
30-40	1.32	1.83	1.66	1.91	2.06
40-50	1.97	2.56	2.44	2.89	2.69
50-60	3.60	4.32	5.17	5.21	6.58

Source: Farr, *Vital Statistics*, p. 503.

City-dwellers were reported by the friendly societies to have lost most weeks 'sick' or 'incapacitated for labour', followed by town-dwellers and then people in the countryside (see Table 5.7).[15]

Table 5.7: Sickness Duration in Weeks

Age	Rural	Town	City
35-45	1.13	1.24	1.37
45-55	1.73	1.88	2.09
55-65	3.65	3.98	4.43

Source: Calculated by T.R. Edmonds from friendly society records for 1840s and early 1850s. *Lancet*, 2 Dec. 1854, p. 454.

These figures again are conservative. They probably represent only weeks for which benefit was claimed, and many funds did not pay benefits beyond the first period of illness within the current year, with a normal maximum of twelve weeks. 'Incapacity for labour' also has a distorting effect: actuaries believed that the illness rates for the country-side and in mining areas were increased by it, while this definition reduced claims among skilled city workers in light trades. On the other hand, comparatively well-paid and independent coal-miners might have been readier to take 'sickies'. There is also the absolute inability to work from exhaustion. An investigation by the Board of Health in London, probably in the 1870s, found that 'every workman or work-woman lost about 20 days in the year from sheer exhaustion'.[16] But the report of the mining inquiry of 1864, giving the number of days lost from sickness in the industry per year between 1846 and 1850 suggests that at the higher age range the sickness benefits were going to at least partially incapacitated semi-retired miners as a form of old age pension.[17]

Table 5.8: Days Lost in Sickness in Mining Industry, 1846-50

Age	Days Absent from Sickness per Year per 100 Living Members
35-45	1,224
45-55	1,946
55-65	2,697
65-75	4,940

Source: Lee, 'Occupational Medicine' in F.N.L. Poynter (ed.), *Medicine and Science in the 1860s* (London, 1966), pp. 166-7.

By the 1890s 1 per cent of the insured lives at age 50 in friendly societies were 'permanently sick', meaning that they had been 'sick and unable to work for two years'. At age 60 the proportion was 3.8 per cent and 19 per cent at age 70.[18]

Although attendance on old people must have comprised a large part of their practice, doctors showed little interest in the irremediable illnesses of the old. ('Geriatrics' is a word of the first decade of this century.) As students they had rarely encountered old people in the teaching hospitals and were denied their one real opportunity to study the disabilities of the old when the profession blocked proposals in the 1860s to allow students to learn in workhouses. The doctors' published lectures and papers refer only incidentally to maladies which they took for granted as widespread among the old. Dropsy in all its manifestations crops up regularly. Cases of oedema of the legs, usually described as being associated with ulcerated varicose veins, were tapped and towards the end of the century doctors also tapped the abdomen in cases of ascites (accumulation of fluid in the peritoneal cavity, associated with a variety of conditions, including liver disease, kidney disease and local cancers). Stomach disorders, diarrhoea and dysentery and lung infirmities were also common.[19] These must partly have been the outcome of sheer malnutrition and hypothermia, although it was laymen who noticed these conditions rather than doctors. Cold snaps always lifted the death rate among the elderly. That of the spring of 1860 in Scotland lifted the rate by about one-fifth; the long severe winter of 1875 caused 5,000 more deaths than average in London, 2,000 of them people over 60, mostly from 'bronchitis' and 'pneumonia'; in the south-west the death rate was doubled among old people — 'firing' had become very dear and they were said to be unable to afford it; in Glasgow in mid-February 1895 a cold snap more than doubled the death rate. The cold winter of 1962-3 also brought about 30,000 deaths above the average. Acute rheumatism was also undoubtedly prevalent, but it is not mentioned as an item of medical investigation until 1888.[20]

Influenza

Severe influenza outbreaks in 1775, 1782, 1803, 1823, 1833, 1837, 1847-8, 1889-94 and 1899 each destroyed aged victims while younger sufferers generally survived. During the epidemic in London in 1847-8 the average mortality of people over 60 was doubled. Deaths from 'bronchitis' increased fivefold, deaths from 'asthma' threefold, and from 'old age' by one-third. The general death rate was worst in the poorest parishes — St George's-in-the-East, for instance, where it jumped from a normal 29 per 1,000 to 73 per 1,000 compared with Lewisham, 17 per 1,000 to 27 per 1,000. In all, about 50,000 deaths in London in 1847-8 were ascribed to influenza: this was about five times the number of fatalities from the cholera of 1849.[21] The death rate among the over-60s during the 1890s epidemic was also much above that of other age groups. Between 1890 and 1893 influenza killed about 16,500 people, mostly adults and the elderly; this was 3,000 more than died in the cholera epidemic of 1849.[22]

In 1833 and 1837 the influenza was said to have had a higher case-mortality rate among the rich than among the poor. Nine lords and ladies died in one week in mid-April 1833. In 1891 it carried off Archbishop Magee of York, while an attack invalided Viscount Arbuthnot for three years before his death in 1895.[23] These notable cases, together with the observation that while males suffered more attacks, females died more often, suggest that medical intervention contributed to the death rate, as Dr Renaud suggested in 1890. (Of course, males reported to be peculiarly liable to attacks, postmen, railway servants, policemen, for example, would have increased the proportion of males who caught the disease in a vigorous period of life.)[24]

Influenza baffled the doctors. For much of the century they could not agree on whether it was a specific disease. In attempts to comprehend the varying symptoms of successive outbreaks, coughing, expectoration of phlegm, muscular pain, shivering and vomiting and headache they variously diagnosed it as 'pulmonary disease', 'acute catarrh', 'fever' and 'a head disease'. Their treatments were on the same comprehensive principles. In 1823, 1833 and 1837 they variously used calomel, digitalis, camphor, bleeding, opium, tincture of henbane and squills, colchicum, rhubarb, James's Powders, Dover's Powder and colocynth. Dr Whiting of the Westminster Medical Society remarked that patients appeared 'to die more after bleeding than those not bled'. By 1899, bleeding and leeches had mostly disappeared as treatments, but most of the rest were still in service, together with some new ones, including strychnine, as a counter to respiratory collapse.[25]

The profession does not appear to have issued public advice during the outbreaks. Indeed, rather than avoiding public gatherings, medical opinion during the epidemics of the 1840s at least seems to have favoured business as usual. During the 1890s doctors emphasised notification and removal to isolation wards and workhouse infirmaries, but by 1909 Local Government Board officials had to admit that influenza outbreaks 'appeared to be very slightly controllable by sanitary measures'.[26] At home, sufferers made up mixtures similar to that used by Mrs Clifton in

Sleaford about 1870: half a pound of treacle, half a pint of vinegar, with 3 teaspoonfuls of laudanum. By the 1890s people who could afford it were giving themselves 'large doses' of quinine three times a day. Among those who could not, Lady Brooke's Fund for the Relief of the Distress from Influenza was distributing bottles of brandy.[27]

Heart Disease

Angina pectoris first appears as a cause of death in the Registrar-General's report for 1856. 'Fatty degeneration', 'cardiac aneurysm' did not appear until 1905. Dr A.D. Morgan, writing in 1968, argues persuasively that most coronary disease would have gone undiagnosed in the nineteenth century, yet that there must have been 'quite a lot of it about' as the outcome of, amongst other predisposing conditions, the high incidence of rheumatic fever and syphilis.[28] Authors of domestic medical manuals implicitly accepted that their readers would have some acquaintance with symptoms of heart disease. Dr Morgan guesses that there was probably a slow increase after 1855. The pathology of coronary disease was described during the 1880s, although effective diagnostic procedures were not discovered until 1912. I have found two investigations which support Dr Morgan's hypotheses. In 1839 the surgeons at the Marylebone Infirmary reported the results of over 500 recent autopsies on poor people. They found the two largest single pathological states to be consumptive lungs, at about 15 per cent, and diseased hearts, at 33 per cent. The dead males had a heart-disease rate of 37 per cent, the females 24 per cent. The heart-disease cases were also concentrated in the 50-70 age group. The surgeons added that their heart disease totals were conservative because of the 'frequent exclusion of aged people from hospitals'. In 1848 Dr Whyte Barclay of St George's Hospital reported on 419 autopsies performed at the hospital during 1846-7. These 419 investigations yielded 79 cases of 'valvular lesion', indicating past syphilis and/or rheumatic fever: of these, almost 70 per cent were aged above 37.[29] It follows that the slow increase of coronary artery disease, which Dr Morgan postulates, was largely associated with the increased longevity of larger numbers of people. Cerebral apoplexy probably increased in the same manner.

There was no cure. Mr John Bury, the local surgeon at Foleshill, near Coventry, who treated George Eliot's father in his decline in 1848, diagnosed 'imperfect action of the *heart*'. He ordered blisters for Mr Evans's chest and complete immobilisation in bed. (Three days later two other doctors diagnosed Evans 'as free from real disease' and they attributed his disorder to repeated attacks of influenza which aggravated 'a wrong

state of the liver and the secretions generally'. They prescribed a change
of air to the seaside and hearty exercise.) Neither regimen succeeded.[30]
In the 1860s Dr Barlow told his students to bleed the patient, keep him
tranquil, on a spare diet of bread and biscuits, with a little lean meat,
very few vegetables and no alcohol. The action of the heart and lungs
could be aided by stimulating the liver and bowels with rhubarb and
other aperients.[31] Barlow also recommended digitalis, but only as an
adjuvant. He, in common with his medical contemporaries, was suspicious of the drug because he could not tell why it worked and knew it
to be a 'cumulative poison'. Its dosage is difficult to control. Digitalis
also carried a bad connotation of folk medicine and quackery.

Although they implicitly recognised the prevalence of heart disease,
writers of domestic manuals tended to dismiss the subject curtly. One
of the few who did describe the symptoms was Dr Spencer Thomson.
He enjoined rest, low diet and regular medical attention. 'Indulgence . . .
in violent passions' was especially to be avoided. But he ended by admitting that the very discovery of symptoms signalled the end.[32] Herbalists
avoided the distressingly intractable disease, too. Dr Phelps Brown in
the 1860s recommended plants with leaves or roots possessing the signature of a heart-like form: balm, mint, parsley and fuller's thistle. These,
he advised guardedly, 'yield medical properties congenial to that organ'.[33]
He did not mention foxglove. Indeed, and ironically, for it is a useful
drug, digitalis seems to have been little used in folk medicine or by
quacks.

Cancer

Superficially, the rising incidence of cancer after 1840 follows a pattern
similar to that of heart disease. The Registrar-General's figures show a
fourfold increase within two generations(see Table 5.9). Most of these
deaths were among persons over 35 with the ratios progressively higher
in each advancing age group. By 1894 cancer was reported as a cause of
death four times more frequently than typhoid fever and it was rising
while the death rate from phthisis had been halved.[34] The contribution
of the larger number of aged people to the increase is illustrated by the
course of the disease in Bath. The town's population remained stationary
between 1860 and 1900. Two-thirds of it was female. By the 1890s 76
in every 1,000 were over 65 against the national ratio of 45 per 1,000.
It was also a wealthier community: 101 persons in every 1,000 were
'living on own means' compared with the national proportion of 36 per
1,000. Deaths attributed to cancer, however, were 50 per cent higher
than the national average, after correcting for age and sex.[35]

Table 5.9: Cancer Deaths in England and Wales, 1840-94

Date	Cancer Deaths	Cancer Deaths per 100,000	Cancer Deaths as Proportion of Total Deaths
1840	2,786	17.7	1:129
1850	4,961	27.9	1:74
1860	6,827	34.3	1:62
1870	9,530	42.4	1:54
1880	13,310	50.2	1:40
1890	19,433	67.6	1:29
1894	21,422	71.3	1:23

Source: *Lancet*, 8 Aug. 1896, p. 427, 29 Aug. 1896, p. 626.

Some medical statisticians and sanitarians, such as Dr Arthur Newsholme, rejected the idea of a massive increase and argued instead that the advance of medical interest in the disease, and public apprehension, had led to better diagnosis, indeed, to an over-simple medical vogue for 'cancer' as a cause of mortality, combined with widespread under-registration before the 1860s.[36] There is some evidence for his opinion. In 1864, for instance, a doctor at Greenwich reported a private patient to have died of 'neuralgia and acute phthsis'. She had died of cancer of the uterus, but the doctor, apparently following medical protocol on this shocking disease, relating to private patients at least, entered a respectable cause of death and informed her sister privately.[37] Female friendly society tables such as those of the Scottish Widows' Fund showed only a very small increase, although by the 1880s doctors performing examinations for medical assurance companies looked carefully for signs of cancer. Newsholme also rejected the belief that the rising incidence was a straightforward result of greater longevity, on the grounds that the increased number of aged was incommensurate with the increased incidence of cancer.[38] But he did not consider age-specific cancer mortality and his argument seems to be mistaken.

Diagnosis of cancer in earlier decades certainly was haphazard. Younger doctors were beginning in the 1850s to use the microscope to exclude non-malignant 'scrofulous growths', but leading practitioners, like Sir James Paget, continued to diagnose by the naked eye into the 1860s. There was no agreement about the meanings of 'benign', 'malignant', 'semi-malignant' and cancroid manifestations of the malady.[39] Of course, only external cancers could be located. Doctors and patients

were agreed that it was an 'incurable, killing disease', and were resigned
to attempting ineffective but severe excisions or applying blisters and
other excruciating palliatives.

Females had a higher reported mortality than males, because of breast
cancers.

Table 5.10: Cancer Death Rate per 100,000

	Male	Female	Sex Ratio
1851-60	19.5	43.4	1:2.2
1861-70	24.4	52.3	1:1.9
1881-90	43.0	73.9	1:1.7
1891-95	47.0	86.8	1:1.6

Source: James Paget, *Lancet*, 19 January 1856, p. 63.

Women, and many doctors, avoided operations as long as there appeared
to be any chance that the growth was non-malignant or remained small.[40]
Dr Graham in the 1830s, for instance, warned that the knife only caused
pain and accelerated death. He recommended iron compounds, iodine
and hemlock, mild diet and sherry, and held out hopes for a 'cure'.[41]
Some doctors treating desperate cases at dispensaries often resorted to
trying to burn out the growth with caustic. Others denounced the practice as useless, and so painful that it 'hastened death'. It seems to have
been abandoned by the 1860s.[42] By the 1850s doctors and patients
seem to have become more resigned to the incurability of the disease,
and readier, now that anaesthesia was available, to resort to the knife.
Drs Druitt and Snow led opinion in pronouncing cancer to be 'a constitutional' disease and therefore beyond medical palliation. Cancer
operations were difficult and expensive and were rarely performed on
the poor. Dr Snow claimed that most operations were in private practice,
on women at 45 or over. James Paget, who built a large practice on
breast surgery, claimed that the average expectation of life for the patient
from the time the cancer was first observed was four years. Those operated upon within two years of the first observation and surviving had an
expectancy of about eight years. The average mortality from the operation itself was 10 per cent in the 1850s. Paget's statistics did not include
recurring cancers: these began to turn up in apparently sizeable numbers
in the 1860s.[43]

For males of this period the detected cancers were more varied. Among
167 of Paget's cases between 1843 and 1861, three-fifths of them private

and two-fifths hospital, the following formed the main groups: tongue — 19 male, 11 female; lips and cheeks — 25 (possibly the outcome of chewing tobacco) and 4; 'bones' — 16.7; 'integuments of limbs and trunk' — 13, 5; lymphatic glands — 10, 6; and testicle — 14.[44]

By 1901 the pattern had changed, with internal cancers much more prominent (see Table 5.11).

Table 5.11: Most Common Reported Cancer Deaths, Scotland, 1901

	Males	Females
Stomach	389	439
Intestines	128	180
Rectum	110	92
Jaw	65	18
Lung	18	15
Arm and leg	18	21

Source: *PP*, 1904, vol. XV, p. xlviii.

The development of abdominal and thoracic surgery through the 1880s, after the triumph of antisepsis, had discovered a new range of cancers. The first mention of lung cancer that I have noticed is in 1869, when Dr Hyde Salter, physician to the Charing Cross Hospital, discovered a case during an autopsy. He pointed it out to his pupils, remarking that it was 'one of the rarer forms of disease and you may probably pass the rest of your student's life without seeing another example of it'.[45] By 1892 Dr C.R. Drysdale was warning against smoking because he was convinced it caused cancer of 'the lip, tongue and larynx'. His observation came about five years after the sudden, enormous increase in smoking of cheap cigarettes made from Virginia tobaccos with a high nicotine content.

Among the many puzzles that cancer presented, the enormous increase among males was a central one. Between 1851 and 1890, reported mortality for males had risen by 167 per cent, compared with 91 per cent for females. Yet over the same period females were living longer than males. One explanation that became popular among some doctors and many vegetarians and health faddists in the 1880s attributed the increase to an increased consumption of meat. This theory had been propagated by A.A. Verneuil, the French surgeon. France had experienced a fourfold rise since 1844 in mortality ascribed to cancer. Dr C.R. Drysdale, sensible and pertinent as ever, remarked that the increase of cancer would have been more uniform among the age groups, had meat-eating been the cause, for young people also ate meat. He argued that the spread of longevity had simply brought more people into the physically degenerative population at risk.[46] In the late 1890s Dr Roger Williams ascribed the increase among males to 'urbanization' which made the lives of men more to resemble those of women, that is, 'excess of food, with want of proper exercise and changed surroundings'. This explanation also covered the higher death rate which women still retained: they still had more 'high living' than men.[47] Most cancer deaths were at ages over 35, and females, mainly because of the incidence of breast cancer, still in 1900 had about 25 per cent more reported deaths than males. But the gap was narrowing continuously, and by 1911 males registered more sarcoma deaths than females.[48]

Advancing Disabilities

'Urbanization' as a factor in the increase of cancer should have provided a clue to further epidemiological investigation, especially as doctors had known for over a century of specific relations between particular deleterious substances and occupations and cancer, as, for example, soot and chimney sweeps' cancer of the scrotum. But these leads, which indicated the need for radical interference in working and living conditions, were abandoned in favour of generalised moral condemnations.

Many occupations were very dangerous, like fork-grinding in the Sheffield cutlery trade, which occasioned what was believed to be lead poisoning in the form of 'grinders' asthma', but might equally have been silicosis of the lungs from inhalation of grindstone dust, and left 'mites' in the eyes, causing blindness. 'Fork grinders go off like dyke water, so quick', one remarked fatalistically, yet sadly. Women grinders also developed grinders' asthma, though only at two-thirds the male rate, except in the needle-making trade at Alcaster, which damaged women much worse than men.[49] Men who prepared black oxide of manganese for bleaching powder could become paraplegic and deaf, with paralysed facial muscles.[50] Bakers were subject to skin diseases, occasioned by 'the flour insect' and weevils, and were notorious for suffering from TB of the lungs and 'bakers' asthma'.[51] Females in the indoor lace-making areas, Newport Pagnell, Bedford and Towcester, and in the cotton-manufacturing and straw-plaiting trades, all had their particular forms of respiratory disease, at up to double the rates of male workers in these industries. Female weavers in the cotton trade, for instance, had extraordinarily bad teeth because they sucked the weft up in the shuttle.[52]

Colliers were said to be old men at 45. They suffered a wide range of disabilities, ranging from 'black spit' (pneumoconiosis), heart disease 'associated with . . . acute rheumatism', renal disease, associated partly with 'habitual intemperance', and skin diseases, which partly resulted from their almost incredible . . . personal uncleanliness'. They lived, according to a doctor who knew south Lancashire, 'almost apart from other men . . . [amidst] an entire absence of intellectual converse and association for mental or moral progress'. Female miners, who numbered 11,000 in the 1850s, recorded a sickness rate about one-fifth lower than males in the lead and tin mines of Cumberland and Wales, but much the same disability rates in the coal villages.[53] Former agricultural labourers were reported to be almost uniformly deaf; a final manifestation of the years of ear infections and 'catarrh' that I described in Chapter 3.[54]

None the less, working and living conditions gradually improved after the 1840s and increasing numbers of working women and men lived into retirement and old age. Doctors noticed in the 1860s that sempstresses using sewing-machines had less of the 'contracted chest, . . . the pallid colour and the weakened eyes . . . of the old sempstress'.[55] Between 1862 and the 1890s an increasing number of coal-miners survived accidents and disabilities and came to draw on miners' permanent relief funds.[56] After all, several of the dangerous and heavy trades were also comparatively well paid. These workers and their families probably ate better than labourers and many artisans. As a police sergeant remarked of children employed at a brickyard:

I often wonder that the children can stand the work as they do [loading barrows and carrying clay], but nothing seems to hurt them; they are as hardy as ground toads; . . . yet I have seen them so tired at the end of the day's work that the men have had to take them up in their arms to carry them home. They are well fed; that is a great thing.[57]

Domestic servants, by contrast, were ill fed and commonly suffered from anaemia.

One legacy of such heavy work and debility was hernia, the protrusion of some stricture in the abdomen through a weak point in the abdominal wall. Early in the century doctors asserted that up to 1 in 10 or 15 of the population suffered from it and that it afflicted about 1 in 9 of the labouring population. The rate among over-35s was double that of under-35s and it was highest in the 50-60 age group and about five times more males than females sought trusses.[58] Bricklayers, stevedores, coal-heavers and general labourers who did heavy lifting constituted the largest single set of victims.[59] Until Sir Astley Cooper, the great surgeon, who himself suffered from hernia, made it an item of orthodox medical interest, hernias were treated by 'rupture doctors' and with trusses supplied by charities or sold by druggists. Rupture doctors pressed the part back, and the trusses were designed to support the weak section of the abdomen and hold in the protuberance. The trusses rotted and the springs rusted and a wearer normally needed to secure a new one every two years. Brave or desperate cases of irreducible hernia submitted to the surgeon, who usually cut off the offending piece of intestine or omentum and sewed up the rest.[60] Queen Caroline died of just such an operation in 1821 when the wound mortified. Until the advent of antisepsis, it was an extremely dangerous procedure.

Eyesight

Doctors enjoyed great success in treating blindness. The incidence of reported blindness declined at every census after 1851, and between 1871 and 1891 it fell dramatically from 95.1 per 100,000 to 80.9 per 100,000.[61] Among the children, the decline was attributed to the diminution of smallpox which accompanied vaccination. Among old people, where the highest incidence of cataract and glaucoma occurred at around 60, surgeons coped brilliantly with cataract. By the 1850s the Liverpool Opthalmic Hospital, for instance, was claiming that two-thirds of the cases regained 'useful vision'. Surgeons could operate without anaesthesia and with small risk of infection.[62] The patients must have shown great fortitude. As Charlotte Brontë wrote of her father, who successfully underwent such an operation in 1846: 'Papa displayed extraordinary patience and firmness; the surgeons seemed surprised . . . The affair lasted precisely a quarter of an hour; it was not the simple operation of couching . . . but the more complicated one of extracting the cataract.'[63]

People with other forms of impaired sight were less fortunate. Until the 1890s there was no control over the making and selling of spectacles. People with poor sight bought them on a rough and ready basis from poorly trained opticians or from quacks.[64] Blindness commonly accompanied other infirmities: in the 1880s, of about 30,000 blind persons in the United Kingdom, only 10,000 were able-bodied and only 800 of these were enabled to work to support themselves. Their plight was worsened by the squabbles between the various blind-teaching charities – each taught its own system of embossed types. Agreement on Braille had to wait until this century. Not surprisingly, the Royal Commissioners on the Poor Law in 1909 found that 33 per cent of blind persons were paupers.[65]

2. QUACKS

The old and the despairing were the natural prey of irregular practitioners. Terrorist quacks purveyed secret remedies, mostly relating to sexual troubles, nostrum mongers fixed their faith and that of their clients on a single substance, specialist practitioners dealt with particular ailments, while counter-prescribers treated patients according to allopathic, homeopathic or other regimens based fundamentally on sympathetic principles. By and large, the more secret, terrorising or specialised the ritual, the higher was the charge.[66]

Cancer, inexorable and terrible, provided a lush field for the unorthodox. Its many victims who were afraid of the surgeon's knife or pronounced inoperable readily turned to quacks. Specialist cancer quacks, who could no more cure cancer than the regulars, nerved themselves with ample effrontery or self-deception, or both. In 1839 Susannah Thomas, of Bridgend in Glamorgan, had had severe stomach pain for four months. She had visited a doctor in nearby Cowbridge 'who .. occasionally prescribed for her', but she obtained no relief. She then read in the local newspaper of the forthcoming visit of Baron Spolasco, the cancer-curer. Upon their meeting, the Baron told her that he knew by her eyes she was very ill and that he would cure her. She would 'bless the hour she first saw the good Baron Spolasco'. He refused to allow her or her aunt to relate her symptoms. He knew them by her eyes. The aunt paid 22s. 6d., upon which the Baron handed her two pills in a paper. The woman took the pills and got worse. The aunt returned to the Baron and beseeched him to visit her niece. The Baron told her to give the woman a wine-glass of brandy and half a wine-glass of wine mulled together: 'that would rouse her.' The woman still deteriorated. The aunt went again to the Baron, who this time, after a short delay, came to his patient. He ordered a spoonful of castor oil to be followed by another and an ounce of turpentine. Susannah Thomas died 15 minutes later. The autopsy revealed that she had a perforated duodenal ulcer. The Baron had treated at least 12 clients in Bridgend, each with the same drastic pills. A coroner's jury brought a verdict of manslaughter against him.[67]

The trade could be very lucrative. John Patterson, claiming an MD from a United States university, set up in Welbeck Street in the 1860s and became fashionable. He treated Mrs Frewen for six months until her death in 1869. He had received 150 guineas and at her death demanded another hundred in unpaid fees.[68]

Henry Delvine got 15 months' hard labour at the Central Criminal

Court in 1914 for taking money by false pretences. His technique was that presently practised by Philippine cancer-curers. He 'treated' the patient and then miraculously produced 'the cancer', fresh and dripping blood, without apparent incision of the body. The 'cancer' was proved to be animal offal. Delvine, an illiterate, had been a soldier, court bailiff and labourer; he was also an abortionist, and must have been an attractive rogue. Shortly before his 'cancer' conviction, he had been acquitted at Downham market of an abortion attempt and had been carried shoulder-high through the town.[69]

Quacks could always distract attention from their failures by attacking the regulars. James Ward, who practised in Leeds in the 1830s, asserted, reasonably enough, that regulars were avaricious, often unscientific and ignorantly pretentious, and that they had learned much from irregulars. Ward's ploy was to challenge the regulars to treat 20 cancer-sufferers with the knife while he cured them with herbs, and see who ended with most survivors. It was a safe challenge which could be endlessly repeated.[70] In the West Country during the 1880s and 1890s a cancer-curer travelled the markets on a cart hung with bottles containing the 'cancers' he had removed. He was accompanied by a woman who would testify that where the regulars had failed, in her case he had triumphed. He rubbed patients with caustic. The skin sloughed. This he scraped off the patient and showed it to him as the cancer. He charged £10 a treatment: £5 down and £5 after the cure.[71] The Reverend Hugh Reed, a clergyman of the Church of England, also professed to cure cancer and ovarian dropsy. He specialised in elderly clergymen and their families who had lost faith in their regular attendants. Reed used mercury externally and internally and chlorine gas to 'neutralise the cancer'. One satisfied patient, the Reverend Erskine Head, even wrote to *The Times* in January 1860 to praise Reed and denounce his former doctors. A fortnight after his letter Head died in agony, of throat cancer.[72]

Other cancer specialists were closer to the traditional folk sorcerers, wise women and herbalists. Israel Ferment (or Firmin) was an astrologer and quack who became infamous at 91 by turning (highly unreliable) Queen's evidence against the Chartists after the Newport Rising in 1839. He then set up in Bristol, undertaking to cure the usual range of the afflictions of the old, the poor and the simple: 'the King's evil, cancers, asthmas, ulcerated sore legs, gravel in the kidneys and sore eyes . . . and cramp in the bones; he also draws pain from the head, without leeching, cupping or blistering, and . . . is also a worm doctor'.[73] In the 1870s the 'White Witch of North Devon' cured patients with arthritic disorders by placing metal rods in their hands and then requiring them to move their arms to make the rods strike a piece of metal. He also secured improvements in patients' conditions by 'ruling the planets on behalf of the sick'. 'Doctress Smith' advertised in Deptford in 1846 that 'By Her Majesty's Royal License and Authority She cures the following disorders . . . Deafness . . . Flux (dysentry) in Old and Young . . . Scurvy in the Gums, Piles, Cancers . . .' She used only roots and herbs, she claimed, in her medicines, so they were safe for even the weakest constitution. At Honiton in 1874 a sawyer's wife who had cancer of the breast for three years finally went to Mrs Fish, a herbalist, after the local GPs had told the wife that they would have to operate. She visited Mrs Fish for eight months. Meanwhile the tumour began to ulcerate. Mrs Fish, finding her herbal remedies failing, rubbed a mixture of neats-foot oil, litharge and acetic acid on the tumour. A few weeks before she died the woman returned to her GP with an enlarged tumour and tetanus. The coroner's jury brought a verdict of manslaughter against Mrs Fish.[74]

The 'Halifax Witch', John Brierly, was typical of many unorthodox practitioners both in his large practice and his simplistic physiology. He cured all diseases. Patients queued all night for his morning sessions, and letters and telegraphs, seeking advice or a charmed letter by return (telegraph messages seem not to have been charmed, probably because they could not carry the witch's direct personal influence) came from all over the kingdom. In 1849 he treated a patient 'whose heart was beating three inches too low, his chest full of water, and his lungs were drowned by the water'. Brierly had two men pull the patient's arms backwards and keep them in motion while he put the heart back in its proper place. He also prescribed anti-bilious pills, plasters and drops. The man died two days later. At the inquest the coroner asked the Witch. 'What are you?' 'A doctor.' 'To what College do you belong?' 'To no college; I do as the Whitworth doctor [about 12 miles from Halifax] does.' 'What trade were you brought up to?' 'I have doctored eight and twenty years, and was brought up to nothing else.' Although Brierly is not reported to have claimed it, he probably came from a family of curers and in this sense, as an inheritor of special knowledge and powers, was a true witch. He had started doctoring when he was 12.[75]

Other witches used straight manipulative sorcery. An old woman treating another old woman who was dangerously ill in Taunton in 1858 ordered her nail clippings to be put into a bottle, with other 'personal bits'. The witch then gave her client mandrake root — a strong emetic, narcotic poison with traditional magical properties. The client died. The witch had charged 'several shillings'. In 1847 a man near Bradford consulted a local 'wise man' who instructed him to obtain the skull of a young woman, not decayed, to pound it small, mix it with treacle and administer it in small doses. It was a 'sure remedy'. The Anatomy Act would have made difficult the purchase of an English skull but, presumably, French ones were available from shops like Mr Venus's in *Our Mutual Friend*.[76]

Jane Lacey, a 'cunning woman' at Penryn in the 1860s, put a spell on Mrs Joanna Bate. Mrs Bate was old and, her GPs said, had 'softening of the brain'. She was also wealthy and respectable and normally beyond the reach of 'cunning women': they customarily worked among their poorer neighbours, sorting out the occurrence of misfortune and relating it to upsets in the moral order. Mrs Bate had deteriorated despite the doctor's ministrations. Her nurse persuaded Mrs Bate's daughter to call in Jane Lacey, who demanded a lock of hair for divination and 2s. 6d. as the preliminary fee. She divined a spell and required 12s. 6d. for its removal and another 12s. 6d. when Mrs Bate was better, together with 3s. 6d. for medicine. Patients expected and witches supplied, just like doctors, tangible medicines as well as the fine words and rituals. Next day Lacey returned for yet another 12s. 6d., to pay for a fresh onslaught on the spell. Her previous wish 'had gone wrong'. It had been concentrated on Mrs Bate's right arm, in order to house the weakness when it was removed from the head, but had travelled on to her leg. Lacey brought liniment for the leg. Mrs Bate died. The slip had occurred because Jane Lacey's powers, she claimed, had been over-extended by the severity of the 'ill-wish' which had fallen on Mrs Bate. Perhaps, too, she noticed on her earlier visit that Bate's leg was mortifying, and certainly it was an unusual opportunity to tap a rich client. The 'ill-wish' had been obdurate because the sun and moon had been 'crossed' (eclipsed? or in some kind of astrological opposition?) over Mrs Bate. Lacey's explanation of Mrs Bate's decline and her failure had an integrated particularity and cosmic invulnerability that the local GPs could not match. Dr Byrne, the main supplanted doctor, initiated the inquiry. Jane Lacey got two months' hard labour.[77]

Existence at the losing end of a hostile mechanistic universe bred defeatism. In 1830 the Reverend John Skinner, vicar of Camerton in Somerset, visited two of his dying villagers.

Frapnell . . . seems going rapidly. A woman of the name of Barr was sitting with him, who had been ill, that is, in a low nervous way for some time.

On my entering into conversation with [him] . . . he began to say that he had been brought to that state by the enemy; that . . . Witch-craft had been practised upon him and that the woman who was sitting with him had also been a fellow sufferer. He told me a man had called upon them and shewn them a paper which said that others had been bewitched like them, and that they would not get well again unless they could undo the charm. I said I had read that paper, and that it was the greatest nonsense I had ever seen, and that the person who gave it him, and received money for thus deceiving him, might be . . . punished by the Magistrate.

This incident involving the paper, together with the 'Gothick' stories from almanacs and other popular prints, suggests that the spread of literacy conserved old beliefs as much as it propagated new ones, just as printing is said to have done centuries earlier. The case of Frapnell and Barr is a late manifestation of tensions in a tight undifferentiated com-munity (Camerton had 1,300 souls in 1830), just before the advent of privatisation among the lower orders. Frapnell and Barr had low status and low self-esteem. Their faith in witchcraft, even as victims, helped them maintain their identities and explain their personal predicaments as against the fates of others in the community. Skinner, a middle-class professional, was already privatised, and formed his identity partly by references to categories and classes that extended far beyond his im-mediate community. He was a hidebound Tory and would have disliked the thought, but his attempt to dispel Frapnell's fears and comfort the incurable with his rival magic and invocation of rational supra-communal authority in the form of the law made him a man of the future.

A fortnight later Skinner returned to Frapnell and again tried to con-vince him he was not bewitched. 'I explained to him about the nature and full meaning of the Sacrament which he never yet has received.'[78]

Many of these quack practitioners and their clients mentally existed in a world of forces quite distinct from Christianity. When Thomas Garbutt, a 'medical botanist', and the parents of one of his deceased patients were involved in an inquest in London in 1882, they refused to take the oath, 'because', they declared, 'they had no religious belief'. 'Madame' Combe was the wife of a carpenter in Southend in the 1890s. She had a large practice among middle-aged and elderly females 'miracu-lously', but without any reference to Christianity, resiting fallen uteruses and other internal organs. When her patients died, as they often did, she and those who had faith in her simply explained it by remarking that the deceased had been 'struck for death'.[79]

Many of the procedures which Mr Keith Thomas recounts in *Religion and the Decline of Magic* in England in the sixteenth and seventeenth centuries were still followed in the nineteenth, among them 'touching' and weapon salve. In 1860 an old man applied to leave the Plymouth workhouse. He had the King's evil in one of his legs. Some years earlier he had been touched and cured; but the wound had erupted afresh. The old man intended to walk to Devonport to visit three sisters at North Corner Street. One was an eleventh daughter, another the ninth, and the other the seventh of the same parents. He had to be touched by one of them on the day of the week on which she was born; both parties had to be unwashed and fasting. No one must pass between the touched and the toucher until he was touched 11, 9 or 7 times. No money was to pass from the 'person relieved' to the toucher but 'relatives and friends may show gratitude'. The chairman of the board of guardians started the local subscription to enable the old man to make his journey. Rural workmen who were wounded by nails, axes or chisels did not swear at the offending tool, but carefully wiped it and laid it away in a safe, dry place where it would not rust. This promoted healing of the wound and forestalled lockjaw.[80]

In 1850 an old woman who specialised in 'charming' away burns came to the attention of the coroner when one of her patients died. Her 'charm' was the one for burns that Pepys quotes in his diary at the end of 1664:

There came three Angells out of the East;
The one brought fire, the others brought frost —
Out fire; in frost.
In the name of the Father and the Son and Holy Ghost, Amen.[81]

Parson Skinner had in the Sacrament his own rival restorative for the non-communicant Frapnell. Claims for cures by Christian prayers became frequent in the 1880s. In 1889 Bishop Ernest Wilberforce announced that he had been cured of a 'dangerous internal ailment' by prayer and anointing with oil. At Birchmoor near Birmingham, a girl afflicted with paralysis of the neck for 20 months lost it immediately in 1884 after members of the Blue-ribbon League prayed around her bed. She got up and dressed unaided. In 1880 a healing clairvoyant, Mary Ann Houghton, was charged with infringing the Pharmacy Act by selling homeopathic pills at 2*s*. 6*d*. a box. The pills came into use after Houghton performed her trance diagnosis under the guidance of William Harvey.[82]

Much cure-mongering, like a lot of orthodox treatment, was predicated on the belief that heat meant life. In an age in which many people passed much of their lives feeling chilled to the marrow, the belief made sense; quite apart from its pseudo-rational medical endorsement, as 'counter-irritation'. And in many cases heat treatment worked. The Taylors of Manchester, a family traditionally associated with healing, specialised in applying and selling a liniment, the 'Whitworth Red Bottle', of which the main ingredient was spirits of turpentine, as a cure for everything.[83]

Captain Ackerley, a cheerful rascal in the 1840s and 1850s, used a lamp to cure slow circulation of the blood. He covered his patients with a table cloth and ordered them to inhale the vapour of the lamp until they got 'into such a heat as to be scarcely able to bear it'. He then turned them out into the cold street, exclaiming to the bystanders, 'That's the way to put new blood into them!' Ackerley also employed lactating women to milk themselves and sold the milk 'to decrepit old men' to drink, to prolong their lives. Ackerley claimed that Lord Stanley had taken his milk regimen and 'experienced considerable benefit'. Moreover, Ackerley's system, he said, benefited the women too for it restored the breasts to their original form. In 1851 at the Glamorgan Assizes, Ackerley was charged with manslaughter. One of his lamp patients had been stripped naked and thrust out an open window. He had died next day. Ackerley was acquitted, to 'loud applause'.[84]

More often, internal heat was supplied by herbal mixtures. The most widespread of these systems was that of Dr J.A. Coffin. He was an American and brought with him to England in the 1840s some of the folk beliefs of the American frontier. They are beliefs which also turn up independently in Britain, as with Ackerley, and doubtless have a common ancestry in the seventeenth century. Coffin's physiology began with the epigram that 'Heat is life and life is heat.' Man was a steam-engine: food was the fuel, the stomach the fire place, the breath the smoke, and the faeces the ashes.

> The fire in the stomach makes the water boil and this heats the lungs, and hence the respiration, while the steam of the boiling water escapes through the body as perspiration, and the steam thus generated sets the limbs in motion.

Disease, therefore, derived from a want of heat, or 'equilibrium of heat', in the body. The remedy was to heat the body internally with cayenne and lobelia, the queen of herbs. Coffin's lobelia was *lobelia inflata*, the 'Indian tobacco', native to North America. The entire herb, dried, and in flower, was used, the root being the best part. It irritates the nostrils, and has a burning, acrid taste, the chief constituent of which is a volatile alkaloid, lobeline, which can be poisonous in large doses.[85]

Coffin set up in Manchester about 1846 and established several Botanic Colleges as centres for training Coffinite curers and distributing cayenne pepper, capsicum and lobelia. The movement took on in the Midlands and the industrial north. Effectively it was a mobilisation of the unlettered resisters to regular medical hegemony, gathered around two new, potent therapeutic agents. The 'faculty' was the great enemy: avaricious, seeking to keep illness as its preserve, callous, ignorant and ever-ready with the scalpel to damage the private integrity of the body. The Botanic Colleges recruited mainly from the traditional independent, often self-employed artisan classes, tailors, cobblers, baker's wives. The chairman of the Birmingham College was a cobbler, in Leeds the College was headed by a woman, Mrs Umpleby, and in Sheffield the local Botanic Society was centred on the universalist Mount of Zion Chapel. At Maryport in Cumberland the agent was a blacksmith, at Whitehaven a foundry labourer, and in the City of London a costermonger. Another practitioner in Limehouse had been successively a gas-fitter, soda-water maker, and blacking manufacturer. Ellis Flitcroft, the Bolton agent, was an American who had been a bricklayer and a policeman. It seems likely that Coffin brought him to Britain as a proselytiser.[86] Their clients came from the same ranks, joiners, boot-makers' wives, grocers and an occasional 'lady of property'.

The heyday of Coffinism was the 1850s and 1860s, but practitioners were still widespread in the 1880s and I have heard that Coffinite dispensaries existed in Oldham and other northern towns until the Second World War. They diagnosed and treated menstrual troubles, difficult pregnancies, lung, heart and stomach disease, constipation and ulcerated legs. The decoction of lobelia was usually administered first, in teaspoonful doses, up to half a pint at a time. This was followed with the cayenne pepper, in half-teaspoonfuls, mixed with treacle. Lung and heart cases were also placed in the vapour baths at the Botanic Colleges. The lobelia strengthened the action of the heart, the cayenne promoted the circulation of the blood in every part of the body and the vapour bath invigorated the lungs and body surface, thereby lessening pressure on the diseased organ and 'affording an opportunity for a coagulum to form around the raptured [sic] vessel'. Lobelia, the College trainees were told, was 'the fire from shavings', cayenne had to be added to keep the blaze going, and the vapour bath was the oven and flue.[87]

The progress of Coffinism can be followed through the numerous inquests on its clients. The lobelia, especially when it was mixed with capsicum and acetic acid, greatly irritated the stomach when taken in such large, unregulated doses. Regular practitioners were keen to bring such deaths to the coroner's notice. But at least lobelia was pure. It was imported directly from the United States, being grown there by the Shakers of New Lebanon. The cayenne pepper, normally adulterated with red lead until the 1860s, presented more difficulties. Either way, Coffinite victims died a peculiarly painful death.[88]

Ordinary Coffinites charged between 1*s*. 9*d*. and 2*s*. 6*d*. for their medicines, while Dr Coffin would ask for £3. 3*s*. 0*d*. In order to evade the law they were careful to charge only for medicine, never for advice.[89] The doctors tried to ensure that Coffinites were indicted for manslaughter after their patients died, but judges and juries normally refused to convict because the Coffinites acted in good faith and did not show criminal negligence. Acquittals were greeted with applause and cheers in the courts, followed by jubilant street processions.

Unorthodox treatments were not restricted to the working classes and the poor. Hypochondriac members of the aristocracy and gentry had from the eighteenth century patronised such fashionable quacks as Sir William Read and Spot Ward. John St John Long, who treated consumption in the 1830s by requiring the patient to breathe hot air through red morocco leather tubes, and to have their chests rubbed with caustic liniment, had an extensive practice among the upper classes, especially among delicate fashionable women. Sir Francis Burdett, the radical, had him touch and brush his liniment on the stump of the leg the Marquis of Anglesey lost at Waterloo. Rumour had it that a toe grew.[90] St John Long's liniment caused extensive excoriation of the skin. The discharge contained the injurious matter. After he was acquitted at his first manslaughter trial, he paid his costs of £250 in cash from a large roll of notes, and rode off with the Marquis of Sligo, followed by the hisses of the crowd. St John Long's recipe for liniment was sold after his death for £10,000. It was said to have consisted of about 50 per cent acetic acid, about 25 per cent spirits of turpentine, suspended in egg yolk.[91] Burdett went on to become a devotee of hydropathy. Mr Justice Tindall also patronised unorthodox curers, as did Earl Ducie and Lord Morpeth, who supported mesmeric healers. Sir Edward Bulwer Lytton and Charles Darwin went to hydropathic establishments while Earl and Lady Denbigh, Lord Robert Grosvenor and the Earl of Wilton patronised homeopaths.[92] Benjamin Disraeli and Viscount Jocelyn were attended by homeopaths at their deathbeds. Thomas Slingsby Duncombe, another radical dandy, was attended by Dr Coffin. In 1858 he tried to wreck the Medical Bill, introduced to protect the orthodox profession.[93] The fact that James Stansfeld, when President of the Local Government Board in the early 1870s, proved such a lukewarm backer of the medical reformers among his officers is largely explained by his long-standing preference for unorthodox healing, especially homeopathy.[94]

Hydropathy and Homeopathy

Hydropathy and homeopathy involved extensive, and therefore expensive courses of treatment. In the 1840s a consultation, to decide whether a patient was suitable for the regimen of showering, wrapping in cold wet sheets, and strict diet, cost 10s. 6d. The subsequent sojourn at the hydropathic establishment, run in many ways like a modern health farm, cost three to four guineas a week. The procedure was introduced to Britain from Germany about 1842. Doubtless it helped chronic patients, as it did Charles Darwin and Charles Bravo, the alcoholic who was to become the victim and possibly also the perpetrator of the celebrated poisoning. Clients were cosseted in a simple way, made to take exercise and moderate their diet, and possibly most important, they were ordered off drugs, and in Bravo's case, alcohol. The hydropathy vogue lasted between the 1840s and mid-1870s, and must have done much good. The scandals about Dr J.M. Gully, the famous hydropathist involved in the Bravo case in 1876, made hydropathy disreputable, but it probably also suffered from competition from the growing private wards in public hospitals and the new private hospitals.[95]

Homeopathy is the practice of curing by the administration, generally in minute amounts, of drugs which would produce in a healthy person the symptoms of the disease being treated. Homeopathic practitioners eschewed cupping, leeching and purging. Actual procedures about the administration of drugs, especially the so-called titrated 'illionths' of a drop, varied widely, as did the choice of drugs. The division between homeopaths and allopaths, vehemently maintained by converts to both sides, was indistinct in practice. Homeopathy must have been beneficial, simply because the treatment mostly left the patient alone. As Dr John Johnston remarked, homeopathy attracted gentle doctors and wealthy patients demanded it from their own reluctant GPs, because they 'were busy and didn't want to be put to bed or bled'.[96] Regulars hated homeopaths for their inroads among the fashionable classes. They snubbed them and refused to consult with them whenever they could, as Dr Quain did during the undignified squabble over the dying Earl of Beaconsfield. Thereafter the RCP ordered its members not to consult with homeopaths, however exigent or distinguished the patient. The

General Medical Council, while it dared not strike off homeopathic converts, did forbid the teaching of homeopathy in British medical schools.[97]

Patent Medicines

During the 1870s reports of cure-mongering by cunning women and herbalists markedly diminish. At the same time there appears to have been an increase in the consumption of patent medicines. The transition was accelerated by clause 27 of the Sale of Food and Drugs Act of 1875. Proprietary medicines were excluded from the Act (and from its successor of 1899) forbidding false claims on the label. The Act had the effect of enabling large manufacturing chemists to make their product a proprietary one, and thereby avoid the stamp duty, by publishing and effectively copyrighting the formula in a trade journal.[98] The small, unorganised medical herbalists were excluded from the trade journals and never managed to mass-produce their concoctions for a national market.

This development was the culmination of a process that began in the 1820s. In 1825 James Morison, a retired Baltic and West Indian merchant, set up as vendor of the 'vegetable universal medicines', which quickly came to be known as Morison's Pills. Morison claimed to have cured himself after 35 years of suffering and failure occasioned by the doctors. He advertised his mixtures as good for everything – fevers, measles, scarlatina, smallpox, consumption, lassitude and debility from old age. In 1828 he established the British College of Health in the New Road, London. He appears to have had close links with evangelical Anglicanism and Nonconformity, and he became part-proprietor of the *Christian Advocate*. Morison conducted 'hygiene meetings' at Exeter Hall, where he extolled the virtues of his pill, preached independence of conscience, and condemned the wickedness of doctors who bled patients into apoplexy and death. By 1834 he was paying £7,000 a year in stamp duty: at 1½*d*. stamp per box, this equals an annual sale of about 1.1 million boxes.[99]

Unlike his rival nostrum sellers, whose remedies were often fairly specific and sometimes mild and usually expensive, Morison's pills were universal, cheap, at 1*s*. a box, and they worked, drastically. Until the 1870s, 'No.1' contained aloes, cream of tartar and gum; 'No.2' these plus gamboge and colocynth. Some patients became addicted. There were frequent deaths from overdoses, but coroner's juries refused to bring down adverse findings. As the foreman of a jury in such a case in 1851 remarked, 'Morison's Pills do no harm. I have a workman who takes 30 at a time.' The coroner capped this. He 'had an old woman at

an inquest recently who used to take 300 a day'. The inquest was upon
a child of five, who had had scarlet fever. Its father, a corn factor's
agent, had bought the pills from one of Morison's sellers after the surgeon had failed; he had prescribed wine and the father was a teetotaller.
The father had fed the child about 20 pills in three days, whereupon it
died. The verdict was 'natural death'.[100]

The consumption of Morison's Pills was immense. They were sold
throughout Europe and the Empire. Between 1830 and 1840 he paid
£60,000 in duty on domestic sales to the government. The medical profession railed against this official recognition of quackery, but at this
level of income no government was prepared to control the contents of
patent medicines, let alone forbid their sale. In 1863-4 a proposal to
legislate to control the proprietary medicine trade was being pressed by
the doctors, but its practitioners successfully stifled it. As their spokesman said, control would 'render valueless two million pounds of invested
property'. They signified their power by subscribing £3,000 to the
defence fund at a single meeting.[101] By 1860, twenty years after his
death, Morison had the largest monument in Kensal Green Cemetery. St
John Long had the second-largest, a huge Egyptian-style edifice.[102] Now
they have been challenged by the great granite head of Karl Marx.

Morison's great rival was Thomas Holloway, who started about 1839.
His pills, too, were cheap and drastic, although they became milder in
the early 1860s after a court action. Thereafter, instead of containing
aloes, ginger and soap, they were composed of lard, wax and turpentine.
He was able to utilise the American T.H. Bishop's patent of 1849 for
compressing artists' paints to increase and vary the output of pills,
cachets and capsules. He improved on Morison's marketing techniques
and made himself a millionaire through mass advertising.[103]

The third great name in the world of pills was that of Beecham.
Thomas Beecham patented his recipe, which was almost identical with
Holloway's, in 1847. His pills were also made of aloes, ginger and soap.
Emulating Holloway, he used saturation advertising to sell his worthless
wares. And like Holloway, who built Holloway College and a mental
hospital before he died, Beecham sealed his respectability by ostenta-
tious public benefactions.[104] Jesse Boot, first Baron Trent, and the last
of the quartet was, like Holloway and Beecham, a Nonconformist. He
learned his herbalism from his mother at his parents' shop in Nottingham
and was launched on his way to becoming the proprietor of the world's
largest retail chemists' company by becoming an agent for Dr Skelton, a
Coffinite. His monument was Nottingham University College.[105]

During the later 1870s, under the protection of the 1875 Act,

Beecham, Holloway and Jesse Boot diversified into other patent medical and retail chemists' products. They were joined in the 1880s by the American interlopers Burroughs and Wellcome and Parke Davis. There was room for all of them. In the 1880s patent medicines represented more than half the business of at least one retail chemist in a poor area in the East India Dock Road. He did very little dispensing.[106] Over 17 million patent medicine duty stamps were sold in the United Kingdom in 1880. In 1887 the people spent over £1½ million on such products. By 1912, three years after the publication of H.G. Wells's *Tono-Bungay*, the people bought over 31 million units of the cheapest patent medicines with 1½*d*. stamps.[107]

Holloway, Beecham and Boot developed export and manufacturing divisions in Europe, the United States and the Empire. They constitute with Nestlé's and other 'health food' companies the earliest multi-nationals catering to the newly literate, would-be independent middle and lower classes throughout the industrialised world, prepared to spend part of their increasing income on the pursuit of well-being through self-medication.

Sudden deaths from swallowing noxious compounds became rarer during the 1880s and 1890s as the big manufacturers began to exclude antimony salts, capsicum, methylated spirits and cannabis, replacing them with the present-day stand-by, alcohol. In 1914 Mrs Lydia E. Pinkham's Vegetable Compound, the subject of the famous ribald song, contained 20 per cent alcohol, plus purgatives.[108] The proprietary men also extended the range of their advertising in the 1890s and developed the headache as a dread ailment. Young girls, mostly 'of the seamstress class', and young men became the targets for the new headache powders made of acetanilide. The maximum dose recommended on the wrappers was three grains. But coroners remarked that few takers knew what three grains were and that they usually swallowed extra doses to be on the safe side. 'Acetanilid' is addictive. By 1898 deaths were reported from overdoses. People often skimped on necessaries in order to save money for their weekly bottle or box.[109] None the less, the amount they spent on dosing themselves would have been less than the sum spent upon equally useless doctors' consultations and prescriptions. It was a dear way to buy alcohol, opium and analgesics, but the buyer had the satisfaction of believing that the purchase was her decision and the wry hope that it might do her some good. As the editor of the *Lancet* lamented in 1870, 'quack medicines will flourish as long as medical men fail to see the importance of paying attention to the little aches, pains, and discomforts to which flesh is heir'.[110]

3. THE MEDICAL PROFESSION AND ITS ENTANGLEMENT
   WITH THE POOR LAW

The doctors' pretensions in the nineteenth century rarely matched reality. They aspired to be regarded as scientific, yet critics frequently dismissed them as humbugs. Doctors wanted to be accepted as gentlemen, when the great majority knew themselves to be parvenus. They dreamed of becoming a united dignified profession sharing the same colleges as defences against outside regulation and as initiates, behaving well to one another; yet their profession was riven with snobberies, jealousies and public rows about competition for patients and recognition. The emerging majority of GPs sought to enter the royal colleges as equals, and the emerging élite of consultant physicians and surgeons used the old privileges of the colleges to enhance their new status and fend off their lowly competitors. The inherited institutional divisions of the profession and the patterns of education they entailed, even after the Medical Act of 1858 and registration of practitioners, never fitted the work being done. Above all, the ambiguities in the doctors' situations were exposed in their treatment of the poor and the old: tradition and their professional aspirations impelled them to act benevolently to people who could pay them little, yet they needed to defer to the wealthy to ensure them the rank they sought and the income required to underwrite it.

In 1830 medicine was the *métier* of outsiders. The sons of Unitarians and Quakers, who were excluded from the law by the education system and the oaths required, and the clever sons of tradesmen, who lacked the connections that promised fair progress in the law, the Church or the armed services, took to medicine.[111] Hospital lecturers admitted all who could pay the relatively low fees. Those with more money and higher ambitions could buy themselves a career by apprenticing themselves at premiums of up to £1,000 to a hospital consultant of high reputation and wide patronage. But the bulk of future GPs, which included high proportions of young Scots and Irishmen, served their apprenticeships with obscure country practitioners. They began at about 16 and were apprenticed for two or three years. Then they walked the hospitals for one, two or three years, paying lecture fees of about £40 a year. Then they faced the world without assured prospects. The length and unsupervised nature of their education made them more akin to Continental students than English undergraduates. The system in Scotland approximated even more closely to the Continental one. Oxford and Cambridge did prepare undergraduates for future top places in the medical hierarchy, with near-automatic entry to the royal colleges, but their graduates numbered only about 10 per cent of the English profession in 1830 and their proportion was to fall to 3 per cent by 1879.[112]

The radicals wanted the examinations to be made more rigorous, but not too hard. They rightly condemned the existing ones as farcical. The Latin translation at the Apothecaries' Hall examination in 1832 could be done in a few minutes and then the examiner asked the candidate to point out a noun, a verb and the genitive case. The candidate did so, whereupon the examiner remarked, 'You appear to be a pretty good Latin scholar.' There were three questions on materia medica, each requiring the common name for a drug, for instance, 'bark' for chinchona and two in chemistry, one of which was, 'what substance forms both acids and alkalis?', to which the answer was 'oxygen'. At Edinburgh, the complete examination took 30 minutes.[113] The radicals looked to new, rational, honest examinations to install promotion by merit in place of the existing corrupt network of patronage. The new republic of merit was not, however, to be universal. Compounding and selling of medicines by practitioners had to be stopped because 'shop pharmacy' degraded the profession. And women had to be excluded from midwifery; if that were not immediately possible, they should be squeezed out by severe qualifying conditions.[114]

These preoccupations were to shape doctors' politics for a hundred years, and beyond. Young medicos, many of them the ablest of their generation, formed the vanguard of the uneasy class. Richard Barrow, James Parkinson and Richard Watson had been active in the London Corresponding Society. Henry Cline, George Knutton, George Pearson and Michael Pearson had been friends of Horne Tooke and Thewall and active in radical politics in Westminster. John Gale Jones and James Watson had been Spencean Philanthropists. Sampson Perry had been a friend of Thomas Paine's. The young Astley Cooper had welcomed the French Revolution and, indeed, had been in Paris in 1792. Richard Webb, a surgeon, told Richard Carlile in 1825 that during his medical training 'infidel opinions were ... freely uttered by lecturers and supported by pupils'. Carlile left his body for dissection to Richard Grainger of the celebrated anatomy school. Surgeon Matthew Fletcher publicly sympathised with the Chartists and surgeon-GP Peter Murray McDouall became famous for his physical force rhetoric. Another surgeon-GP, William Price, was deeply implicated in the Newport Rising. Marshall Hall, who began the revulsion from blood-letting and discovered 'reflex action' and a system of artificial respiration, also helped to abolish open railway carriages and worked to stop the flogging of soldiers, and slavery in America.[115]

As men of the future, they dismissed the exclusive 'College of Physicians' (they never used the word Royal) as 'a relic of the ignorance and barbarism of the century which gave it birth'. They wanted a 'Medical Republic' expressed in a 'National College to embrace all branches of medicine'. Once the 'hideous monster — MONOPOLY' was destroyed, then the new era of national health would begin. The profession had to be unified. Examinations in physic and surgery were to confer a double qualification, allowing the holder to practise in all branches of medicine as a member of a 'National Faculty' conserving the national health.[116]

It was a tragedy for the evolution of the profession, its relations with the state, and its pauper patients that this noble ambition was distorted by the wrangle over Poor Law medicine. Medical trade unionism was already taking its peculiarly defensive, pharisaical attitude before 1834; but the New Poor Law hardened what might still have been a tractable set of ideas.

In 1830 the GPs won a major legal victory when James Handey, a surgeon-apothecary, succeeded in an action in the Court of King's Bench for recovery of fees for 'attendance'. The jury's verdict reversed earlier decisions and 'rescued' GPs 'from the ranks of the Hucksters and Quacks' with whom they had been hitherto linked because they had been permitted to charge only for medicines and services, and not for 'attendance', as did a physician. The decision, 'One of the Committee' announced in the *Lancet*, showed that a 'general practitioner [was] not a surgeon only — he [was] more — he [was] *superior* to a surgeon . . . with "superior consequence . . . by his general utility" because he could also prescribe for internal disorders'. Country practitioners were jubilant. They suggested a public dinner to honour Handey and a collection for a piece of plate. 'Omicron' of Hoxton suggested that a permanent organisation of GPs be formed before the enthusiasm ebbed. This was the germ of the idea of the British Medical Association. It was also indicative of the straitened means of GPs, and their pettiness, that only 20 tickets were sold for the dinner. There was also a squabble over the toasts. Handey was excluded from the main list of speakers who were to be headed by Joseph Hume and Daniel O'Connell. The dinner was abandoned.[117]

Some members of the committee which had tried to organise the dinner had meanwhile adopted 'Omicron's' proposal and formed the Metropolitan Society of General Practitioners in Medicine and Surgery.

Their first object was: 'Such alteration of existing laws and customs as shall promote the prosperity and respectability of the general body of practitioners'. This was followed by a carrot for prospective members in a projected 'benevolent fund'. By 1833 similar bodies had been established in Lincolnshire, south Hants, Essex and Sheffield, and an activist signing himself 'Thorough Reformation' was busy urging them to amalgamate into a national body. 'They were', the Metropolitan Society declared, in a typical example of their querulous rhetoric, 'perplexed by multifarious duties – threatened by extensive responsibilities – oppressed by physical exertions – disturbed by conflicting interests – assailed by jealousies – harassed by intrigue and envy – injured by corporate privileges – insulted by legal enactments – and degraded by an opprobrious mode of remuneration.'[118]

Thus, well before the advent of the New Poor Law in 1834, the GPs were mobilising to increase the stipends of charitable foundation and Poor Law medical officers, as a means of protecting the whole profession against the rate-cutting of its weakest members. They appear to have had some success with the charitable foundations, as in Exeter and Bath,[119] but their battles with tight-fisted vestrymen usually ended in defeat, as at Horsham, in 1833. There, in a sequence of events that prefigured many a declension after 1834, the vestry cut the rate and extended the parish bounds when advertising for a new medical officer. Unemployed medical men were numerous, augmented by half-pay armed services medical officers. The Horsham vestry was flooded with applicants.[120]

At Southam in Warwickshire, at Lymington in Hants and at Southwell in Nottinghamshire, the Poor Law doctors, in league with the local Anglican clergy, developed ways of guaranteeing their income which were to become influential models for the New Poor Law. The doctors at Southam, for example, ran a dispensary for the poor. It was supported by the parish landholders from the poor rate, together with contributions from its members: 'the Independent Poor' or 'better . . . sort of labourers' paid 3s. 6d. a year per adult and 2s. for each child. The dispensary was open for one hour every day except Sundays. The doctors do not appear to have made home visits. In 1827 their joint dividend was £18. 14s. 0d. As at Lymington and Southwell, the non-independent poor, who corresponded to the 'undeserving' poor, got nothing unless they were lucky or persistent.[121]

Against this background it is hardly surprising that the doctors were outraged when Chadwick and Nassau Senior produced their scheme in 1834 with its effective reduction of Poor Law medical officers' incomes and its increase of their work-load.

Chadwick's Poor Law report of 1834 was an elaborate piece of propaganda. Its recommendations did not arise from its impressive-looking but essentially shoddy research findings. Chadwick was concerned to strengthen social discipline, to cut the redistribution of wealth to the non-working population and to enlarge the national economy by forcing the poor to work in it. As Dr Henriques points out, his 'principles' of less eligibility and the workhouse test for relief were acceptable to many rural landowners because they promised a method of controlling the rural proletariat after the 1830 risings and the sporadic incendiarism and animal maimings which followed after them.[122] Chadwick himself appears to have been obsessed by incendiarism; unexpected references to it crop up throughout his life. Town ratepayers, faced with rising costs occasioned by increasing numbers of immigrant paupers whom the laws of settlement could not stem, saw deliverance in the New Poor Law. Otherwise, such an irrelevant, damaging and callous plan would never have won the assent of the propertied. The few radicals and Tories who cared about the poor opposed it.

Chadwick purported to base his scheme on direct evidence from the countryside. His thorough-looking questionnaires elicited widespread instances of cosseting and extravagant expenditure on the poor: these formed a dramatic contrast to the reports of careful austerity at Southam, Southwell and other model places. In all the massive volumes, there is little on London or the new towns, and throughout there is little convincing evidence about anything. The basic terms of the inquiry were never defined. 'Able-bodied' sets its meaning only negatively against 'impotent', which is also undefined, but carries the notion of being unable to participate in the work-force. The partially or short-term disabled have no existence at all. The word 'impotent' was adopted from the statute of 1601; there was no attempt to discover the categories it encompassed: the old, the sick, and widows encumbered with young children. Indeed, the production of such information would have interfered with Chadwick's and Nassau Senior's simplistic conception of 'able-bodied' destitution as the result of a lazy refusal to join a labour market that was simultaneously being freed to receive new workers. Their sets of 41 questions for towns do not even include a question about 'the impotent'. Nowhere in the five volumes of returns are the 'able-bodied' presented as a proportion of the total number of paupers relieved. To have done so, on my hesitant calculations on Chadwick's own evidence, would have shown that the 'able-bodied' were neither a numerous nor significant constituent of the problem of the destitute.

The calculations must necessarily be dubious because Chadwick's questionnaires were badly formulated. They evoked many ambiguous replies or, frequently, baffled the respondents and were returned blank. Even in Essex and Kent, where there was high unemployment, I have counted a majority of parishes reporting that no 'able-bodied' were receiving relief. In Essex, of those parishes which answered the questions and whose replies can be interpreted with reasonable assurance, 4 were supplementing the wages of 'able-bodied' paupers, while 15 were relieving only the old and infirm. In Kent 10 parishes helped the 'able-bodied', and 17 helped only the aged and infirm.[123]

Consideration of the problem of the old and infirm entered the planning for the New Poor Law only as an inescapable afterthought.[124] There are four pages on the 'impotent' among the 260 in the *Report*. 'Impotent' does not appear in the index. Yet the 'impotent' formed the vast majority of paupers. In fact the New Poor Law, while intended to constrict medical relief, had the effect of legally recognising it for the first time. Chadwick had determined to confine to the workhouse all paupers in receipt of medical relief and had recommended this to the Cabinet. But the Cabinet had perceived the utter practical and political impossibility of the suggestion and had quietly rejected it, although Chadwick was still pressing it in 1837.[125] Even after the Poor Law Commissioners were installed, the creation of policy about the sick and poor was not part of their brief.

By attempting to regularise an already harsh, but often haphazardly generous system, Chadwick contracted to the destitute the medical relief hitherto widely available to the poor. 'Extras' such as midwifery or accident surgery which formerly the poor might have received from the parish, they now had to obtain from a dispensary, or sick club, save up for, or go without. And Chadwick made galling the conditions for obtaining medical relief.

His model was Lymington, as described by the vicar, the Reverend Peyton Blakiston. This medically trained hard evangelical product of Eton and Trinity had already separated males and females in his workhouse and he looked forward to 'a more extensive subdivision'. 'The class of female occupants', he reported, 'consists of very aged and infirm persons, children of various ages under 16 and occasionally prostitutes in a diseased state, or mothers of bastards, of which they are generally delivered at the workhouse.' The males were also mostly aged and infirm, 'together with boys under 14, together with one or two imbeciles, who are often very mischievous, grossly offensive and obscene in their language'. Outdoor pauper sick were treated at the discretion of the guardians, who each had 40 pauper tickets at his disposal. Once the tickets were exhausted, treatment ceased. Presumably their relatives were then compelled to do their duty and care for them. Blakiston thought this scheme, together with his provident dispensary for those who could pay, much preferable to indiscriminate poor relief orders for medical attendance. In inclusive systems the contracting surgeons were neglectful and the arrangement produced on the poor 'a sullen and rooted antipathy to the higher orders'. Blakiston's great ambition, and this is at the core of the movement to reform the Poor Law, was to tame a community of squatters at Boldre, near Lymington. They were 'smugglers and deer-stalkers' living on waste land and subject to no man. Their present income derived from selling kindling gathered in the New Forest. In 1830 they had demanded a parish allowance to raise their wages from 6s. to 9s. per week, and had been implicated in incendiarism. Blakiston believed that if they were compelled to enter the workhouse before they received relief they would learn their lesson.[126]

George Rawlins, the Clerk to the Overseer at St Martin's-in-the-Fields had similar ambitions. St Martin's was overrun with able-bodied vagrants. Rawlins believed that the onslaught would only be stemmed by 'due management of a workhouse, by which I mean a receptacle for the able-bodied and not for the impotent and aged ... The diet should be low, the work severe, and the restraint such as to be irksome'. The 'impotent' were to be sent away. St Martin's already separated pauper children from their parents and deposited them at an establishment at Norwood. Mr Smith, the Beadle of nearby St Clement Dane's, casually revealed why St Martin's was beset. At St Clement's they turned away casual able-bodied applicants, whose condition proved their 'indolence and misconduct'. Besides, St Clement's workhouse was always 'filled with impotent poor'.[127] In this context 'less eligibility' and the 'workhouse test' were meaningless.

The New Poor Law made no provision for classification of the sick. The chronically disabled were not distinguished from infection cases, lying-in cases or the insane. Chadwick had made no recommendations about the manner of treating the sick. Only in the general orders of 1842 and 1847 did the Commissioners vaguely permit the provision of medical and surgical attendance and the supply of medicine and surgical appliances. But the poor had to wait until the Poor Law Amendment Act of 1868 until this provision became mandatory, in the limited sense that the central authority, if it chose, could order such provision over the heads of the guardians. The Metropolitan Poor Act of 1867 finally enabled the establishment of asylums and dispensaries for the sick poor in London, but provision elsewhere remained permissive. Only in 1885 under the Medical Relief Disqualification Removal Act – the title is indicative of the chaos which obtained – was the definition of 'relief' enlarged to include food ordered by the medical officer. Hitherto he had been able only to recommend it, and the guardians frequently balked at the cost. Chadwick had made no suggestions about indoor medical relief. Thereafter the Commissioner ignored the problem, except occasionally to reiterate that expensive surgery cases should be directed to the charity hospitals.[128]

Even the 'able-bodied' were not 'able-bodied' when they sought relief. In the eastern counties between 1842 and 1846 two of every three able-bodied adult males receiving outdoor relief were reported as receiving it because of sickness or accident, attested by a medical order.[129] By 1900 the 'able-bodied' had come to be defined as those who in the workhouse master's opinion, were 'capable of a full day's work' and were therefore placed on the Number 1 or worst deterrent diet. In London on 1 January 1906 only about 20 per cent were on Number 1 diet and 60 per cent of these, workhouse masters reported, were probably incapable of completing a full day's work.[130] But the overwhelming majority of 'able-bodied' in the nineteenth century were female adults and children under 16. In 1865, for instance, the adult females were three times as numerous as the males and the children, usually dependants of the females, were seven times as numerous.[131] Throughout the period it was the mothers who clung to the children and bore the brunt of the increased family disruption that apparently accompanied industrialisation and greater mobility. Adult able-bodied female paupers were still almost three times the number of their male counterparts in 1877 and 1887, despite the savage pruning in their numbers during the early 1870s. Throughout the 1890s around 13 per cent of these 'able-bodied' women were classified as sick on New Year's Day, the day of the annual Poor Law returns. By 1906 the Poor Law authorities had ceased to count as able-bodied women who were incapable of earning a living for themselves and their dependants. The indolent able-bodied vagrants, who loomed so large in the original scheme, formed but a tiny portion of the whole, while the 'able-bodied' constituted only about one-quarter of the pauper population.[132]

Females were also about 11 per cent more numerous among the outdoor pauper sick in the 1870s: there were more old females than males, they were more deprived, and more of the males were in friendly societies. Among the indoor poor, 42 per cent were over 60, with another 33 per cent aged 40-60. Many of these were chronic 'permanents'. In agricultural counties these percentages were even higher. Cold weather regularly raised the percentages, too, as old people and the sickly succumbed to respiratory diseases. Over half the men over 65 applying to enter Manchester workhouses in the early 1890s had previously slept in common lodging-houses and other workhouse vagrant wards.[133]

In Scotland the situation appears to have been worse. Under the Scottish Poor Law the 'able-bodied' as such had no right to relief. Able-bodied persons who presented themselves at the workhouse with some 'slight disablement' were sent to the stone-yard and quickly died, according to the Secretary to the Board of Supervision in 1892.[134] There was also no provision for outdoor medical relief. Rural parishes were slow to levy themselves for the rate (they had generally not done so before 1834) and the slums of Edinburgh and Glasgow were swelled by destitute newcomers fleeing from unassessed parishes, especially in the Highlands.[135] The Board of Supervision which controlled the Poor Law until 1894 had very limited powers and used them mostly to save expenditure. In 1845 it made the appointment of a medical officer mandatory in every parish, but did nothing to ensure that the officer was resident or actually treated the poor in the workhouse, assuming the parish had built one. Outdoor medical relief existed *de facto* in the Lowlands, where it was supplemented by the doctors' private charity and customary relief, but Highlanders were terribly ill served throughout the century. In 1892, 30 per cent of Scottish paupers were over 60.[136]

In Wales the New Poor Law had the effect of bringing the treatment of the poor under the control of orthodox medicine for the first time. Before 1834 there was no system of poor relief: some parishes collected the rates and employed a surgeon, others did not. At Dolgellau in Merioneth, the surgeon had an 'informal' arrangement with the overseers and parishioners by which they paid for his requests of relief in kind or extra payments when he treated fractures or other serious cases. In Llandovery in Carmarthenshire before 1834, 'hardly any poor person was attended by ... the medical men except in very desperate cases, such as fractures of the skull'. When the poor became ill they went to local quacks, and 'in cases of fractures or contusions ... and the frequent cases of retention of urine, colic' they were attended by 'old women'. Relief in kind, which included cash, persisted after 1834. The cash was frequently used to pay one of the traditional healers whom the people continued to trust. None the less the Poor Law compelled people to visit the orthodox practitioners and the practitioners were convinced that this marked a great advance. Certainly it marked a new stage in the

Anglicising of Wales. The poverty of Welsh education meant that Wales produced very few doctors and even fewer Welsh-speaking ones. The Poor Law service opened Wales up to English-speaking Scots and Irish GPs. Crickhowel, in Brecknock, for instance, a totally Welsh-speaking parish, had a Poor Law medical officer appointed to it in 1842 who had no Welsh. Wales remained short of doctors through the century. The Welsh National School of Medicine, for which there had been agitation since 1886, did not commence until 1910.[137]

As part of his general object of reducing expenditure on the poor, Chadwick intended to make the Poor Law medical officers salaried servants of the guardians, rather than independent contractors. The sum the local guardians allocated for their salaries and other medical expenditure was to be limited by the central Board. The size of medical districts was to be increased, salaries were to be reduced, open tender for contracts was encouraged and medical officers were to be made subject to the orders of the guardians, without appeal.[138] Payments for treating non-parishioners on suspended orders, which constituted a valuable loading on the contract salaries before 1834, were implicitly forbidden. Chadwick achieved none of these aims in full, but each was implemented in sufficiently large part to trammel the system for the next eighty years.

The subjection of the medical officer to the relieving officer and the guardians hurt the doctors' pride and, as I suggested in Chapter 1 when discussing Poor Law midwifery, stretched the waiting time and deepened the humiliation of the injured and sick poor. Medical salaries were severely cut in the countryside, although in London and other cities the Commissioners did not dare interfere with the local authorities. In 1835 the Wycombe Union adopted a 'liberal contract' but Mr Sub-Commissioner Gilbert compelled them to reduce it. No local GP would accept the new terms: Gilbert imported three men to do the work formerly handled by sixteen. At Tunbridge Wells, Sir Francis Head, the Assistant Commissioner, notified the local GPs that the contract for the ten scattered parishes of the district would be £250 a year, instead of the former £470.[139] The arbitrary enlargement of East Rudham district in Norfolk effectively cut off the existing contractor from his private patients. In 1837 John and Thomas Prince, father and son, tendered for Balsham in Cambridgeshire for 3,614 paupers at £105 a year. They had between them treated the poor there for fifty years. Mr Howard, a new man at neighbouring Linton, tendered for both Balsham and Linton, at £90 for 7,902 paupers, and won. Paupers now had to walk up to eight miles to seek his attendance. Other districts were similarly enlarged and rendered unmanageable, especially for the paupers. Leighton Buzzard in Bedfordshire stretched 8 miles in one direction from the surgeon's residence; Okehampton in Devon was the same; Hereford stretched in two directions 10 miles from the surgeon's house and Westhoughton in Lancashire 11½ miles.[140] Kingsthorpe in Northamptonshire was extended much less, but it illustrates the real distances and time-lags involved. Kingsthorpe was part of Northampton district. In the 1870s the relieving officer lived in Northampton, the Poor Law surgeon lived five miles from Northampton and two miles from Kingsthorpe. The villagers were fortunate that the guardians did not insist, as was common in towns, that pauper applicants appear in person. So a villager had to walk five miles for an order, timing his arrival to coincide with the hour or so a weekday when the relieving officer was available. He then walked five miles to the doctor, who, if he decided to see the patient, travelled two miles. If the doctor prescribed for him, the patient had then to send back two miles to the doctor's surgery for the medicine. As Dr Rumsey remarked in 1844: 'the appointment of distant medical officers acts powerfully as . . . it was intended to do, in restricting the number of applicants.'[141]

The Poor Law Amendment Act of 1834 not only made the medical officers subject to the guardians, but it transferred from the magistrates to the ratepayers the power of ordinary relief. Power over the rates and the paupers was passed from the relatively disinterested, in the sense that they were spending other's money besides their own, to men wholly interested in saving expense. Their meanness shaped the pattern of Poor Law medical expenditure. Payment by case in the form of 'extras' for surgery, fractures and travel was often blocked, while the guardians permitted the relieving officer to issue indiscriminate relief orders for attendance by a doctor on a fixed salary.[142] Woodbury, for instance, was over 10 miles from Exeter, yet the guardians ordered in 1860 that all fractures had to go to the hospital as charity cases. Otherwise Poor Law surgeons had either to treat them as private patients or gratis. The surgeon, Mr Pratt, refused. But parents feared leaving children in the hospital. Throughout 1861 fractures among the poor in Woodbury went unset.[143]

The limits on salaries had the effect of excluding able, well-qualified practitioners and drawing in unqualified and disreputable transients. J.A. Sherwell was brought in as a cheap unqualified officer at Plympton St Mary, in Devon, in the 1830s. He broke promises to see pauper patients, he was rude to anxious patients, and ignorant in his diagnoses. The vestry ignored all complaints about him. As Commodore Brucks, a concerned local landowner remarked, 'the farmers [do not] . . . care one pin about the poor'.[144] The fact that Poor Law doctors had to provide medicines out of their salaries, long after the Board recommended that Unions pay for them, meant that patients got only the cheapest stuff, when they received anything at all. Chalk mixture, in those unions which permitted it, was made without 'aromatic confection', which must have made it taste vile. The authorities at Portsmouth in 1871 simply did not give medicines to the 14,000 people in their charge. Even so, the outcome cannot have been wholly bad. At Nottingham in 1867 patients received 'antimony that would not nauseate, aloes and senna that would not purge, cantharides that would not blister'. Special firms of 'union druggists' developed to supply this lowly but extensive market. In Carmarthen in 1871 the poor were found to be uniformly dosed with peppermint and water.[145] The quinine, cod-liver oil and other expensive medicines recommended in 1866 to the local authorities as a charge on the rates were still uncommon in the 1880s. The Poor Law dispensaries on the rates permitted by the Metropolitan Poor Act of 1867 were very slowly adopted; there were only 37 by 1872.[146] William Rendle, the parochial surgeon to St George's, Southwark, could not afford to use leeches, although he preferred them. Indeed he tried to send to St Thomas's or Guy's the patients he believed needed leeching as return for the incurables who came on to his books after being dismissed from the hospitals. But generally he ended by using the lancet.[147] The result must have been a higher infection and death rate.

Not surprisingly, conscientious medical officers were grossly overworked. In 1836 Mr Wagstaffe of St Mary's, Lambeth, with a total population of 110,000, claimed to have seen over 6,000 cases of illness, made 20,000 visits, sent 16,000 mixtures, 12,000 powders, and 30,000 pills. He received £105 a year, which was supposed also to cover leeches, midwifery, bandages and operations.[148]

The work-load claimed by Wagstaffe was only possible because he, like most busy practitioners, employed assistants. As Rendle, at St George's, Wagstaffe's neighbour, explained, his unqualified assistant saw all minor cases, drew teeth, dealt with chronic and aged patients, and handled 'severe' cases after Rendle's initial treatment. This arrangement, Rendle said, left him time for his private patients: he spent twice as many hours on his private practice as he spent on his Poor Law rounds.[149]

The assistantship device made Poor Law and cheap private practice possible. As one Plymouth guardian remarked, doctors only accepted workhouse practice 'to get premiums for apprentices'.[150] Premiums for two or three apprentices of up to £300 each with a parochial surgeon

made the lowly £60-£100 salary for a workhouse post a lesser consideration. Other assistants were hired as straightforward employees. In the
1840s the best rate for a qualified live-in assistant was £50 a year, less
than the wage of a journeyman carpenter or a policeman. Even a gentleman's footman got £40 and all found.[151] The numbers of would-be
doctors were such that the going rate was £15-20, 'in these times of
competition', R.T. Webb declared, 'when iron-hearted capitalists, Poor
Law Commissioners, and political economists rule the world'.[152] By
1851 the rate had edged up to £30-40 and in 1858 it reached £70, a
navvy's income, although it had fallen back to £30-40 by the 1870s. An
assistant's board in the 1830s cost about £12. 10s. 0d. a year.[153] The
interlude of the mid-1850s was occasioned by the Australian gold rushes.
As one assistant boasted in 1852, they were 'finally finding emanci-
pation'. 'The new yellow fever . . . has thinned, is thinning, and will yet
thin the medical ranks of this country more than the ranks of the other
learned professions.' Four of his friends had left recently on a single
ship. They were going where 'salary *is* an object'.[154] (These founding
fathers built well – the medical profession in Australia still holds their
values.)

Assistants ate with the servant, opened the door to private patients,
delivered medicines to private patients, and treated the paupers. But as
one MD pointed out, many of them were 'so devoid of gentlemanly
demeanour' as to be unfitted to attend a gentle family. Many came
from trade and should have stayed there.[155]

But they must have had some native intelligence, because the number
of bad diagnoses and lethal treatments reported as being traced to them
is surprisingly small – about two a year on my rough count.[156] I have
found only one protest from patients against them, at Shott's Ironworks
in Lanarkshire, in 1882.[157] But the popular esteem for 'Dr' Smith in
Poplar, the unqualified assistant of a doctor who practised in Leyton, is
probably more typical. In 1897, a woman died under Smith's incompetent management. Her relatives and neighbours who gave evidence
were stoical about it and did not blame Smith. Like most patients now,
they were in no position to judge his formal qualifications or lack of
them. Realistically, and deferentially, they expected little of him: orders
about a regimen of doses rather than to be let into the secret of his
diagnosis, palliatives rather than cures. The coroner remarked that 'the
people who came before him seemed to think more of getting a bottle
of medicine than of being told what was the matter with them'.[158]
Certainly assistants must have been productive money-makers for their
employers because few doctors seem to have been without one. Not

until 1887 did the courts decide that a qualified doctor could not legally claim fees for attendance by unqualified assistants on patients he had never seen. The GMC did not extend 'infamous conduct' to include the employment of unqualified assistants, or the 'covering' by a registered practitioner of an unqualified employer until 1897, despite several notorious scandals.[159]

The Poor Law surgeons and later the vaccination contractors found themselves subject to the very classes of men from which they had sought to escape. Guardians and relieving officers insulted them and arbitrarily rejected their medical recommendations. The St George's guardians consistently humiliated Rendle by never supplying anything on the same day that he ordered it. Sometimes, when he ordered medicine or wine and bread, it was 'entirely refused' without his being informed. Rendle fought back and returned the cancelled order with 'not ill but starving' written across it.[160] Mr Small of Radford and Lenton Union near Nottingham was dismissed by the guardians for disobedience about 'too great liberality'. He had ordered beef-tea and wine for old people.[161] In 1875 the Axminster guardians advertised for a new parochial surgeon at Worle at £30 and medicines. There were no applicants. There was a suggestion to raise the salary to £40; but the reverend chairman (the most flint-hearted guardians often turn out to have been clergymen) opposed the move. It 'bore so close a resemblance to going down on their knees'. He preferred to seek 'some retired physician, who wants a little work to fill up his time, with no pay'. The guardians finally on a narrow vote decided to advertise again at £40.[162] In 1891 the Thetford guardians supported the relieving officer when he rebuked a doctor for seeking an order for a desperately ill patient on a Sunday.[163]

The hard-used poor were equally contumacious of the doctors, and the town ones at least showed it openly. As William Rendle confessed, they swore constantly at the receiving officer and the Board, and 'had no sympathy with medical men . . . for they know nothing of our contracts . . . They feel their own necessities, not ours.'[164] When the out-patients' wards developed at county hospitals those who could among the poor voted with their feet. By 1909 they were known to walk 'long distances' to hospitals at Sheffield, Birmingham, Bootle and Sherborne, rather than be healed by their local Poor Law man. They 'did not trust him'.[165] The aged and the isolated rural poor necessarily were more passive. By the twentieth century, they had 'absolutely all complaint knocked out of them', according to Dr Cecil Stephens, Poor Law medical officer for North Witchford in Cambridgeshire. Their relatives did not complain either. 'Agricultural labourers' were, Dr Stephens said, 'rather . . . selfish [men] in many things of this sort'.[166]

The doctors' subordination was the more galling because their Poor Law employers were much better paid. While their own incomes had been cut by one-third to a half by the New Law, the salaries of the bureaucrats had not been touched and the number of 'jobs' had been increased. One of the Poor Law Commissioners in the 1840s was George Cornewall Lewis, who succeeded his father in the post. Lewis perfectly expressed the outlook of the Commissioners when he explained that

> medical care is one of those things which each person provides for himself according to his class in society. The highest class provide a better sort of . . . attendance than the middle class, and the middle class better than the poorer classes. I do not see how it is possible for the State to supply medical relief to the poor of as good a quality, and to as great an extent as the richer classes enjoy.[167]

He could rest more easily in this belief because his salary as Commissioner was £6,000 a year. The Secretary to the Commissioner, Edwin Chadwick, at £1,200, also did quite well out of his brain-child. There were also two Assistant Secretaries, at £1,100 each, 33 clerks who cost £4,000, and 21 Assistant Commissioners who cost £32,000. In 1837 the Poor Law bureaucracy cost over £52,000; the total expenditure on the 2,000 medical officers in that year was about £130,000, around £65 each. By 1868 the Board was costing £60,000 a year but still had never met. The senior Commissioners signed documents automatically as they were brought to them. There were difficulties each winter, when distress was worst, because the senior Commissioners usually departed for the south of France.[168] The opponents of the New Poor Law had predicted that the Commission would perpetrate Old Corruption and they were right: jobs for idle aristocrats and pushy briefless barristers.

At the local level, the relieving officer, a local patronage appointment, got about £150 a year in London in the 1840s and about £160 in 1908. In rural parishes the rate in 1908 varied between £90 and £130. But in all cases he received more than the medical officer. He was also registrar of births and deaths and vaccination, and received the fees from this. The clerk to the guardians was usually a solicitor with a private practice and local political connections. In Greenwich in the 1840s he received £350 a year. He also had 'some emoluments from elections' (he got ¼d. per head for voters) and was the vestry clerk, at £300 a year. The clerk did no Poor Law work personally but employed two under-clerks to do the job at £150 and £80 a year respectively.[169] The provisions in the

New Poor Law for local audits do not appear to have been very effective. Moreover, the Commission and the Local Government Board had a policy of never publishing the salaries of officers. Successive Select Committees and Royal Commissions never got very far in trying to elicit the figures. In 1895 Robert Elcock, a guardian of the Wimborne and Cranborne Union, claimed that the officials of his Union cost 2s. 3d. for every 1s. 9d. spent on the poor. The two relieving officers each received over £110 a year. About another £680 went on other officials' salaries.[170] At Huddersfield the clerk got over £300, yet the work was done by the registrar and guardians' assistant clerks. At the same meeting, at which the guardians raised the clerks' salary by £75, they refused the paupers an extra 6d. a week for coal, when the price had risen during a colliers' strike.[171] By 1909 the clerk to the Liverpool guardians was receiving £1,000 a year. His was a 'political appointment' and the work was done by subordinates. The figures for 1904, which are the only ones we have in print, are unclear, but they suggest that by the twentieth century about 23 per cent of Poor Law expenditure on medical relief was going to 'administration'.[172]

These sums indicate that the local management of the Poor Law was much more political than historians have hitherto assumed. There were rates to be protected, spoils to be had and spoiling to be done. The structure of local Poor Law authority also suggests that the opposition to the New Poor Law, which has been generally characterised as irrational, backward-looking and emotional, had a sound basis in the desire to allocate resources rationally and humanely. It is time we looked again at what paternalist Tories and Chartists actually said and did against the Poor Law. Their predictions about it were better borne out than those of its advocates. Hitherto the opposition has been naïvely and superficially appraised through the reports of the Poor Law entrepreneurs. These reports might well turn out to be as unreliable as their research.

Contemporaries and historians have accepted the Metropolitan Poor Act of 1867 as a great advance. Within six years £4,500,000 was spent on building and renovation, or nearly as much as was spent on Poor Law building in the thirty years after 1834.[173] Wash-basins replaced buckets, hairbrushes, towels and looking-glasses were installed. But, as Dr Joseph Rogers protested, 'architects, surveyors and builders gobbled up the money meant for the poor'.[174] The real needs, Poor Law dispensaries and better nursing, were thrust aside. Quite apart from all the other weaknesses in the published returns of numbers of paupers (the difficulties begin with the varying seasonal dates at which figures were collected) amounts of expenditure and the rest, the question of who got what and how much out of the £600,000,000 said to have been spent on the Poor Law between 1834 and 1908 seems to me to cry out for research.[175]

As with the case of sanitary improvements, there is also a question of who actually paid for what. The poorest districts bore the heaviest rates and carried the largest numbers of paupers, and apparently provided for them best. In 1856-7 St George's, Hanover Square, relieved 210 casuals while Shoreditch relieved over 13,000. The poor fled St George's for less austere treatment in poorer parishes. St George's expenditure on the poor equalled 6½d. in every pound of tax while in Shoreditch it equalled 2s. 10¾d. The *Lancet* implied in 1858 that poor parishes were effectively subsidising wealthy ones.[176]

From the early 1850s the medical men gradually improved their income from the Poor Law. In 1847 they had succeeded in obtaining an Order that only qualified contractors be employed. While the number of paupers remained at around 900,000-1,000,000, the number of parochial surgeons increased from 2,300 in 1840, to 4,000 in 1870, to 5,000 in the mid-1880s.[177] Their work-load, or at least that of their assistants, must have lessened slightly, especially as new, more compact districts were created. Their share of the total expenditure remained steady until the 1890s at about 3.6 per cent, but as the total increased at a greater rate than the increase in the number of medical officers, their remuneration must have increased, especially after dispensaries spread in the 1870s and 1880s and the duty of supplying drugs out of their salaries was removed. In 1834 the nominal *per capita* expenditure on paupers was £6; by 1908 it was £16. After superannuation for medical officers was introduced in 1891 their salary share improved again, possibly to as much as 17 per cent of the expenditure.[178]

4. AN ESTIMABLE PROFESSION?

The BMA, formed from some of the provincial GP protest associations in 1836, had by the 1850s become the united and respectable organisation of the bulk of the profession. In 1838 it had amalgamated with the Glasgow Medical Association and in 1839 incorporated bodies in the north of England. Through the 1840s the BMA fought the Poor Law Commissioners, winning small concessions, but losing the main battles over greater medical independence. In 1848 it defeated John Simon, MOH for the City of London, by refusing to supply him with statistics until he agreed to pay each reporting GP £50 a year for the job.[179] The

Royal Colleges' membership rules were liberalised during the 1850s and the Medical Act of 1858 generally satisfied GPs, although they were denied direct representation on the GMC created by the Act.[180]

The GPs' growing professional confidence and the continuing irritations of Poor Law practice strengthened the interest of many of them in 'state medicine'. At the core of the system was the resolve to win individual clinical freedom with a guaranteed income. Even before 1834, Thomas Wakley had called for the division of the country into medical districts, served by publicly paid medical officers, under the direction of regional Officers of Health directed by a National Faculty of Medicine. All properly qualified men would be members of the National Faculty and eligible to nominate and vote for the national directorate. There was to be no political interference: Parliament's duty was simply to raise the taxes and make the payment set by the National Faculty. The state, after all, was already involved in medical care through the army and naval boards, while the *ad hoc* Boards of Health established during the cholera epidemic of 1831-2, however badly they had been chosen and had performed, showed that the state henceforth would be involved in civilian medical provision. The way was open, the doctors hoped, for the development of a rational harmonious relationship between the state and the profession, on the profession's terms.[181]

Chadwick's New Poor Law destroyed this possibility, for the nineteenth century at least. Superficially, his plan was not dissimilar from the doctors' schemes. He, too, wanted a national full-time publicly paid service, but a service that was subject to bureaucratic inspectorial control rather than one that was autonomous.[182] After 1834 doctors' schemes for state medicine were developed as piecemeal criticisms of the New Poor Law, rather than thoroughgoing conceptual innovations.

The doctors' proposals mostly collapsed (in the nineteenth century at least, for they partly succeeded in the twentieth beginning with the National Insurance Act of 1911) on the problem of *per capita* fee-for-service payments as against payments for total numbers of listed patients. Proponents of voucher-for-service schemes were usually poor country practitioners outside the Poor Law with relatively small numbers of patients. They were willing to retain the power of the overseer to issue vouchers or 'medical cheque books' to the poor up to a set total, in the expectation that free competition between the neighbourhood doctors would bring them some voucher patients who otherwise were monopolised by the parochial surgeon. The voucher was to be received by the doctor for the treatment and then cashed on the parish. 'Corvinus', of Corwen in Merioneth, suggested as a further refinement that a list of paupers and their families unable to pay for assistance should be drawn up annually after public discussion between the doctors and guardians and prominently posted. This could limit the list to the truly needy who could then be treated at 4*d*. a head in the country and 10*d*. in the towns, that is at about double the rate that often obtained. 'A doctor', 'Corvinus' remarked, did not expect 'to *fatten* by means of *poor patients*', but treating them helped 'increase his connections and reflects his duty to the "chain of society" '.[183]

   The weakness in these schemes was pointed out by Dr J.C. Yeatman, one of the more zealous among the progenitors of the BMA. The Poor Law Commissioners and local guardians always ensured that *per capita* fees were paid only to a very low total ceiling. At Wexcombe in Wiltshire these sly and parsimonious managers paid participating doctors 2*s*. 6*d*. a head for 100 patients up to £10. The doctors apparently agreed before doing their arithmetic. The working of the scheme is unclear, but it seems that the doctors' claims, which would have been made after 80 patients, were not met until 100 had been treated; the last 20 were free. Meanwhile the doctors bribed relieving officers to send them patients quickly, before the 80 was reached. Yeatman admitted the defect in the simple covering salary system which obtained: overseers thoughtlessly flooded the doctor with patients who were not '*fully* sick'. The only solution was full independence for the salaried doctor to decide whom he would treat and when.[184] The BMA recommended that the salary be set by assessors, partly chosen by doctors, partly by the local authorities, drawing on a national scale which weighted the total number of cases, the density and size of the district, costs of medicines, the prices of 'extras' and value of time and skill of the doctor. In an attempt to solve the most intractable problem of all, the costing of treatment of the incurables, the BMA proposed an annual *per capita* payment of £5. 5*s*. 0*d*. a year.[185]

   The most visionary state medicine advocate was the now forgotten Dr H.W. Rumsey, a provincial surgeon and sanitarian. He looked to a system of national medical attendance provided on the model of the national Church. The state endorsed the Established Church but did not interfere too much. Every Briton had a duty to sustain the church financially and every Briton had the right to receive spiritual sustenance from its priests. Yet paupers seeking medical sustenance were disfranchised and Poor Law doctors were humiliated. Already state vaccination had been inaugurated without pauperising its recipients: state medicine should be the same. Justice was not administered on a discretional, variable, parsimonious basis by ill-chosen local incompetents: why should medicine – 'the application of general hygienic laws' and the science of epidemiology – be so treated?[186] In 1846 Parliament allocated £61,000 towards payment of half of the Poor Law doctors' salaries, but the state never moved beyond this concession. Ministers rejected proposals for a Central Medical Office in the 1850s and 1860s and refused to consider the amalgamation of the various sanitary, Poor Law and vaccination authorities.[187] These bodies themselves vigorously resisted all proposals that threatened to force them together.

Rumsey and Chadwick, from their respective extremes, continued to press through the 1860s and 1870s for a united state service on the Prussian model; but in vain. Parliament and the Treasury found it easier to ignore them because the BMA's attitude had changed. Now secure in their private practices, doctors scorned state medicine. Dr Stallard predicted that it would only attract the 'young and the old incompetents'. It would also duplicate existing private services and exclude 'the local man from the influence that accrues from local . . . cordiality'. In 1872 the *Lancet* editorialist opposed a move by the President of the Local Government Board, James Stansfeld, to appoint specially qualified medical men as advisers. Such appointments 'would take confidence away from general practitioners'. Moreover, there was no longer any need for a 'State Church of . . . sanitary bishops . . . [forcing] housewives . . . to spend their money freely on every new-fangled scheme these said bishops may devise'. The recent success of antiseptic clinical 'scientific' treatment had made extension of rigorous sanitary law unnecessary.[188] By 1900 'State medicine' had been narrowed to cover the lately demeaned medical aspects of legally controlling infectious disease and poisons. Other aspects, water supply, sewage disposal and food adulteration, were passing to the newly developing 'paramedical' services, staffed by engineers and laboratory technicians.

Medical education reflected these changes in professional ideology. The Bill of 1858 had almost suffered the fate of its numerous predecessors because it originally included a clause giving the GMC power to regulate the curricula and standard of qualifying bodies. This clause was quietly dropped. Thus the existing enormous variation between qualifications was preserved. Men passed by some institutions were rejected as medically ignorant when they applied to the army and navy medical boards. Oxbridge retained its gentlemanly but patchy Latin.[189] Effectively, the distinctions between physicians, surgeons and apothecaries were erased while the emerging differentiation between consultants and GPs was confirmed. Members of the BMA had called themselves 'doctor' since 1837.[190]

The GMC carefully avoided becoming an advisory body to the government on health and disease, and instead busied itself hearing but not settling quarrels of rival professors and vice-chancellors and playing at lawyers while they studied the squalid minutiae of 'infamous conduct' cases. When in 1876 John Simon tried to make 'public health and hygiene' an essential subject in medical courses, the GMC thwarted him. The Council did nothing to assist the growth of clinical teaching, especially at the bedside, as it developed during the 1870s, and refused to inspect or set standards of conduct for it. Post-graduate medical courses began in the late 1890s, but again they seem to have been created despite the GMC rather than with its encouragement. And the GMC always blocked moves to teach in workhouse infirmaries although, as Dr John Johnston of Glasgow pointed out in 1900, only in workhouses would students see many of the conditions they would later encounter among older patients,

> apoplexy, advanced renal disease, alcoholic poisoning, meningitis, epilepsy . . . bronchitis, heart failure . . . pneumonia . . . To the senior student, the end of the hemiplegic or paraplegic, helpless and dirty for months or years is unknown . . . He might . . . see the man whose hernia had been operated upon two months ago, and healed (no drainage-tube used) by first intention, die of purulent peritonitis . . . He would see irritable stumps from old amputations, persons permanently demented from the shock of injuries, ulcers of all ages, sizes, and origins.[191]

From the 1860s the profession gradually became wealthier, higher in status, and conservative in ideology. In 1860 Drs J.S. Gamgee and Robert Barnes collected money and medicines from the faculty for Garibaldi, but that was the final radical flourish.[192] The improved standing of the Poor Law surgeons, who constituted about one-quarter of the profession throughout the century, damaged their radicalism and that of their colleagues. At the beginning of the reign a medical journalist had remarked that 'a young Tory practitioner or a Tory medical student [was] a real *rara avis*'.[193] Sixty years later the *Lancet* reported that Haverfordwest in Pembrokeshire had six doctors. Each was a Tory. The *Lancet* man added:

> Of course, as Herbert Spencer has shown . . . medicine and the priest-hood went out one time hand in hand, so naturally a medical man bears the interior instinct of Toryism. The essence of good medicine

is not to be meddlesome, not to upset existing institutions as long as they work well . . . whereas Radicalism — but we are a non-political paper.[194]

The doctors' improved status derived from the higher profits they were able to command. In 1831 one Bermondsey general practice with several extras — for instance, a contract for the police in 'R' division — was sold for 300 guineas. The net income, presumably after bad debts were written off, was £91 a year.[195] A country practitioner in 1847 (whose horse, incidentally, at £35 a year cost him more than his assistant, at £30) complained that his annual outlay of £465 left him too little profit for an annual 'long holiday'. But twenty years later, 'a good practice' grossed £700-1,000 annually and a young, energetic GP, even one 'without connections', in a respectable London suburb could expect £300 profit a year. The discovery in the mid-1860s that nearly all of the 300 doctors who died in 1861 had bequeathed property was sufficiently new to excite remark.[196] My patchy survey of biographies of medical men suggests that more sons of doctors, and certainly more sons of successful ones, went into medicine from about the 1860s.

Fundamentally, the higher medical incomes rested on the growing mid-Victorian economy, although the profession made several innovations to enable them to enlarge their share. Their incomes seem to have grown steadily, with a pause in the late 1870s to mid-1880s, and thence on towards the high level they achieved in Edwardian Britain.

The innovation that underpinned the rest was the doctors' ability to control their numbers in relation to their market. This development was partly fortuitous, but mainly resulted from the doctors' resolute efforts. The fortuitous factor was the emigration of assistants that set in during the 1850s and, possibly a little unforeseen, the effects of stiffer examinations. But the introduction of the registration hurdle in the 1858 Act and the continued refusal to recognise foreign qualifications were the doctors' own work. Over all, while the population of England and Wales grew by over 13 per cent between 1851 and 1871, the number of doctors increased by only 1.9 per cent.

The stiffer examinations helped greatly: the number of students enrolled for medicine increased steadily, but the number graduating remained almost stationary. In 1861 961 registered, in 1871 777, in 1881 about 1,200. In proportion to population the 9.7 doctors per 10,000 in England and Wales in 1851 fell to 7.8 per 10,000 in 1871, or one practitioner to every 1,276 men, women and children. By 1886 this proportion had improved, from the doctors' standpoint, to one to 1,662.

(The NHS currently projects 2,000 patients per doctor as the optimal number for efficient practice.) Even so, British doctors remained vigilant. In 1886, F.H. Alderson, the president of the West London Medico-Chirurgical Society, called for the reintroduction of Greek and longer medical courses 'to limit the number of doctors and stop the decline of incomes, and to stop the easy registration of Irish doctors'.[197]

The distribution of GPs generally increased their scarcity value. In 1861, the census, relying on a wide definition of 'doctor', reported 1 per 514 persons in London, compared with 1 per 1,769 in Wales. By 1886 only two 'unhappy places' were reported to be over-supplied: Brighton, with 1 per 726 and London, with 1 per 939. Below these, the distribution ranged from Bristol 1 per 1,232, Liverpool 1 per 1,564, Glasgow 1 per 2,209, Sheffield 1 per 2,593 to insalubrious Salford with 1 per 3,908. But these averages must hide grossly uneven distributions between rich and poor places within those cities. In 1914 Shoreditch had 1 per 5,000 compared with Kensington's 1 per 500.[198]

Recognition of foreign qualifications might well have transformed the market and returned it to the free-for-all that had obtained with the influx of Scots and Irish in the 1820s and 1830s. But by the 1840s the GPs were sufficiently powerful to destroy a series of medical bills, including Sir James Graham's sensible measure of 1845, partly because they opened the way to registration of foreign practitioners.[199] Even so, a steady trade continued on the mail-order sale of genuine MD certificates from such universities as Rostock and Erlangen. Their local agents sent circulars describing the various grades of certificate and prices to young British licentiates. In the 1860s an MD *in absentia* from Rostock cost £60. 6s. 0d. inclusive. Dr Pritchard, the poisoner, had bought his MD *in absentia* from Erlangen.[200] There was also a public trade in the British certificates of deceased practitioners. They could cost up to £30, depending upon the repute of the issuing institution.[201]

The transition to wealth and respectability was also underwritten by the increased numbers of propertied elderly valetudinarians who could afford a daily visit from a responsive gentlemanly practitioner, and by the families who could pay for those lengthy bedside vigils awaiting the crisis, or death, which became dramatic set pieces of medical care during the second half of the century. The Harveian lecturer for 1898, Dr W. Ewart, congratulated his colleagues on lately being supported by 'a wholesome dread . . . [which had] seized the educated classes . . . The medical man's advice [was] anxiously expected.'[202] The doctor developed an intimate relationship with the family, he enhanced his self-esteem as the indispensable chief of the sick-room, and he did well out of the bill. In practical terms he could do little to help the patient, except issue opiates and perhaps perform a tracheotomy on diphtheria victims. But it was his presence that counted; probably its importance increased while that of the vicar counted for less. Slum-dwellers, by contrast, who received only the medicine and perhaps only the curt attendance of an assistant, were not much worse off; the more fortunate among them received free from kin and neighbours the comfort the upper classes had to buy from the doctor.[203]

The emergence of the consultant-specialist also depended upon increasing numbers of valetudinarians and chronic cases. Originally in the 1830s and 1840s a consultant, summoned by the patient or the GP and acting jointly with him, shared the GP's fee and, excepting a handful of very great men, was hardly distinguishable from him in qualifications, experience or standing. This loose arrangement, in an age of boisterous behaviour and rhetoric, produced endless rows and accusations of 'kidnapping' and levying of secret fees.[204] Specialists liked to rip off bandages applied to patients by GPs; patients with fractures splinted by one man, who then consulted a specialist, were liable to have the first GP return to tear off the new splints. A woman in Chelmsford lost the use of her arm after one such incident in 1840.[205] After a suggestion from a GP the BMA established a 'court-medical' to handle such 'unprofessional conduct' and keep unsavoury episodes out of the courts and newspapers. But the 'court-medical' lacked authority and took months to cajole the parties into accepting its compromise judgements. Still, it created three precedents for the later GMC tribunal: the tribunal refused to hear charges of 'incompetence', and 'incompetence' was never incorporated into 'infamous conduct'; the court-medical also tried to institute the rule whereby the patient was precluded from summoning the consultant; and it permitted the building of a separate fee structure for consultants and GPs.[206] These two latter developments remained shaky until about the 1880s, partly because wealthy patients insisted on calling and dismissing anyone they liked.

By the late 1850s consultants were charging £3. 3s. 0d. and more per visit, to distinguish their advice from that of the humble GPs, at 5s. to 10s. 6d.[207] During the following decades the consultants gradually defined their caste. They formed specialist societies and dominated the GMC. By the 1870s a consultant was expected to be a lecturer in a hospital with a big following of pupils or a man of outstanding reputation in fashionable lay circles, a standing he achieved only after 10-20 years' practice, unless he had good connections. He now charged at least £5. 5s. 0d. a consultation and made about £5,000 a year, while the top

10 or 20 doubled that.[208]

During these same decades the GPs raised their fees in the wake of the consultants. Their usual charge for a visit to a respectable patient increased from the old 2s. 6d.-7s. 6d. to the newly 'customary' 7s. 6d. to 10s. 6d. to £2. 2s. 0d. and for a poor patient from 2s. 6d. to 5s. Money had fallen in value, they asserted, while their fees had remained stable, and the costs of the new medical courses had jumped by 300 per cent.[209] The advent of less interventionist therapeutics also necessitated a change in pricing. Educated patients now balked at taking several large draughts a day and instead sought only teaspoonfuls of the mixture with water. The GP's income from drugs had fallen sharply. Young 'Rusticus', from North Lonsdale in Lancashire, showed his colleagues how the difference could be more than adequately supplied. He had doubled the charges set by his elderly old-fashioned rival and he added 1s. 6d. to the fee for every visit.[210]

The GPs also enlarged 'the dignity of our . . . profession' by raising their fees for sick clubs. Generally they achieved this without much friction, although there were isolated instances of fierce opposition. The clubs had been created by doctors and local bigwig philanthropists in the 1820s and 1830s and, excepting the miners' clubs, had run on the doctors' terms. The guaranteed return from the club for treatment of the labouring classes who formed the bulk of the membership was higher than the sum the doctor would otherwise have obtained from them as private, pauper or charity cases. Many clubs, those at Oldham, Gloucester and Yarmouth for instance, were subsidised from the poor rate as a means of keeping down the rate.[211] But the terms of trade had changed by the 1860s. Doctors to miners' and iron-workers' clubs in Cornwall and Shropshire were becoming openly restive about the club committees, elected by the workers, who advertised for and chose the doctor and defined his duties.[212] At Southampton in 1868 the doctors struck in an attempt to make the clubs pay 5s. per head per year instead of the traditional 2s. 6d.-3s. The doctors at Wednesbury successfully squeezed the wealthy clubs there — although they already paid contracting doctors £2,000 a year — by blacklisting them and threatening potential strike-breakers.[213] By 1869 the doctors had generally instituted the 5s. minimum. This was for them an excellent rate, given that treatment was provided by assistants.[214] Thereafter, despite occasional rows with miners who demanded personal service from their doctors, the clubs continued to satisfy both members and doctors. By the 1890s the average doctor to a miners' club was receiving about £190 a year for comparatively easy work. GPs competed eagerly for election by the clubs. Some even issued handbills — 'Vote for Dr— the Genuine Working-man's Friend' and promised their personal attention.[215] Chronic sufferers and the old, who were unrewarding, time-consuming cases, were usually removed from the books of sick clubs after one year's treatment, pro-vided they had retired while in good standing. Some, like the Durham coal-miner who broke his leg in 1889 and defaulted on his payments (the mining companies usually took them out of the miners' weekly wages) after a fortnight away from work, were expelled and forfeited all entitlements. They usually ended up on the parish.[216]

In the 1890s GPs began to charge £1. 1s. 0d. for a sickness certificate under the Workmen's Compensation Act, while consultants examining candidates on behalf of insurance companies demanded £2. 2s. 0d., pre-sumably from the candidate.[217] Their probity as assessors, the doctors argued, required greater recognition; probity in this instance not being its own reward. The cost of the certificate, which has been ignored by both contemporaries and historians when discussing the statistics of industrial accidents and insurance, must have considerably diminished the numbers of reported accidents and claims.

Among the more respectable reaches of the profession, the change to less heroic dosages and consequent fall in income heightened the attrac-tiveness of the ethical 'custom' of charging for 'the prescription', which was then taken by the patient to a chemist, rather than for actual medicines dispensed by the doctor himself.[218] But lower-class patients were disgruntled at having to pay for a piece of paper and thus 'pay twice' for medicine from the chemist. Moreover, many poor patients clung to the traditional understanding that they need not pay the doctor for treatment if they queued at his home, but only for the medicine he dispensed.[219] In cheap practices profits from the sale of medicine formed the largest single item of income for many GPs. There was a continual temptation to overcharge. These GPs continued to sell medicines to their poorer patients and often won patients from doctors who had gone over to issuing only prescriptions. From the 1860s young men in 'good respectable practices' were careful to charge only for 'attendance and advice' while reprobates in the slums continued to sell medicines until the First World War. The royal colleges had long had rules against the practice (which is why radical Lydgate in *Middlemarch* had done his own prescribing), but they rarely enforced them.[220]

By the 1890s respectable GPs followed a 'widespread custom' of sending only an annual bill, at Christmas. The bill covered the whole family and was not itemised. The 'custom' (I have been unable to find when it began — or whether indeed it existed widely before the 1890s) was to charge high for the first case in a 'good' family and lower for subsequent ones.[221] In 1907 'Only a Beginner' refused a demand from 'a landed proprietor' in his village for a detailed bill. The 'Beginner' obtained a written agreement from his fellow local GP not to treat the proprietor – but the other GP secretly broke the agreement – and the Beginner's bill remained unpaid.[222]

'Good' families who did not pay were rarely sued. In the confused state of the law there was always a chance that the doctor might lose or have his claim halved. Judges and juries were notoriously unsympathetic to doctors. The good families' patronage helped the doctor's local standing among other 'good' families. Moreover, a doctor's reputation was harmed when he became a dun and the 'good' family turned to a rival practitioner.[223] Debts among unprestigious families in the earlier part of the century were sold to local attorneys, who could distrain the debtor's goods, put the debtor in prison and put the family on the parish.[224] Later in the century specialised, little-publicised agencies such as the British Medical Protection Society emerged to collect debts for GPs. They worked on commissions of around 12 per cent and claimed a total reclamation in about 45 per cent of cases.[225] 'In the case of persons in lodgings, birds of passage, those who are not rate-payers, and many *employés*... also ... doubtful people, and invariably in venereal cases', the rule, as it had traditionally been, was instant cash. 'We must discriminate', one provincial surgeon explained, 'in the case of substantial ratepayers, heads of families it would hardly do.'[226]

Our present knowledge about the proportion of private income spent on medical care is skimpy. Indeed historians of the 'standard of living' notably avoid it. The host of varying considerations affecting medical expense make generalised averages almost useless. Yet the scraps of disparate information we have suggest, first, that expenditure on care took a sizeable part of middle-class income; second, that the onset of serious illness could be economically catastrophic in working-class families; and third, that the casual labouring poor, just above the level of the destitute, may well have been unable to afford medical help, at least during the first half of the century. Dr Patricia Branca has unearthed two annual budgets for lower 'middle-class' families on £150 a year, one for 1828 and another for 1874. Medical expenses in both, lumped with amusement costs, at £3. 14s. in the first budget and £10 in the second, equal the total outlay on groceries and slightly more than the wages of the servant.[227] These probably are ideal budgets for healthy families because there are indications that families hit by illness spent much more than this. In 1831 a GP in Scotland charged a family that was 'not indigent'

£29. 9s. 6d. for one week of 'visits and detention, bloodletting, blister and applying ditto, anodyne, evening visits and opiate'. In England in the same year a GP charged a 'poor' patient £17 for nine weeks of visits and purgatives.[228] Also in the 1830s a hospital surgeon charged a widow in 'very moderate – nay, straitened circumstances' £80 to remove a breast cancer. He had made a concession, he said – his usual charge was 110 guineas. Under threat of legal action the widow's relatives, as must frequently have happened, jointly contributed to meet the bill.[229] In 1854 at Mildenhall in Suffolk a servant-housekeeper broke her leg. Her annual wages were £12. The doctor charged her £11. 0s. 6d. for setting her leg and subsequent visits. In the late 1860s at Cwm Harrold near Haverfordwest a surgeon charged a carpenter 13s. 6d. for a one-night visit. This represented roughly half the carpenter's weekly wage.[230] The court reduced the fee to 5s.

George Howell, the London radical politician and foreman-bricklayer, was earning £2. 10s. a week in the first three months of 1868. In that period he spent £1. 10s. on medicines for his sick son, or equal to one week's full housekeeping money.[231] His total savings for 1867 had been £6. Shortly after, he accepted a secret subsidy from the Liberal Party – an act for which he has been criticised by historians. In the mid-1870s at Wellington, near Hereford, a surgeon sued for a fee of £12. 15s. for treating the fever-stricken family of Woodhouse, an 'ordinary labouring man', at the rate of 3s. a visit plus 1s. travel. The judge upheld the charge as fair, to the *Lancet*'s gratification. This probably represented one-quarter of Woodhouse's annual income.[232] Similarly, in the 1890s the surgeon's fee for a 'minor operation' on a 'clerk . . . in lodgings' was 20 guineas, a special reduction from the usual 60-80. This represented an appalling sum to a man who was probably not insured, on an annual income of about £70.[233]

Pharmacists' fees were also hurdles for the working and lower middle classes. Doctors who gave 'free advice' to poor clients recouped by directing their scripts to particular chemists with whom they were in partnership. These medicines in the 1850s cost 4s. 6d. instead of the usual 6d.-9d.[234] By the 1870s, as the opportunities for adulteration lessened, chemists' charges in London had become 'so exorbitant as to render it useless to give a prescription to any even moderately poor person'. A reporter from the *Globe* took round two simple everyday prescriptions, for two compound rhubarb pills, and for a mixture containing 24 drops of sulphuric acid, 1½ ounces of syrup of acid, 1½ ounces of syrup of poppies and 8 ounces of water. The estimated real cost of the pills, mixture, box and bottle was 5d. altogether. The reporter

tried chemists' shops from the East End to the West End 'and a reduction from the price first demanded was in nearly every case asked and
obtained, on the score of the poverty of the sick person'. Yet the prices
actually paid ranged from 8*d*. in the East End to 3*s*. in the West End.
The prescription required the medicine to be renewed three times
weekly. The total outlay would have been prohibitive for families outside the West End.[235] Below this level, families who did not wish to
become paupers, or who could not obtain free treatment or even meet
the charges of a 'sixpenny' GP, probably went without. In Bolton during
the depression of 1842, a family comprising a man, wife and four
children, receiving 26*s*. 6*d*. a week, spent only 4*d*. a week on 'medicine
and attendance'.[236] Probably the expenditure covered penny opiates,
and no 'attendance'. In 1864 'An Old Practitioner' remarked that agricultural labourers, 'even those on 16*s*. a week . . . [could] not keep a
doctor'. He proposed a special low fee of about 1*s*. 6*d*. for a total treatment: it was more than the doctor would get if they went untreated or
turned to a local wise woman, or if they became pauper patients.[237]

Among the higher ranks, the more rapacious of the doctors visited as
often as was seemly and charged as high as they dared. We have rather
more evidence about this area because the doctors' lawyer-patients
frequently challenged their bills in court. At Shrewsbury in 1842, Mr
Keate, a practitioner of 15 years' standing, attended a wealthy man (he
left £14,000 at the conclusion of Keate's ministrations) and charged the
estate £97. 15*s*. 6*d*. for six months' attendance and medicines. Keate
kept no proper records and could not prove his claim, but the jury
awarded him the money.[238] In London in 1845 Mr Baker visited a half-
pay captain 437 times over what was apparently a period of a few
months. Baker's bill, after his treatment had failed and the captain
sought other advice, was £193, for visits at 7*s*. 6*d*. and medicines at £13.
The captain protested against the number of visits, and the jury decided
to cut the 7*s*. 6*d*. to 5*s*.[239] Mr Cochrane charged and received £100 for
crushing a stone in the bladder of a rich old man in Wickham Market in
Suffolk in 1858. Ten years later Dr Fookes, a specialist in rheumatism
and paralysis, got 300 guineas for a year's unsuccessful treatment of a
solicitor.[240]

The doctors' reference group was the legal profession. They saw the
lawyers as having achieved the standing and income that they still lacked.
The lawyers' better-controlled entry to their profession excluded riff-
raff. The fashionable surgeon, Richard Quain, who married a viscountess
and left £75,000 in 1887, lamented in the late 1870s that underbred
persons could so easily enter medicine and remain in it. After 1858 a

doctor paid £5 on registration and nothing more, whereas a lawyer paid £80 on his first admission to articles, £35 when admitted as a solicitor and up to £9 annually for his licence to practise. A barrister, looking to becoming a gentleman and mixing with gentlemen, had to possess sufficient private means to cover his education and lean early days at the bar. A GP, by contrast, could start with less and begin earning immediately: he had no incentive to further professional self-improvement.[241] An attorney's lowest fee was 3*s*. 4*d*.; a Poor Law medical officer sometimes received one penny a case and 'sixpennys' did little better. Professional ethics prohibited lawyers from dispensing advice gratis; 'foolish' medical tradition led doctors to provide it often. Lawyers engaged by charitable organisations always sought and took their fee; hospital doctors did the opposite. The overcrowding of medicine by persons of humble origin was partly the outcome of the unlimited right of GPs to take apprentices. A solicitor was restricted under a law obtained by the lawyers themselves to two apprentices. Attempts by unqualified persons to practise law were severely punished; unqualified persons practised medicine with impunity.[242]

The doctors' standing was poor in relation to the Church, too. Prison chaplains, at between £100 and £300 a year in the provinces, were generally receiving twice the salary of parish surgeons: at Lincoln Gaol it was £200 against £25. Governors of gaols, who were never chosen from the medical profession, received about twice the chaplains' salaries.[243] The clergy were also rivals in the field of treatment. In the countryside, especially in Scotland and Wales where doctors were scarce and, before 1834, Poor Law medicine rare or non-existent, the local clergy, like the Reverend Sydney Smith at Foston, near York, had supplied the poor with nostrums, wine and advice. The doctors waged an unrelenting campaign to force the clergy from the field. By the 1860s they had largely succeeded and the nagging anti-clericalism that marks medical comment in the earlier part of the century died away. None the less there were still fastnesses, villages like Langtoft in the Yorkshire Wolds, for example, where the vicar attended 'all ordinary cases', made poultices and lanced abscesses in 1900.[244]

The lawyers' professional advantages resulted from their superior connections with the aristocracy and parliament. The doctors never had more than two or three representatives in the Commons and, for most of the century, none in the Lords. Chief Justice Lord Denman was the son of an *accoucheur*, but he had turned to the law to better himself. In 1872 Dr William Gull received a baronetcy after successfully tending the Prince of Wales, and Sir William Jenner a KCB, but neither was made a privy councillor, as equivalent lawyers of their distinction would have been. Medicine had no great figurehead among the chiefs of state, as did the law and the Church.[245] The government nominated aristocrats and lawyers to the Board of Health between 1848 and 1854 but ignored the claims of medical men. This continuing slight, after the fiasco of the cholera committee of 1831-2 and the Poor Law Commission, bred in GPs an undying hatred of central government interference in medicine. Only in 1892, when Sir Walter Foster was appointed parliamentary secretary to the Local Government Board, did the doctors have one of their number at ministerial level. Even when Lister was created a peer in 1897 at least one aristocrat expostulated because a mere sawbones had been placed among them. A month previously, for 5 guineas Lister had performed a digital exploration of the noble marquis's rectum.[246] The Lords need not have worried. Lister emerged as a rabid Tory.

'Medicine is not looked upon as the profession of a gentleman', 'Self-Respect' lamented in 1858; doctors 'are not visitable . . . our wives are not visitable . . . the great body of the profession is looked upon by the upper classes as about a shade better than respectable tradespeople'.[247] Army and navy surgeons were frequently snubbed by their brother officers. The English Club at Rome excluded doctors in the 1840s. In 1850 the ladies' committee of the newly opened Establishment for Gentlewomen during Illness, in Chandos Street, Cavendish Square, ruled that GPs were to report on their cases to the committee and not to the senior medical officers, while consultants (unpaid) were only to be summoned by the ladies 'in their discretion'.[248] Doctors rarely became magistrates. In 1850 one local gentleman discussed with Lord Hatherton possible names for the bench in the Black Country. They did not consider GPs and they eliminated one possible nominee because he did not 'move in Society higher than those who generally surround the Middle Class table at Dr Day's'.[249] Novelists in the first half of the century portrayed doctors as ignorant, coarse and grasping: Dickens' Jobling and Parker Peps, Lord Lytton's Squills, Thackeray's Sir Lapin Warren, Trollope's Fillgrave and Rerechild, and Scott's Gideon Gray. Surgeons still engaged in public fisticuffs in the 1850s.[250]

'Self-Respect' must have been gladdened by developments during the 1860s. Deputations of local worthies began to present retiring GPs with writing desks, sets of silver plate and engraved epergnes. Charity hospitals had already begun to allow doctors a stronger voice on policy. Consultants began in the 1860s to establish 'country residences' and presumably improved their acquaintance.[251] At the same time the spread of trained nurses enabled lowly GPs to renounce as unprofessional certain unpleasant jobs they had hitherto performed. As one surgeon remarked in 1864 during a dispute over who was to give an enema: it was no more his task

> than it [was] his duty to administer the medicine he . . . sent . . . or to make or apply a mustard plaster . . . to apply leeches and to attend to their bites; to draw breasts; or to perform any of the other thousand obvious duties of the nurse.[252]

In fiction too the doctors' stocks were rising. Mrs Oliphant's Dr Marjoribanks (1866) is a wealthy, leisured cultivated man at the top with local gentry and retired generals of Carlingford society, although he has somewhat obscure Scottish origins and retains links with some not well-off and not completely genteel relatives. By the 1890s it is nothing untoward that a gentleman of independent means like Sherlock Holmes should have a Scottish doctor as his confidant. In 1890 a man qualified both in medicine and dentistry asked the *BMJ* whether he should call upon the other doctors and dentists in the district where he proposed to practise. The ambiguities in his question made the *BMJ* writer careful to spell out the rules: if the inquirer intended to practise only as a doctor he must not call on the dentists and must not perform even occasional dentistry. If he proposed to do only dentistry he must leave his card only with the dentists.[253]

The profession had so closed ranks that when in 1890 Dr J.B. Russell, the irrepressible MOH for Glasgow, informed the city sanitary committee and thereby the newspapers about gross incompetence in diagnosis and management during a typhus outbreak, his colleagues were furious. They appealed to instant 'custom' and facile 'ethics' to defend their irresponsibility. Russell's action was, Dr Hamilton said, 'a very glaring transgression . . . of the most fundamental professional ethics'. Dr Erskine thought that 'the most objectionable thing . . . was the way in which this information had been brought before the public. Dr Russell's report should have been read before a medical society; the public were not qualified to judge medical practitioners.' The row continued for a year and ended with Russell being censured by his colleagues.[254] Doctors never acquired the complacent confidence of their legal brethren. When in 1898 the loftily conservative *Saturday Review* referred to medical students as 'cads' possessing a 'maximum of ill-breeding with a minimum of sobriety', the *Lancet* editors were still insecure enough to notice the provocation and to claim that doctors belonged to the 'same class as . . . the church, the navy and army, the law, literature, science and journalism'.[255]

The quest for respectability served to narrow clinical practice and the medical imagination. Bakery cobwebs had been demonstrably successful as a styptic on wounds and as an aid to quick, sound healing; doctors, especially army and navy surgeons, had used them as such. But by 1860 medical resort to cobwebs had become an unprofessional resort to folk mummery. The common people continued to use them, despite the doctors. In 1861 a poor man came to Dr Strachan of Dollar in Clackmannan to have his ulcerated legs treated. 'He had been at many doctors, and had tried all the Holloway's ointments and other infallible remedies.' Strachan found that he was half-starved and

> with great difficulty . . . got him a larger allowance from the poor's funds, and some of his friends assisted him . . . As soon as the system got into good condition the ulcers began to heal and . . . the poor man was restored and fitted for his work.

Six months later Strachan asked him how he was getting on.

> Weel, doctor, I maun tell you what it was that cured my legs, and it will maybe be usefu' to ither folk. It was just moose wels [spider's webs]. Jenny Donald advised me to try them, and they cured my legs at once.

Had the procedure continued as part of the orthodox armoury, recognition of the potentialities of penicillin might have come earlier in this century.[256]

Acupuncture was occasionally used in the first half of the century to relieve lumbago, rheumatism, oedema of the legs and trismus (spasm of the jaw muscle, an early symptom of tetanus), after the conventional aperients, blisters and bleedings had failed. It does not appear to have been used as an anaesthetic in surgery. The practice had been known in Europe since the seventeenth century. By the nineteenth century in Britain it was regarded as unorthodox and it was not formally taught in hospitals (except by the great Robert Graves in Dublin): presumably apprentices picked it up from those GPs who independently practised it, some of whom had learned it in France.[257] The procedure varied greatly and was completely empirical. Some practitioners used triangular glovers' needles, others used silver round ones, some drove the needles inches deep, others, ¼ inch; the needles were sometimes driven in at the seat of the pain, on other occasions they were spaced along the limb.[258]

In the 1820s acupuncture had been taken up by Dr John Elliotson at St Thomas's Hospital. He was also later to embrace mesmerism as a diagnostic aid. His subsequent disgrace after the mesmerism frauds in 1838 (his mediums, the Okey sisters, were deceiving him and were exposed by a group of radical, rationalistic doctors, led by Thomas Wakley probably helped discredit acupuncture and drive it further underground as a pseudo-scientific procedure.[259] In 1837-8 doctors were still reporting good results with acupuncture in cases of sciatica and hydrocele, but by 1842 Mr Toogood Downing was condescendingly dismissing Chinese acupuncture as primitive superstition.[260] None the less acupunture continued on the Continent and British doctors with foreign experience still resorted to it, after customary procedures brought no alleviation. But officially acupuncture did not exist. By 1860 'Trocar' was asking publicly how acupunture was performed.[261] Yet it persisted, if unheralded. Lister used it, probably in the 1860s. In 1871 Mr T. Pridgin Teale reported that although acupuncture was 'almost forgotten' it was 'still commonly used in the Leeds Infirmary' to relieve muscular disability and pain.[262] Research in hospital records might well reveal similar situations elsewhere. However, by 1889 one prominent surgeon was confusing acupuncture with puncturing to draw off pus and it seems really to have been passing into oblivion. The exceptionally well informed William Osler was recommending it in 1892 at Johns Hopkins Medical School but apparently without effect. The procedure has since been so forgotten that a recent historian of acupuncture described it as 'new' in Britain.[263]

Given acupuncture's good results in cases of rheumatism, why did it fall from sight? Apart from Elliotson's fatal patronage, its similarity to quack medical galvanism cannot have helped it with the orthodox, who preferred a comfortable static conception of body function to venturing empirically among allegedly dynamic body forces which no one understood. From the 1880s the keen young men who embraced germ theory would have found acupuncture unspecific and non-experimental. Dr Ogier Ward in 1858 preferred an explanation complementary to these two hypotheses and probably more valid. He had used acupuncture with great effect on patients with neuralgic and rheumatic pains but he implied that he, like other practitioners, had had to abandon it because of resistance from patients. They feared the pain and found it difficult 'to believe so trifling an operation can produce such powerful effects'.[264] Among the common people cobweb styptic and antisepsis continued because of its foundation in folk medicine: acupuncture had no folk medical tradition to sustain it.

Fear of the quackery taint also kept GPs aloof from chiropody. Corn doctors deserved their reputation of being avaricious crooks. Dr Wolff, an itinerant chiropodist in the 1840s, charged £6 a treatment. He told patients that corns grew on the feet bones in the manner that leaves proliferated on twigs. He could extract and 'show' up to 25 hitherto unperceived corns from a single foot, at 2s. 6d. each. The minimum charge for fashionable patients in the 1850s was £1.1s. One itinerant worked in Hull for three months in 1846 and took about 10 guineas each day.[265] Those who could not or would not pay the tariff used ivy leaves soaked in vinegar. A leaf was wrapped over the corn each day. Gradually the corn, it was said, would disappear.[266]

Spectacles were commonly sold by itinerants at fairs. This association inhibited respectable doctors from prescribing and supplying them, although the lower ranks continued to do so into the twentieth century. The practice finally became 'unethical' about 1908 and the field was left to the paramedical opticians.[267]

Just when the profession was becoming respectable in the late 1850s and ready at last to achieve a Medical Act designed in its interests, women sought to join it. The earlier bantering dismissals of allegedly unskilful female practitioners now became fearful rebuffs on moral grounds. Prudery and physiological determinism were now invoked to reassure the faithful. Female students' attendance at the dissecting table or at the lock wards of a hospital would 'violate every feeling of decency and propriety . . . in men having mothers and sisters, for whose sex they wish to return respect'. Such coarsened women could have no 'social position' if single, and if married they must necessarily neglect their husbands and children and thereby lose caste.[268]

'Foolish virgins' who wanted to become doctors outraged 'the simple, pre-ordained law of Nature'. They were neither physically nor mentally 'stern' enough to cope with the endless medical round. Only a man could 'brave . . . the revolting scenes of childbirth'.[269] As the Obstetrical Society explained in 1875 after again rejecting female candidates, women were 'not by nature qualified to make good midwifery practitioners'. The work was arduous and required firmness of mind. Only 'vulgar females' would be attracted to it and they would only 'lower the profession'.[270] Woman's admirable character and delicate sensibility perfectly equipped her for home nursing as the ' "handmaids" of doctors', who

With lenient arts extend a mother's breath,
Make languor smile, or smooth the bed of death.

After all, women were not besieging the law or the Church.

Despite the doctors' opposition, the 'nasty Yankee invasion' began in 1859 with American-trained women led by Dr Elizabeth Blackwell. She began lecturing on 'Physiology and its applications to the wants and duties of women' at the Marylebone Literary Institution. The *Lancet* reporter did not attend the lectures but he knew they must be worthless because of the 'meagreness and imperfections which must mark the physiological protusions [*sic*] of a lady'.[271]

The higher ranks of the profession in the teaching hospitals were less uniformly hostile than the GPs and obstetricians. In 1860 the authorities at the Middlesex Hospital permitted Miss Elizabeth Garrett to take courses in materia medica. But when she applied to enter the anatomy and physiology courses a row erupted. The students protested that 'no woman [ought to] . . . hear discussions of organs etc. unfit for a mixed audience'. They petitioned their lecturers, a majority of whom acquiesced, and Miss Garrett's enrolment was terminated. She then applied to the London Hospital, but there the staff decided unanimously against admitting her. She was later excluded from the universities of Edinburgh and St Andrews, again mainly at the instigation of students.[272] Left to themselves, the teachers would have given in fairly quickly. In 1862 the College of Physicians of Edinburgh and the Senate of the University of London decided, by very narrow majorities, against admitting women.[273]

The hard-line opponents used the threat of student unrest to frighten waverers. The staff at Edinburgh quietly decided to admit women in 1870 but again the students took the offensive by physically stopping the women, Sophia Jex-Blake among them, from entering the lecture theatres. The students later mobbed the women in the street.[274]

The women's champion was the great Dr C.R. Drysdale, who supported their cause throughout. In 1868 he sought their admission to the Farrington General Dispensary and Lying-in Hospital, with which he was associated, but was thwarted by his colleagues.[275] Still, the major barrier of registration had been breached in 1858 when Dr Elizabeth Blackwell was admitted by virtue of holding a diploma from the Irish College of Physicians. Once the women discovered that possession of the Irish diploma meant that the Society of Apothecaries could not refuse their examination, the problems of finding somewhere to train became easier, although the obstacles to gaining experience in anatomy and physiology remained serious and hurt their prospects as future surgeons. By 1866 Dr Garrett had her own dispensary for women and children in Marylebone. By the mid-1880s her colleagues had opened similar institutions in Edinburgh, Bristol, Leeds, Birmingham and

Manchester.[276] None the less, their numbers remained small during the nineteenth century (see Table 5.12) (indeed their numbers are still disproportionately small) and their practice was largely confined — partly by necessity, partly by choice — to women and children. This was a splendid advance, especially for female patients, but it had the unfortunate effect of limiting the women's general influence in medicine. Perhaps, too, it bore out the critics' prediction that male patients would not trust them.

Table 5.12: Numbers of Female Doctors (England and Wales)

8 in 1871
25 in 1881
101 in 1891
212 in 1901
477 in 1911

Source: 'Physician and Surgeon, General Practitioner' — Female — as reported in census returns.

5. WORKHOUSE HEALTH

The abatement of medical radicalism lost the workhouse inmates their one chance of amelioration. The doctors were the one organised group with both the information and power to create the social knowledge which might have moved the government and the guardians. The metropolitan doctors did cause a flurry in the mid-1860s when the *Lancet* commission exposed conditions in London workhouses, but thereafter the majority of doctors increasingly drew their income and self-esteem from the ratepaying classes, while the minority who tended the paupers identified themselves with their professional colleagues and private patrons and remained uncommitted to the poor. As the big workhouses were built and rebuilt they increasingly became unknown to the outside world, while the outside world of novelists, journalists and social critics was content not to know. Enlightenment came only from a new breed of historically minded non-medical investigators, Charles Booth, Miss B.L. Hutchens and Sidney and Beatrice Webb.

The New Poor Law and its workhouses had not been designed to provide for aged paupers. They must have comprised a large proportion of both indoor and outdoor paupers before 1834, yet Chadwick's questionnaires ignored them. Between 1830 and 1848 28 per cent of the deaths at ages over 50 in St Bride's parish occurred in the work-house, about one-third of them from 'debility, decay or decline'.[277] The exclusion of the 'able-bodied' women and dependent children seems to have become progressively stricter through the middle years of the century, as separate boarding-out establishments were built for the children and the women were forced on to outdoor relief. Indeed, the costs incurred in building workhouses apparently compelled econo-mies elsewhere. In London even before the 24 new workhouses were built after the Metropolitan Poor Act the workhouses had become effectively barracks for the infirm and closets for the dying. In 1865 the *Lancet* commissioners found over 85 per cent of inmates to be 'infirm'. Nearly all of them were 'permanents', leading a 'vegetable' existence. A parliamentary return of 1861 had shown that the largest single group of adult impotent 'permanents' suffered from 'senility' and that the majority of them had been incarcerated for at least 10 years. The next-largest group comprised the insane.[278]

After 1871-2 the proportion of old and infirm inmates increased to about 70 per cent as the number of younger 'able-bodied' paupers was further diminished by administrative action.[279] During these years James Stansfeld, the responsible Minister, abetted W.E. Gladstone, Robert Lowe, Chadwick, Florence Nightingale and his permanent officials in converting the Poor Law Board into the Local Government Board. The Public Health Department of the Privy Council was also absorbed into the division of the new Board. Henceforth health officers were subject to the parsimonious bureaucrats of the LGB, R.B. Caine, John Lambert and Henry Fleming. At LGB meetings Fleming and Lambert now sat next to their Minister, while the medical officer, Sir John Simon, sat at the end of the room. G.J. Goschen, Stansfeld's predecessor, had excluded Fleming and Lambert from meetings. Simon himself had been tight-fisted and hard in Poor Law matters, but he was prodigal compared with Lambert and company, with the Treasury bearing on them. Their purpose, expressed in their Public Health Act of 1872, was to reduce expenditure by imposing more rigorous Poor Law rules for relief and increasing responsibility on to local guardians, whom they could trust to be thrifty.[280]

Goschen in 1870 had already begun an austerity drive and Stansfeld took it up enthusiastically. Between 1870 and 1873 the number of paupers in England and Wales was cut by 18½ per cent, or 194,000. The great majority of these were outdoor paupers, 183,000, but some-how the guardians, pressed by the LGB 'to a more vigilant administra-tion', found 11,000 paupers whom they dismissed. The guardians were keenest in the north; there they eliminated paupers at twice the rate of the rest of the country. The drive was directed against 'vagrants', but these, as always, despite the Commissions' and LGB propaganda, had formed a minute proportion of the pauper class.[281] In fact the number of vagrant paupers rose during the 1870s. The pruning was done simply by reclassifying infirm as 'able-bodied' — about 100,000 of them between 1871 and 1877, and sending children out to boarding establishments, foster homes and work. At some places, Liverpool for instance, the healthy marriage partner of an aged senile person, who formerly commonly also entered the workhouse when the senile one was received, was now excluded. Over all, the Liverpool guardians proudly reduced their costs by nearly 100 per cent between 1871 and 1872: the numbers of 'outdoor sick' were reduced by the same proportion.[282]

The proportion of nominally able-bodied inmates remained at between 13 per cent and 18 per cent until 1905.[283] It is not surprising, although contemporaries seem not to have noticed it, that this savage reduction in Poor Law relief coincided with the new pressure on the out-patient wards at hospitals, new pressure on private charities and the rise of monitoring bodies such as the Charity Organization Society. True to the principle of 1834, Goschen, Stansfeld and Lambert believed against all the evidence that poverty could be diminished by forcing able-bodied loafers into a free labour market. Their solution was no solution: it merely shifted the problem and temporarily made it less obvious. In the 1880s the problem surfaced again as 'unemployment', and in the 1890s as 'destitution and old age'. At Manchester Township Workhouse in 1894 over half the male inmates over 65 had previously dwelt in common lodging-houses and vagrant wards.[284] By 1912 there were more people in workhouses than ever before. Only when the ruling classes had to reorganise the economy during the First World War did the number drop decisively — by 100,000. But the reorganisation was temporary. By 1926 over a quarter of a million were back in workhouses and 2½ million were on out-relief.[285]

Charles Booth's investigations in the late 1880s and 1890s finally revealed the extent of deprivation among the old and made it into social knowledge. He calculated in 1894 that 30 per cent of all persons over 65 were paupers. The Royal Commission on the Aged Poor in the following year estimated it at over 40 per cent. (The LGB had been careful, like the Poor Law Commission before it, not to collect statistics by age group which might have shown this.) 'The national conscience', Booth wrote, 'has not realized how the old live.'[286] The proportion of aged paupers was reported as highest in the eastern agricultural counties and lowest in the industrial north. The Reverend W.J. Blackley obtained returns in 1895 from clergy in 70 rural parishes spread through the country which showed that since 1884 42 per cent of persons aged 60 or above had been buried as paupers.[287] Country people had greater longevity, resulting probably from their relative isolation from killing infectious diseases and freedom from major disabling accidents, together perhaps with better nutrition than their urban counterparts, but they were less well paid and less able to save against old age. Friendly societies and the Post Office Savings Department had failed to build effective superannuation schemes. The trade unions had done best at superannuation but their funds were too limited to provide full coverage.

However, in terms of the proportion of inmates who were aged and infirm, rural workhouses were indistinguishable from urban ones. Cardiff had above 50 per cent over 60, Birmingham about 40 per cent, Enfield 72 per cent, King's Norton (Warwickshire) 50 per cent, while rural workhouses such as Okehampton (Devon), Kendal (Westmorland), Newhaven (Sussex), Ashby-de-La-Zouch (Leicestershire) and Machynlleth (Montgomeryshire) each had about 50 per cent.[288]

The poor still called the workhouses the Bastilles in the 1890s and in one sense the name was more apt than they knew. At Newhaven over half the inmates had had no visitors in the twelve months before 1908; at Okehampton, 40 per cent had had no visitors; at Kendal and Machynlleth almost 80 per cent; while at King's Norton, 351 of the 460 aged inmates had no visitors and 104 'never' went out.[289]

In the 1880s an urban workhouse surgeon had listed their main infirmities as 'chronic ulcers, chronic bronchitis, chronic gout, chronic rheumatoid arthritis, forms of paralysis in old people, and . . . bed-ridden . . . senile decay'. In 1909 Dr McVail added diarrhoea and heart disease. These were the incurable masses the hospital authorities refused to treat. Already in the 1890s, the London workhouses provided nearly three times as many beds as the hospitals.[290]

Many more aged people died in workhouses and workhouse infirmaries than in hospitals. In 1893 about 27 per cent of all reported deaths in London occurred in institutions, and half of these occurred in workhouses and workhouse infirmaries. The voluntary hospitals had only 9.6 per cent of the deaths. In Bristol 20 per cent of all deaths occurred in the workhouses and in Liverpool and Manchester 19 per cent. The poorer the place, the higher the percentage of deaths in the workhouse: Stepney 36 per cent against Hampstead 8.4 per cent, and Westminster

31.6 per cent against Woolwich 14 per cent. In 1902 the deaths in London workhouses and workhouse infirmaries equalled the total deaths in all the voluntary hospitals in England and Wales.[291]

The plight of the overburdened workhouse infirmaries was ignored by the medical profession, by nearly all charitable organisations and by the LGB. The doctors' main concern was to ensure that the workhouses did not become teaching institutions (one repeated objection was that they were sited too inconveniently for 'the leading consulting physicians and surgeons to attend') and to protect their investment in their profession. In 1866 St George's Hospital had beds for 350 patients. The hospital was staffed by four consultant surgeons and four consultant physicians, who were each supposed to visit three times a week, two resident apothecaries, three resident house surgeons and one dresser for each surgeon. There were also the paid nurses and scrubbers. The Shoreditch Workhouse infirmary contained 220 'sick', 140 'insane, epileptic and imbecile' and 240 'other inmates'. It was staffed by one non-resident medical officer at £120 a year. He was supposed to visit for two hours each morning, private practice permitting, 'during which he [had] to perform the combined duties of medical officer, dietist and dispenser'. There was no trained nurse and no night nursing. The patients were simply locked in their wards. Conditions were almost unchanged in the 1890s. The Paddington Workhouse infirmary had the same number of patients as St Mary's Hospital. St Mary's had 9 resident and 9 visiting doctors, and students to help. Paddington Workhouse had 3 residents, no visiting doctors and no students.[292] Moreover, the paralysed and 'nervous' cases required more time and nursing than the surgical and medical cases in the hospital.

In theory the medical officer was supposed amongst other duties to examine every case on admission, perform vaccinations, classify the sick, perform surgical operations, report defects in sanitary arrangements in the building, keep his medical relief book, and compile annual lists of the sick. In practice he rushed through as much as he could in the time he allowed himself. Very few kept their books up to date. Medical case-records were 'almost non-existent' in 1908, partly, as a doctor explained, because 'so many [were] old, chronic cases' and therefore uninteresting. Dr St J.T. Clarke of the Leicester Workhouse was commended in the early 1870s because he was 'one of the few officers who present an annual report'. (The rules required annual reports.) When the visionary Dr B.W. Richardson proposed in 1869 that Poor Law medical officers gratuitously contribute weekly returns towards a national register of morbidity he was icily rebuffed. After all, no precise rules about the duties of the medical officer, his hours, procedures or records were ever issued by the Poor Law Commissioners on the Local Government Board.[293]

Mr Baldwyn Fleming, a general inspector from the LGB, timed officers in several West County and Surrey workhouses in 1908. He found that they were 'rarely there more than half an hour, and usually "only a few minutes", which they mostly spent with the master and matron. They had no time to examine inmates bodily.'[294] In 1895 an old man in the Stepney Workhouse was taken ill on a Friday and died 'from syncope' on the following Monday. He received no medical attention, although a succession of workhouse inmates was sent to bring the non-resident medical officer. The old man was finally seen by the medical officer's assistant on the Monday, but he had to wait another 4 hours before the assistant got round to prescribing medicine. This was then supplied from a stock 'already made up and ready for giving out'. Another case indicates the degree of attention that the medical officer and the local magistracy thought necessary. An old woman died in the Southport Workhouse, Lancashire, in 1886. Friends of the deceased alleged that the medical officer had been negligent and had not visited her as frequently as her case required. Mr Moore, the Poor Law surgeon, explained death was general decay, accelerated by bed-sores, and the shock of the accident (the old woman had been 'run over' while outside the workhouse), and that the case being of a kind 'requiring nursing, etc., more than medical aid, the patient had been seen quite as often as was . . . needed'.[295]

The basic confusion of function in the workhouse system is vividly illustrated by the Bethnal Green infirmary in the 1890s. Among 335 female inmates, there were 65 over 80, 10 totally blind and 26 crippled, and another 100 infirm, yet there was only one nurse, whose title and function was 'the labour mistress'. She was appointed 'for the elimination of that perennial presence, the sturdy beggar' — of whom there were none. Meanwhile it was 'utterly impossible for this one person to keep the women clean and wholesome'.[296]

The rules about nursing in workhouses were few and vague. In 1847 the General Consolidated Order recognised the use of paupers as nurses to their fellows, both indoor and outdoor. The sole direction about their qualifications required that if they were to be paid they should be able to read 'written directions upon the medicines'. In 1865 a second circular ordered the employment of paid professional nurses and the discontinuance of nursing by paupers. In 1878-9 the LGB claimed that the transition was complete, yet by 1897 it was still ordering guardians to end pauper nursing and still not enforcing that order. Moreover, the guardians evaded the order by employing underpaid, improperly enrolled 'probationers'.[297]

The Order of 1847 allowed the master of the workhouse to employ the semi-able-bodied as nurses. They were cheap and biddable. They seem to have scrubbed and tidied competently enough but the dozens of accounts which reached print through court inquests suggest that workhouse nursing remained a harrowing compound of neglect and mindless cruelty. The cases which follow are a representative selection from one five-year period of better than usual reportage. Pauper nurse Brutton at Rotherhithe Workhouse infirmary in the 1860s used to beat and drug patients after getting at the infirmary opium supply. She specialised in dragging dying patients to the WCs and leaving them there. At Devonport Workhouse in 1868, the sole nurse for 180 patients was 70 and insane. She was 'most unkind' to them. In 1864 her predecessor had lifted an old patient roughly and broken her arm. The nurse had hidden it from the surgeon. When he discovered it the arm had mortified. Catherine Dawben, 'a sullen girl' and 'an imbecile', was a nurse at the Wigan Workhouse in 1868. In a case I can match with many others she was set to bath a seven-month-old infant; Dawben killed the child by pouring boiling water over it. She was acquitted at the Liverpool Assizes as unfit to plead. At Wigan, as in most workhouses, only the old and the imbecile were permitted to nurse: the rest were sent out to work or to oakum-picking and stone-breaking. One of the two nurses in the men's ward at Tavistock Workhouse in the late 1860s, for instance, was 73, and his partner was one-armed. On the demise of the one-armed nurse, his place was taken by an imbecile.[298]

There had been attempts since the 1860s, backed by Florence Nightingale, Dr Joseph Rogers, and Louisa Twining, the leader of the Workhouse Visiting Society, to introduce trained professional nurses from the respectable classes into the workhouses on the pattern of the nurses in the charity hospitals. A few heroines had accepted the call and made some impact, notably Agnes Jones, the workhouse nursing martyr, at Liverpool. But the movement remained weak. The LGB and the guardians begrudged the money and were unhelpful.[299] (Chadwick and the Poor Law Board had in 1855 already thwarted an attempt by Dr John Snow and others to supply trained nurses to outdoor paupers.) The nurses also loomed as a force which would upset existing arrangements and demand more expenditure. As a master of a workhouse in West Sussex warned his guardians: 'They defy the authority of the master and the matron, and find fault with everything.' In 1897 there were only 130 places on offer for trained nurses in the 700 workhouses of England and Wales. And the Workhouse Nursing Association had only 73 nurses to fill them.[300] Miss E. Julian, nursing matron of the Croydon Workhouse infirmary, attributed the shortage of trained nurses in 1899 to the 'loss of status, lack of adequate assistance, the monotonous home life, and uncongenial surroundings'. The 'popular idea' was, she said, that nurses in workhouses comprised 'those not refined enough to go into hospitals'.[301] The religious sisterhoods, for example, showed no interest in workhouse nursing. The general nursing associations also made difficulties by setting 200 beds as the minimum number for recognition as a training institution: only 10 per cent of workhouses had 200 beds.[302]

Workhouse infirmaries were, moreover, still dangerous places. The guardians and masters steadfastly resisted attempts at isolation of infectious cases. Special wards were not always fully occupied and were therefore a luxury. In the early 1890s many unions, like Dewsbury, still admitted smallpox cases to the general workhouse wards, even though the LGB had 'threatened' to order them 'to desist'. By 1905 only 32 of 695 unions had begun to isolate consumptives.[303] Not surprisingly, Louisa Twining's Workhouse Visiting Society remained 'unpopular among ladies'.[304] The Society did not gain permission from the LGB to visit at any time and to make suggestions to the LGB for new rules until 1893. Miss Twining's retrospect of her achievements, written in old age, in the 1890s, is too rosy.

The vagueness of the rules about nursing was but part of the general vagueness enveloping the administration of the aged poor. The Poor Law Commission's and LGB's control of them exhibits a resolute absence of mind. In 1836 the Commissioners first recognised their distinct existence by allowing people over 60 'something extra' in the dietaries. The Order of 1847 provided for classification of 'infirm' men and women and grouped the aged with the infirm. The medical officer was also permitted to 'recommend' food and nursing as part of relief, but he was not enabled to 'order' it until 1885.[305] There were no clear rules about the qualifications of the old for admission to the workhouse or about their treatment as inmates.

Medical men put people in the workhouse when they were no longer able to earn a living. They were also got 'rid of as cases' by doctors and relieving officers as an economy measure, on the theory that incurables cost less time and money inside than out. As Dr John Beddoe, of Clifton Workhouse, said, he lost valuable time in 'tracking them out in their garrets and hovels'.[306] The removal of a bedridden husband could also enable the wife to work, and thereby lessen the rates. Families with aged parents often welcomed their removal. They took up room that might otherwise be let.[307] Many liberal guardians defied the principles of 1834, the Commission and the LGB by giving relief in cash, for victuals and rent.[308] This too was saved when the old people were placed in the House.

Of course, the majority of old people among the working and upper classes lived out their lives, especially if they kept their health, in their own houses, or they resided among kin and servants who looked after them. At present we know very little about these matters and good evidence is not easy to find. I have emphasised the workhouse aspect of dealing with the aged partly because evidence about it is more immediately accessible but mainly because students of the Poor Law neglect it.

The old people feared the workhouse and sought to avoid incarceration. As workhouse infirmaries developed into separate buildings through the 1870s and 1880s the people began to distinguish them from the workhouse proper and were readier to enter them. There was, A.R. Jephcott of the Birmingham Trades Council told the Royal Commission on the Aged Poor, 'a stigma on one and not on the other'.[309] There was also a popular though unfounded notion that entry to the infirmary did not legally pauperise the patient. The LGB had ruled some years earlier that the infirmary was to have an entrance separate from that of the workhouse, but after numbers in the infirmaries grew during the early 1890s the guardians sought to stop the flow by compelling people to enter the workhouse formally before their removal to the infirmary. As Mr S.D. Fuller, the chairman of the Paddington Board of Guardians explained, 'it deters the sick from applying.' In practice, the cases in the infirmary beds were indistinguishable from those in the workhouse wards.[310]

On admission, the inmates were supposed to be bathed and thereafter were bathed once a month. The people were unused to body-washing and hated it. The water had usually to be carried and the nurses skimped it. At Bethnal Green the same water was used for each batch of newcomers.[311] After a fresh series of scaldings in the 1880s the LGB issued directions about the bathing procedure: the bath was to be filled with cold water and hot water was to be added, until the temperature was between 98° and 80°. But in 1909 Preston-Thomas, the LGB inspector, confirmed that 'many attendants in workhouses simply did not know how to bath' patients.[312] Verminous newcomers were usually fumigated with sulphur fumes. At Bolton Workhouse their clothes were put in the oven, immediately after the bread had been baked. The heat killed the fleas but the nits survived.[313] Sick patients, because they were not subject to the deterrence rules, were not always put into workhouse uniform. At Bethnal Green, for instance, while their own clothes were being washed or fumigated, they changed into the (unwashed and unfumigated) clothes discarded immediately before by those newcomers sent to the able-bodied wards.[314]

The rules had provided since 1847 for private bedrooms for couples over 60, but in practice they were separated and sent to the male and female wards. By 1895 only 200 couples were accommodated together in English and Welsh workhouses. Preston-Thomas alleged that aged husbands and wives were often glad to be separated, especially when one partner was infirm and the other tired of nursing him. Married quarters were rarely occupied in workhouses. Given the fear and loneliness of most inmates, this assertion looks implausible, especially as Preston-Thomas does not say whether many workhouses had married quarters.[315]

The wards of a typical metropolitan workhouse contained 24 to 30 beds arranged 17 inches apart in two rows. There was usually only one row of small windows, set high to prevent escape. Direct sunlight rarely penetrated. Most wards faced north, because the masters' and matrons' quarters occupied the southern frontage. The walls were painted half way up with 'drab' and the rest was whitewash. It was rare to have pictures or mottoes on the walls: they harboured vermin. Moreover, the walls of new workhouses were frequently made of 'rough irregularly set brick'. These could not be pierced easily, or cleaned. The bedsteads were iron by the 1860s and long enough; but the mattresses were a standard 4' 6". The mattresses were flock; only Paddington ran to horsehair. Each bed was supposed to have one sheet. But some workhouses did not provide any sheets and others, like St Pancras, 'rarely' changed them, even after smallpox cases had died in the bed. Each bed had a chamber pot under it; bedridden patients habitually washed their hands and faces in it. Normally there was one round towel provided for each 8 patients. There were no screens or bed-pulls for partially paralysed patients in the wards, and despite requests to the LGB for an order, no easy chairs. The benches had no backs. Marylebone was unique in having WCs that flushed efficiently. The rest, the *Lancet* man found, were 'horrible'. St Pancras Workhouse infirmary had one nightstool per ward. An observer in 1867 counted 37 people who used it in the night. The one pauper nurse for the ward was aged 78. Fireplaces, where they existed, even in 1908, were 'tiny'.[316]

Marland Workhouse near Rochdale was a representative economically run provincial institution in the 1870s. It had been built in 1864,
and was designed to contain 210 inmates, at two to a bed. In 1870
there were 194 paupers, not one able-bodied. Forty-seven of them were
imbeciles, mostly bedridden. Medicines were administered by paupers
who could not read. The diets ordered by the medical officer were
rarely provided. Infectious cases wandered at will through the wards.
There were few means of washing clothes, utensils or bodies. The institution's records were ill kept and some books were missing. In the
wards there were no shelves or cupboards. The medicines were kept in
unlabelled bottles, together with blacking and firewood, in a box. All
inmates urinated into a tub in the corner of each ward. The urine was
sold by the guardians for scouring cotton. (The corporation leased the
town public urinal for the same purpose.) The inmates had head sores
and the itch. 'All had been dosed with sulphur, brimstone and cod-liver
oil' for eight months but the scratching had not stopped. The medical
officer found this 'most distressing'. Diarrhoea was endemic. All the
milk was skimmed. There was no butter. Saturday was special pudding
day: suet and currants, 'as firm as a rock'. Monday was 'lobby' day:
'mutton and potatoes, frequently sour'. The lobby was retrieved from
Thursday's weekly meat dinner, after Friday's pie 'ten to one', that is
ten potatoes to one piece of meat, had been made from it. No other
vegetable but potatoes entered the House. All the food was steamed.
The piggery was next to the children's yard. The pigs were fed on what
the inmates could not eat and were in 'superb condition'. Of course, the
guardians and master were breaking the Poor Law Commission's rule
that pauper nurses had to be able to read. But the guardians effectively
met the Commission's complaint. They pointed out that the medical
officer never wrote prescriptions, and he did not need to, because the
only medicine in the unlabelled bottles was cod-liver oil, as the illiterate
nurses well knew. Indeed, the illiterate nurses only came to the Commission's notice because the master was charged in court with an assault
on a female inmate. But to the relief of the master and the Commission,
the court found that the master had suffered 'great provocation' and let
him off with a minimal fine.[317]

A small rural workhouse, such as Alderbury, near Salisbury, had 86
inmates, 23 of them 'sick' in 1868. They slept two to a bed. Female
venereal cases were allowed only coconut fibre mattresses, without
bedsteads or sheets. There were no wash-basins, and no ventilators in
the infectious wards. There was no paid nurse, and incontinent cases
were not supplied with a bed mackintosh. Mr Hawley, the Poor Law

Board inspector, reported 'perfect satisfaction' with the arrangements after his visit. The Sheffield Workhouse was old and ricketty with damp, uncovered stone floors. The guardians agreed in the late 1860s that a new one was required, but refused to build it because they did not wish to upset the ratepayers.[318]

Careful guardians refused to supply inmates with spectacles and ignored the LGB's mild suggestion that paupers be given regular dental treatment.[319] Fires were forbidden in the old men's ward at Chelsea in the 1880s. George Catch was the psychopathic master of a succession of London workhouses. As soon as he was removed from one house after some unusually blatant torture episode he was appointed to another house. The guardians found him and his wife, the matron, great economisers. At Lambeth he forbade the night porter to summon the relatives of any dying pauper between 9 p.m. and 6 a.m.[320] Dumbarton Workhouse still had no fires at night in 1898. The two night nurses, one 73 and the other an epileptic, slept in the kitchen, while the inmates were locked in their wards out of earshot.[321] At Toxteth in the 1880s bodies, after being left all night in the wards, were jammed into special small cut-price coffins in the mornings. Women's stays, in places where the guardians permitted them, were bought by contract, in a small range of sizes. The inmates were made to fit the stays. Menstruating women were forbidden fresh linen.[322]

Workhouse food was supplied on contract. In 1890 it was still never sampled for adulteration, despite findings in 1872-3 that 90 per cent of London workhouse milk was adulterated. James Fecit [*sic*], who supplied the West Derby Workhouse at Walton, was one of the first dealers to be prosecuted for this offence in 1890. In nearly all of the samples he had removed over half the cream and added up to 10 per cent water. He was fined £10.[323] The masters and matrons of workhouses were frequently caught further watering the milk, and the wine and spirits ordered for the patients. In 1875 the Liverpool Select Vestry let a contract for port wine for sick paupers at £16 per pipe, that is 10*d*. per bottle. They rejected other tenders at around the usual price of £28. Midst great merriment the 'lowest priced wine was selected as being the best'. One vestryman remarked that 'on one occasion we had, in consequence of feeling a little faint, tasted a drop of the port wine supplied to the workhouse patients', and that he did not recover from its effects for the remainder of the day.[324]

Drugs were similarly contracted for and were often of a similar quality. The cod-liver oil was bought cheap from manufacturers who had rejected it for retail sale because it was rancid. Even the peppermint water was made thin.[325] It can have given little relief when it was poured down the throats of patients suffering agonies of fever or rheumatism.

> Whatever my God ordains is right:
> He taketh thought for me;
> The cup that my physician gives
> No poisoned draught can be.[326]

This verse from Louisa Twining's *Readings for Visitors to Workhouses and Hospitals* must have reassured the lady callers more than the inmates.

In 1894 the LGB ordered that women in workhouses might be permitted to make their own tea. Guardians at Birmingham, Withington in Gloucestershire, Salford and elsewhere moved quickly to avert extravagance. At Birmingham the ration of 1¼ ounces of tea to every gallon of water was raised to a permissible 1½ ounces, and the accompanying 4 ounces of sugar was increased to a possible 5. The one ounce of salt put into every 15 ounces of pudding was raised to two ounces. The guardians discussed the possibility of introducing fish and cheese, but rejected the notion. The *Lancet* reporter thought that none the less the 'paupers ought to be . . . very satisfied'.[327] At Withington the guardians apparently decided to increase the amount of tea placed in the canvas bag and normally stewed for 4¼ minutes 'to get the full flavour'. At Salford the usual one ounce to one gallon ratio was also to be slightly improved. The move would slightly increase the cost of each brew from its present ¾*d*. Sugar was to be added, but no milk. The paupers were also to have 'buttered' bread, for the first time. In 1894 the guardians had thoughtfully snapped up 18,000 pounds of substandard margarine at 6*d*. per pound.[328]

Bad teeth were near universal among paupers. They had never known good teeth, but their condition was worsened by the refusal of most unions to supply dentures. The old people could not masticate the pea soup and salt puddings, quite apart from the inedibility of much of the stuff put before them. As Dr C.M. Jessop of Redhill Workhouse in Surrey remarked in 1896: 'workhouses, especially the well-run ones, had to keep pigs nearby to consume the leftovers from the pauper compulsory rations' because a LGB order prohibited the use of leftovers for the next meal. In 1868 the Poor Law Board, on the advice of its medical officer, Dr Markham, had rejected a suggestion that old people be given more tea and bread instead of pea soup and suet. On the other hand, five ounces of bread at each meal was too much for most old people. Chorlton Workhouse in the 1890s had a surplus of 80 pounds of food every day.[329] Lady John Manners had sought to grapple with the problem in 1885. She was opening a bazaar to raise funds for a chapel for the Melton Workhouse in Suffolk. She 'showed', the *Lancet* reported,

> how possible it is for a lady with all the means of comfort and luxury to put herself sympathetically into the place of the inmates of a workhouse, and, as it were, feel their loneliness, their hopelessness, and the dreary monotony of their lives. It is the virtue of such sympathy as that of Lady John Manners that it does not evaporate in mere words and sentiments; it takes a practical form. One of the very last things that would occur to mere benevolent dreamers is the condition of old toothless people in workhouses, and their difficulties with a piece of tough meat, which often means that they go almost dinnerless. . . . Lady John Manners has given kindly thought to the case of poor paupers who have indifferent or inadequate teeth, and who cannot hope to be helped by a fashionable dentist. . . . She proposes the more systematic introduction of mincing machines to do the work of teeth for them.[330]

Some middle-class well-wishers and guardians were generous and some were both generous and concerned. But many concerned guardians were preoccupied with propelling the feckless paupers upwards to independence and saving the rates. Others, possibly the majority in rural unions and slum districts, were small farmers and tradesmen who were at once careful of the rates, intermittently generous, but confined by their own crude expectations of daily work and cleanliness. So far as I have found, with one exception, they reveal that they were rather pleased with themselves for having gained office and being permitted to order other people's lives, and honestly but complacently puzzled that paupers should have allowed themselves to sink into poverty.

The Wisbech guardians in Cambridgeshire were among the generous ones. Around 1883-4 they defied the LGB and spent 3s. 3d. on toys for the workhouse children. The LGB lawyers had previously ruled that expenditure on toys or entertainment was prohibited by the New Poor Law and subsequent Poor Law Acts. The President of the LGB, Sir Charles Dilke, also defied his officials and upheld the expenditure, thereby apparently allowing the guardians to escape retribution.[331]

On the other hand, the LGB, as I have already suggested, was slow to intervene when local guardians defied an order to spend money. In 1885 the LGB reiterated the order that couples over 60 might live together in workhouses, but it made no attempt to ensure that the order was obeyed. Similarly, the Board ordered in 1892 that inmates might be allowed tobacco and snuff, either by purchase or by gift from the guardians. Some guardians, at least, simply ignored the innovation.[332]

The obsession with economy which had characterised the measures of 1834 continued through the century. Albert Pell, MP and his fellow guardians at both Brixworth, Northamptonshire and St George-in-the-East (Pell, like Chadwick, was preoccupied by the incendiarism of 1830 and the need for local control) instilled self-help by simply abolishing outdoor relief: in 1871 there were 381 cases and in 1881 there was none. He and his friends also cut medical relief for indoor sick paupers. Pell's coadjutor, Canon W. Bury, boasted in 1895 that the abolition of medical relief had made 'medical clubs universal throughout the Union'. According to Bury, 'general prosperity [had] increased'. Sidney Ward, a collector for the Liverpool Friendly Society and a member of the Salvation Army, had a different view. The Brixworth people now had to walk 6 miles to Northampton to get relief. The aged poor, 'forced away from friends and furniture' into the Northampton Workhouse, died earlier than they would have done, Ward believed, at home in Brixworth on outdoor relief. The Canon provided a 'refutation' of Ward's allegations. But none of Ward's claims is shown to be false and Bury adds details which only confirm them. The guardians never met formally. Applications for relief were secretly decided by Bury and the 'almoner' who turns out to be Mrs Bury, presumably on a relieving officer's salary. Among the cases that were rejected on the grounds that the applicant and his family had shown too little self-help and too much immorality was that of Walter Austin. Bury describes this and over 20 other cases in detail, to show that he and his wife did their work conscientiously. Austin was 23. He had a diseased hip, and abscesses (bed-sores?) on other parts of his body. Austin's father had 'one arm off and two fingers off his hand'. He worked regularly on the roads for 10*s*. per week. On Wednesdays and Saturdays he also got 'good wages' as a drover. The applicant's mother drank and was 'unfit to look after' him. The Austins' cottage consisted of one room downstairs.

Small, dark, and dirty (in this the applicant lay day and night), and two equally small and dirty rooms upstairs; besides the father, mother, and sick son, there [lived] with them two grown sons, a daughter aged three, and an illegitimate grandchild, and sometimes its mother.[333]

William Vallance, the clerk to the Whitechapel guardians, also headed a group which included Canon Barnett, keen to help the poor to help themselves. They had reduced outdoor medical relief cases between the early 1870s and 1887 from 3,000 to 21.[334] The fate of these rejects is indicated by what happened to those at Stepney and St George-in-the-East. At Stepney, C.S. Loch of the Charity Organization Society got to work. He found that 44 per cent of the inmates over 65 had had a previous 'pauper incident in their life'. This proved their propensity to laziness and the necessity to make them learn to sustain themselves. Somewhat inconsistently, Loch also made the holding of savings a ground for refusing relief. His investigations ignored sickness. Pell was as busy at St George's as he was at Brixworth, reducing outdoor and medical relief. The rejects simply walked to overburdened Poplar.[335]

Guardians at Whitechapel, Paddington, Fulham, Greenwich and Bradford, after various attempts at sick clubs had failed, introduced loan systems for medical relief. It was not provided for in the New Poor Law or the LGB regulations and was only doubtfully legal. Some paupers, as at Fulham, had either to pay 1s. in advance for a visit from the Poor Law medical officer, or 'prove' that they could not pay. Whitechapel sent collectors after the case had been treated 'to shame the people into paying something', usually by getting it from their relatives. Only about half could pay something, but the system had the virtue, the guardians believed, of making people think twice before they sought relief. As William Vallance remarked, an application for medical relief was the first step to pauperism and people ought to be deterred before they took that step. And it did help the rates: at Paddington and Greenwich the number of applicants had fallen by half.[336]

The economists of the Charity Organization Society had in their journal in the 1870s the equivalent of the modern weeklies' competitions. The 'Difficult Cases' clues were printed one week and readers' solutions the following week. 'CD's' case is typical and 'AGC's' response provides an insight into the COS mentality: not unkind, but involved with 'cases' which threatened waste and social dislocation, not human beings in need; contriving 'solutions' which perverted the ostensible aim of the exercise by building fantasies of 'independence' for their producer while imposing control and conformity on the 'object'. The game was to save the case, or at least the case's family, from indiscriminate charity and if possible from pauperism:

> CD, aged 51, is a ropemaker with four children six months to nine years. Wife aged 40, earns 8-10/- a week — washing. Husband's sight has been gradually failing over last four years — finally had to give up work completely eight months ago — medical certificate says optic nerve is failing and there is no hope — He used formerly to belong to his Trade Club — No relatives able to assist — would it be worth the family moving to Hampstead, instead of their present 'low neighbourhood' where more washing is available?

'AGC' gave the fullest answer. The case was a knotty one and 'AGC' was somewhat defeatist:

> it does not seem to me to be a case for a pension. First, it seems to me that unless there are other circumstances of providence and desert besides that of the man having belonged to his trade club, the case should be dealt with by the guardians. The man should enter the infirmary, whence he might be removed to a blind asylum when eligible, at the expense of the rates, and that number of the children which the wife cannot maintain should be taken into the District schools. Ropemakers are not usually of a sufficiently high class to have any fair objection to such a mode of assistance.
>
> Secondly, presuming that the circumstances of the case do make it incumbent on private charity to deal with it, I do not see that any permanent allowance is required. The almoner for the Society for the Relief of Distress might assist the family through the winter to supplement the better work, which will, it is expected, be obtained for the wife. The case might during the summer be helped directly by some private person or from the funds of the Charity Organization Society, and directly the man becomes eligible for an asylum, his maintenance should be paid for by the guardians.
>
> As to the children, it is possible that the wife might be enabled to support them all; if not, the elder ones might be placed in an orphanage, and a lump sum paid for their maintenance until of working age, or some charitable person might be found to allow a sum for the same period.
>
> It occurs to me as just possible that the wife might obtain work with which her husband though blind, might be able to assist; and, if so, there would be no advantage in separating them, unless it were possible for the man, though 51, to learn at a blind institution some

means of earning a livelihood.[337]

The office of guardian provided local worthies with endless opportunities to spite their enemies, while pursuing the paupers' higher good. In 1895 a guardian of Billericay in Essex proposed that the workhouse chapel be used for entertainments. Two others immediately said, 'the dining hall'. But the Billericay Workhouse had no dining hall. The move to use the chapel, presumably from a Dissenter, was defeated. The chapel, a guardian said, was an 'emblem dear to Church people', and an entertainment in it would upset them. The paupers were not reported as being mentioned.[338]

Preston-Thomas, the LGB inspector, recalled that many guardians' meetings were 'like bear gardens', and that many were 'very unbusinesslike'. The Earl of Kimberley, chairman of the Wymondham guardians was, according to Preston-Thomas, a despot. Preston-Thomas had once had to ask the guardians to spend money on improving the bathing and sanitary arrangements, which were 'most primitive'. But Kimberley objected to 'baths as dangerous to health'. He ignored Preston-Thomas and refused to allow any expenditure.[339] When a lady was elected to the Board at Dorchester, probably during the 1890s, she was horrified to learn that inmates did not sit at table to eat, but sat on the day benches around the wall, eating food out of their bowls with their fingers. They had no night-clothes, and there were no baths. When the lady spoke up for baths one male guardian objected, and pulled back his sleeve, saying: 'white as a hare's tooth and hasn't been washed these forty years'.[340] The usual entries during the 1860s in the guardians' visiting book at Bermondsey Workhouse were 'verry good' and 'all appeors quiet'. The quality of guardians only really began to improve after 1894, when Fowler's Act extended the franchise for voting for guardians, abolished monetary qualifications, and prevented JPs from being *ex officio* members. Even so, the Act had little effect in the countryside, where the local farmers and gentlemen remained in charge.[341]

Evidence about the daily routine in a workhouse is scanty. The most complete that I have found is George Lansbury's account of the Poplar Workhouse in the mid-1890s. Lansbury became a guardian in 1892. The total impression is akin to that conveyed by the COS's Difficult Cases exercise. There appears to have been little intentional ill-treatment, but workhouse life was pervaded by a painful austerity exemplified in systematic stinting of clothes, food, warmth and affection. The pervasive smell was a mingling of sour potato and stale urine, the prevailing noise a mingling of intermittent groans, oaths and screams from the idiots, the howling of babies, syncopated by the clinking keys carried by the matron and taskmasters. Everybody in the Poplar Workhouse, except the bedridden, had to rise at 5.45 a.m. in summer and 6.45 a.m. in winter. Breakfast was at 6.30 a.m. in summer, 7.30 a.m. in winter. Dinner was at 12 noon and supper at 6 p.m. There was nothing in between. Meat was served to everybody although 'many [could] not masticate it'. Everybody also received 14 ounces of suet each day. There were no vegetables except potatoes and onions. The doctor never remarked on the diet except occasionally to order beer or stout. He did 'not like to inconvenience the cook'. The meal was badly cooked. The tea was always stewed. Friends were permitted to visit on one Monday in every month. The meeting was supervised. The inmates had no flannel underclothes, only cotton, through winter and summer. They had one thin coat each. There were no overcoats in winter.[342]

Miss Octavia Hill, the philanthropist and stalwart of the COS, spent much energy in the 1890s opposing state old-age pensions because they endangered thrift. In 1895 she told her fellow COS enthusiast Albert Pell, at the Royal Commission on the Aged Poor:

> I think we ought to think for them (the poor) very much.
> Pell: Would you think it desirable to take the opinions of patients in Guy's Hospital as to the treatment of diseases?
> Hill: Hardly.
> Pell: Is there not something almost parallel in taking the opinions of the very poor on Poor Law relief?
> Hill: I should have felt it so; the very people who cannot see far enough to say that it is doing them harm, I should think.[343]

None the less, George Lansbury did produce a pauper to give his opinion. The former inmate, T.H. Walker, is very likely unique in the nineteenth century in being recorded in print. Walker was not a typical pauper: he had started higher, slipped further and possibly felt his declension more keenly. But the petty tyrannies, humiliations and boredom he suffered he must have shared with tens of thousands. Walker had been a hat manufacturer, but had lost his business after prolonged illness followed by a lawsuit. He had been placed in Wandsworth Workhouse in the summer of 1894. He was over 60, but classed as 'able-bodied'. The able-bodied men under 60 broke stones all day. The over-60s 'have to go and pick oakum for eight hours a day, in twisting little pieces of corded string for eight hours until the people nearly become inbecile; they do not know what to do.' Whenever the taskmaster was absent the people swore wildly, and tried to speed the time in intricate personal operations, cutting beards and trimming corns. The hours were 8-12 a.m. and 1-5.30 p.m. Walker tried to read a newspaper that his daughter brought to the House, but was threatened by the task-master with bread and water for 24 hours, so he gave up. He had a perpetual sore throat and wore a red scarf over his blue workhouse uniform. This angered the taskmaster: 'I will pull those rags off you . . . You must not wear such things . . .' Walker replied, 'I have a sore throat.' . . . 'I don't care whether you and your father and your grand-father had sore throats.' Walker's father had, he said 'died of starvation through his throat growing together, and he suffered with sore throat'. Walker did not complain to anyone: there was 'not the slightest good in doing that'. One day the workhouse doctor examined him. The doctor was formerly a neighbour and Walker's private GP. 'Halloa! are you here? . . . oh, you have got to do some hard work now.' Walker did not tell the doctor about his sore throat. That, he claimed, would have been 'useless'. Indeed, Walker owed the doctor 7s. 6d. for an unpaid bill. Finally Walker's daughter arranged his release from the House. As he left, the taskmaster snatched at the scarf. The Royal Commission asked him to verify this allegation — what was the date? Walker could not say. As he explained, once he lost his newspaper, he never knew the date. Walker's evidence nonplussed and irritated the Commissioners; but only temporarily, it seems, because their report reveals no sign of having been affected by it.[344]

In general, inmates gave the public impression of becoming what Octavia Hill and Canon Bury wanted them to be, apathetic, acquiescent and diligent, if somewhat slow and ungrateful. Within the workhouse younger paupers were frequently rebellious and violent but their pro-tests rarely got through to the world outside. In 1909 the paupers at Lutterworth roused themselves to petition the guardians (unsuccess-fully) against the appointment of Mr J.C. Buttachargi as medical officer — they wanted a doctor of their 'own race and colour'.[345] But the majority of the old and the impotent, helplessly caught in a system both grudging and never designed for them, just mouldered into second childhood and mere oblivion — sans teeth, sans eyes, sans taste, sans vote, sans everything.

Notes

1. Calculated from B.R. Mitchell and Phyllis Deane, *Abstract of British Historical Statistics* (Cambridge, 1962), pp. 12-13. Laslett, by noticing only the stable *proportions* of the elderly in the nineteenth century, misses the point, which is the increase in *absolute numbers*. His definition of 'old' at 65 is misleading, too (Peter Laslett, *Family life and illicit love in earlier generations* (Cambridge, 1977), pp. 192-3).

2. Edwin Chadwick, 'On the best Modes of representing Accurately . . . the Duration of Life . . . amongst different Classes of the Community', *JSS*, vol. VII (1844), pp. 4-16.

3. William A. Guy, *L*, 9 Aug. 1845, pp. 147-8.

4. Quoted by C.R. Drysdale in *BMJ*, 20 Aug. 1887, p. 409. Cf. Registrar-General's tables, comparing Farr's, Ogle's and Tatham's tables, in *L*, 9 Jan. 1897, p. 115.

5. *JRSS*, vol. L (1887), p. 288.

6. *L*, 1 Sept. 1888, p. 428.

7. P.H.J.H. Gosden, *The Friendly Societies In England 1815-1875* (Manchester, 1961), pp. 73-84.

8. Reuben Watson, Actuary to Manchester Unity of Oddfellows, to RC on Aged Poor, *PP*, 1895, vol. XV, Qs. 11380, 11395, 11513, 11568-70.

9. J.D. Grout, wire-worker, Finsbury, to RC on Aged Poor, Qs. 13142-7.

10. RC on Aged Poor, Qs. 11568, 13127; Michael Anderson, *Family Structure in Nineteenth Century Lancashire* (Cambridge 1971), p. 107; Alex Mair, *Sir James Mackenzie, M.D. 1853-1925* (Edinburgh, 1973), p. 45.

11. *Charity Organization Reporter*, 27 Mar. 1872, p. 63.

12. *L*, 19 Nov. 1881, p. 886.

13. RC on Poor Laws, *PP*, 1909, vol. XXXVII, p. 257.

14. Farr, *Vital Statistics*, p. 503.

15. *L*, 2 Dec. 1854, p. 454.

16. Helen Bosanquet, *Social Work in London 1869-1912* (1914, reprinted Brighton, 1973), p. 173. For comparable figures for 1971 see Michael H. Cooper, *Rationing Health Care* (London, 1975), pp. 15, 67.

17. Lee, 'Occupational Medicine' in Frederick N.L. Poynter (ed.), *Medicine and Science in the 1860s* (London, 1966), pp. 166-7. Lee's reference should be *PP*, 1852-53, vol. C.

18. E.W. Brabrook and William Sutton, Chief Registrar and Actuary to Friendly Societies' Central Office to RC on Aged Poor, *PP*, 1895, vol. 15, Qs. 11093-4.

19. Charles Ritchie, *GMJ*, vol. I (1828), p. 372; John Smith, *Edinburgh Medical and Surgical Journal*, vol. XLII (1834), pp. 342-3.

20. E.g. Keir Hardie to SC on Distress From Want Of Employment, *PP*, 1895, vol. VIII, Q. 737; *L*, 1 Sept. 1860, p. 226, 16 Jan. 1875, p. 98, 1 May 1875, p. 622; Alan Armstrong, *Stability and Change in an English County Town* (Cambridge, 1974), quoting D. Gould, p. 242; 'Acute Rheumatism', *Westminster Hospital Reports*, vol. IV (1888), pp. 206-7; for a recent estimate of the ravages of this condition see Office of Health Economics, *Rheumatism and Arthritis in Britain* (London, 1973).

21. Henry Jephson, *The Sanitary Evolution of London* [1907] (reprinted New York, 1972), p. 43; *L*, 3 Dec. 1847, p. 612, 25 Dec. 1847, p. 683; *JSS*, vol. XI (1848), pp. 167-8.

22. *L*, 31 Dec. 1892, p. 1507; F.A. Dixey in *Sheffield Medical Journal*, vol. I (1892-3), pp. 120-1.

23. *L*, 27 Apr. 1838, p. 145, 9 May 1891, p. 1061; *Truth*, 26 Dec. 1895, p. 1570.

24. Frank Renaud, 'Reminiscences of the Influenza Epidemics of 1837 and 1847', *Medical Chronicle*, vol. XII (1890), pp. 89-90; Charles Creighton, *A History of Epidemics in Britain* (London [1891-4]), vol. II, p. 377; Samuel West, *St Bartholomew's Hospital Reports*, vol. XXVI (1890), p. 195.

25. Dr John Hume, *Quarterly Review of Foreign and British Medicine and Surgery*, vol. V (1823), p. 462; *British Annals of Medicine*, 10 Feb. 1837, p. 229; *L*, 18 Mar. 1899, p. 778.

26. *L*, 3 Dec. 1847, p. 612; *Medical Chronicle*, vol. XI (1889-90), pp. 450-4; Herbert Preston-Thomas, *The Work and Play of a Government Inspector* (London, 1909), p. 213.

27. Mrs Clifton's Recipe Book, MS in Menzies Library, Australian National University; *BMJ*, 30 Jan. 1892, p. 250.

28. A.D. Morgan, 'Undiagnosed Coronary Disease in Nineteenth Century England', *Medical History*, vol. XII (1968), pp. 355-6; Registrar-General, 19th Report, *PP*, 1856, vol. XIX, p. 144.

29. John Clendinning in *JSS*, vol. I (1839), pp. 144-8; A. Whyte Barclay in *Medico-Chirurgical Transactions*. vol. XXI (1848), pp. 186, 208-12.

30. George Eliot to Mrs Henry Houghton, 17 and 20 Apr. 1848 in Gordon S. Haight (ed.), *The George Eliot Letters* (New Haven, Conn., 1954), vol. I, pp. 257-8.

31. George Hilaro Barlow, *A Manual of the Practice of Medicine* (1861), pp 348-9, 355-9.

32. Spencer Thomson, *A Dictionary of Domestic Medicine* (1853), p. 274.

33. O. Phelps Brown, *The Complete Herbalist or the People Their Own Physicians* . . . (London, 1867), p. 16.

34. W. Roger Williams, 'The Continued Increase of Cancer', *Medical Chronicle*, vol. V (1896), p. 322.

35. W.H. Symons, MOH Bath, in *L*, 26 Nov. 1898, p. 1402.

36. *Proceedings of the Brighton & Sussex Medico-Chirurgical Society*, vol. I (1894), p. 47.

37. *L*, 30 Apr. 1864, p. 511.

38. *Proceedings of the Brighton & Sussex* . . . (1894), p. 48.

39. *L*, 17 Dec. 1853, pp. 585-6; *Medico-Chirurgical Transactions*, vol. XLV (1862), pp. 390-1.

40. W. Roger Williams in *L*, 20 Aug. 1898, p. 482.

41. Thomas J. Graham, *On The Diseases Peculiar To Females* (1834), pp. 14-16.

42. W.R. Rogers, *L*, 2 May 1857, pp. 464-5.

43. *L*, 17 Dec. 1853, p. 586, 19 Jan. 1856, p. 63, 20 June 1863, p. 691.

44. *Medico-Chirurgical Transactions*, vol. XLV (1862), p. 390.

45. Sir Spencer Wells, *L*, 15 Dec. 1888, p. 1192; *L*, 17 July 1886, p. 144, commenting on *Report of Registrar-General for 1884*; *L*, 3 July 1869, pp. 1-4; Drysdale in *BMJ*, 2 Apr. 1892, p. 737.

46. *BMJ*, 5 May 1888, p. 993.

47. *L*, 8 Aug. 1896, p. 427; *JRSS*, vol. LXI (1898), pp. 560-4.

48. *PP*, 1916, vol. V, 77th Report of Registrar-General, pp. 35, 39.

49. Children's Employment Commission, *PP*, 1865, vol. XX, pp. 9-10.

50. John Couper in *British Annals of Medicine*, 13 Jan. 1837, p. 41.

51. *L*, 30 Dec. 1854, p. 553.

52. *Sanitary Review*, vol. V (1858), pp. 216-17; Allen Clarke, *Effects of the Factory System* (London, 1899), pp. 43, 52.

53. William I. Cox in *Journal of Public Health and Sanitary Review*, vol. II (1856), pp. 40-3, 374-6.

54. Preston-Thomas, *Work and Play*, p. 286.

55. *L*, 18 June 1864, p. 716.

56. William Steele, Secretary to Northumberland and Durham Miners' Permanent Relief Fund, to RC on Aged Poor, *PP*, 1895, vol. XIV, Qs. 9151, 9234, 9238-40.

57. Police-Sergeant Ilsley to Children's Employment Commission, *PP*, 1866, vol. XXIV, Q. 14.

58. Miss A.M. Anderson, Factory Inspector, to Physical Deterioration Committee, *PP*, 1904, vol. XXXII, Qs. 1514-15.

59. *Medical and Physical Journal*, vol. XVII (1807), p. 584; vol. XVIII (1807), p. 33; *London Medical and Physical Journal*, vol. XXXVIII (1817), p. 336.

60. B.B. Cooper, *Life of Sir Astley Cooper*, 2 vols. (London, 1847), vol. II, pp. 48-9; *L*, 15 Aug. 1835, p. 648, 4 July 1846, p. 9; *Edinburgh Medical and Surgical Journal*, vol. LXXI (1849), p. 145; *St Thomas's Hospital Reports*, vol. III (1872), pp. 246-8; *L*, 13 Apr. 1889, p. 756.

61. *BMJ*, 9 Sept. 1893, p. 594.

62. Farr, *Vital Statistics*, p. 55; *Opthalmic Hospital Reports*, vol. I (1857), pp. 2-5; *Liverpool Medical and Chirurgical Journal*, vol. I (1858), p. 98; *Medico-Chirurgical Transactions*, vol. LXIV (1881), p. 348.

63. Elizabeth Gaskell, *The Life of Charlotte Brontë* (Folio Society edition, 1971), p. 255.

64. Minty, *Legal and Ethical Aspects*, pp. 167-8.

65. Bosanquet, *Social Work*, pp. 191-3; RC on Poor Laws, *PP*, 1909, vol. XXXVII, p. 283.

66. B.W. Richardson, 'On Phases of Quackery . . .', *Medical Times and Gazette*, 26 Apr. 1879, pp. 446-7.

67. *L*, 23 Feb. 1839, p. 822.

68. *BMJ*, 30 Jan. 1869, p. 105.

69. *L*, 9 May 1914, p. 1346.

70. *L*, 10 Feb. 1838, pp. 699-700.

71. *L*, 20 Apr. 1895, p. 1031.

72. *L*, 14 Jan. 1860, pp. 41-2, 21 Jan. 1860, p. 67.

73. *L*, 16 May 1840, p. 287; for Ferment's extraordinary earlier career see D. Williams. *John Frost. a Study in Chartism* (London, 1969), pp. 243-4.

74. *L*, 27 Oct. 1877, p. 637, 11 Apr. 1846, p. 423, 9 Jan. 1875, p. 65.

75. *L*, 26 May 1849, p. 572. On the problems of understanding sorcery and witchcraft in illness and healing see John Middleton (ed.), *Magic, Witchcraft, And Curing* (New York, 1967), especially the opening essay by E.E. Evans-Pritchard and M.G. Marwick, *Sorcery In Its Social Setting* (Manchester, 1965).

76. *L*, 3 Apr. 1858, p. 346, 20 Feb. 1847, p. 216.

77. *L*, 16 Apr. 1864, p. 444.

78. John Skinner, *Journal Of A Somerset Rector 1803-1834* (Bath, 1971), pp. 400-1.

79. *L*, 7 Jan. 1882, p. 26, 15 Apr. 1899, p. 1042.

80. Keith Thomas, *Religion And The Decline Of Magic* (Penguin ed., 1973), pp. 225, 237-42; *L*, 3 Mar. 1860, p. 227; *Once a Week*, 28 Mar. 1863, p. 374.

81. *L*, 2 Feb. 1850, p. 161. Cf. Latham and Matthews edition of Pepys' *Diary*, vol. V (1664), p. 362.

82. *L*, 18 May 1889, p. 1008, 23 Feb. 1884, p. 364; *BMJ*, 16 Oct. 1880, p. 629.

83. J.T. Slugg, *Reminiscences of Manchester Fifty Years Ago* [1881] (reprinted Shannon, 1971), pp. 55-7.

84. *L*, 8 Apr. 1848, pp. 405-6, 15 Mar. 1851, p. 312. Faith in the restorative powers of human milk is very ancient, as is faith in the milk of exotic animals. 'Elephant's Milk' was a good seller in the early nineteenth century: 'Under the Caveat of Government, an effectual cure for debility, blindness, faded complexion, grey hairs, nightly disturbance, spasmodic complaints, certain diseases, bald head, noise in the ears, stiffness of joints, premature waste, watery eyes

... [guaranteed] by P. Campbell, Senior Surgeon of the Royal College of London, late of Middlesex Hospital.' The milk cost 10s. per bottle. It was obtained in Africa. The elephants were attracted by crackers and drums, lassoed, raised on pulleys, and milked. 'Her natural strength accounts for its giving strength to the infirm and aged. Her long age for its powers of prolonging ... life. Her mildness, for its ... soothing powers; the sweetness of her breath, for its purifying qualities ... Shallow draughts only palliate, but drinking largely completes the cure and regenerates the constitution.' The milk also came in pill form. 'To guard against imposition, each bottle is sealed with the impression of an Elephant, in the act of being milked on the one side, the Doctor's initials P.C., on the other.' The milk consisted of 'spiritous varnish, water and a little mercury'. *Gazette of Health* (June 1817), pp. 523-6.

85. William Fox, *The Working Man's Model Family Botanic Guide; or, Every Man His Own Doctor* (Sheffield, 1909), pp. 20-31.

86. *L*, 1 July 1848, p. 19 (Birmingham), 11 Sept. 1847, pp. 280, 288 (Leeds and Sheffield), 8 Sept. 1849, pp. 275-6 (Maryport), 6 July 1850, p. 31 (Whitehaven), 30 Aug. 1851, p. 209 (City of London), 10 Apr. 1858, pp. 375-6 (Limehouse), 17 Apr. 1846, pp. 4-9, 22 Apr. 1848, p. 454 (Bolton).

87. Fox, *Working Man's ... Family Guide*, p. 35.

88. *BMJ*, 1 July 1882, p. 23; *L*, 30 Apr. 1864, pp. 509-10, 2 Feb. 1867, p. 154; *Examiner*, 19 Feb. 1853, p. 124; Report of Analytical Sanitary Commission on cayenne pepper, *L*, 3 July 1852, p. 18, 12 July 1884, p. 80, on sources of lobelia.

89. *L*, 16 Feb. 1856, p. 191.

90. *L*, 13 Nov. 1830, p. 251.

91. *L*, 30 June 1838, p. 485.

92. *L*, 3 Feb. 1844, pp. 623-4, 1 Aug. 1846, p. 133.

93. *L*, 1 May 1858, p. 449.

94. *L*, 17 July 1852, p. 67, 24 July 1852, p. 87.

95. *L*, 12 Nov. 1842, p. 254; Elizabeth Jenkins, *Dr Gully* (Harmondsworth, 1974).

96. *L*, 12 Nov. 1836, p. 258.

97. *L*, 7 Jan. 1882, p. 22; Minty, *Legal and Ethical Aspects*, pp. 138-9.

98. SC on Patent Medicines, *PP*, 1914, vol. IX, pp. v-vi.

99. *L*, 12 July 1834, p. 569, 27 Feb. 1836, p. 880; *Dictionary of National Biography*, 'Morison' [London, 1894] (reprinted Oxford 1963-4).

100. *L*, 18 Feb. 1837, p. 764, 20 July 1839, p. 635, 18 Apr. 1863, p. 450, 25 Oct. 1851, p. 405.

101. *L*, 23 Oct. 1841, p. 139, 2 Jan. 1864, p. 26.

102. *L*, 25 Oct. 1862, p. 455.

103. *L*, 14 Mar. 1846, p. 305, 6 Dec. 1862, p. 627, 17 Jan. 1863, p. 76, 5 Jan. 1884, p. 29. For an example of Holloway's early advertising methods, see Louis James, *Print And The People 1819-1851* (London, 1976), p. 233. Holloway claimed to have discovered his recipe in Algiers, where he had cured the populace of plague.

104. J.C. Umney to SC on Patent Medicines, *PP*, 1914, vol. IX, Qs. 9509-12.

105. S.D. Chapman, *Jesse Boot of Boots the Chemists* (London, 1974), pp. 35-6; *Dictionary of National Biography*, 'Boot'.

106. Chapman, *Boot*, pp. 29, 37.

107. *BMJ*, 26 Nov. 1881, p. 884, 26 Oct. 1912, p. 1171; *L*, 15 Dec. 1888, p. 1193; SC on Patent Medicines, *PP*, 1914, vol. IX, Q. 2618.

108. *L*, 9 Feb. 1884, pp. 262, 278; SC on Patent Medicines, *PP*, 1914, vol. IX, Q. 6188.

109. *BMJ*, 11 June 1898, p. 1539; Dr Alfred Cox to SC on Patent Medicines, *PP*, 1914, vol. IX, Q. 2616.

110. *L*, 24 Dec. 1870, p. 902.

111. See S.W.F. Holloway, 'Medical Education in England, 1830-1858', *History*, vol. XLIX (1964); Ian Inkster, 'Marginal Men . . .' and Ivan Waddington, 'General Practitioners and Consultants . . .' in J. Woodward and D. Richards, *Health Care and Popular Medicine in Nineteenth Century England* (London, 1977).

112. Charles Newman, *The Evolution of Medical Education in the Nineteenth Century* (London, 1957), p. 46; G. Burrows to SC on Medical Registration, *PP*, 1847, vol. IX, p. 51; Lyon Playfair to SC on Medical Act, *PP*, 1878-9, vol. XII, Q. 175.

113. *L*, 23 Feb. 1833, p. 695; Andrew Wood to SC on Medical Act, *PP*, 1878-9, vol. XII, Q. 4011.

114. *L*, 23 Oct. 1830, p. 147.

115. I am indebted to Dr Ann Hone for help with this list. Cline Parkinson, George Pearson, Perry, Robert and James Watson are in the *Dictionary of National Biography*. See also *Medical Gazette*, 17 Feb. 1843, p. 752 (Grainger); R.C. Brock, *The Life and Work of Astley Cooper* (London, 1952), p. 6; *Republican*, 30 Dec. 1825 (Webb); J.T. Ward, *Chartism* (London, 1973), pp. 69 (Fletcher), 135 (Price); Hunt, *Medical Society of London*, p. 72 (Marshall Hall).

116. *L*, 6 Jan. 1827, p. 455, 26 Sept. 1835, p. ii, 18 Nov. 1837, p. 265.

117. *L*, 16 Jan. 1830, pp. 539-40, 20 Feb. 1830, pp. 701, 711, 6 Mar. 1830, p. 807, 8 May 1830, pp. 212-13.

118. *L*, 19 June 1830, p. 451, 24 July 1830, p. 653, 2 Oct. 1830, p. 52.

119. H.W. Rumsey to SC on Medical Poor Relief, *PP*, 1844, vol. IX, Qs. 9103, 9116.

120. *L*, 9 Nov. 1833, p. 263.

121. *Medical Gazette*, 22 Dec. 1826, p. 56, 27 Dec. 1827, p. 57; Rev. Peyton Blakiston to Poor Law Commission, *PP*, 1834, vol. XXXVII, p. 3c.

122. Ursula Henriques, 'How cruel was the Victorian Poor Law?', *Historical Journal*, vol. XI (1968).

123. *PP*, 1834, vols. XXX, XXXI, XXXII, XXXIII, XXXIV.

124. Rogers claims in his *Reminiscences* that C.P. Villiers, a Commissioner in 1834, told him that 'the question of sickness, as a factor in the production of pauperism was not referred to them, and if it had not been for the pertinacity of Dr G. Wallis and some others, that important subject would have been passed over altogether' (Joseph Rogers, *Reminiscences of a Workhouse Medical Officer* (London, 1889), p. 250).

125. John Walter, *The Times*, 24 Feb. 1843; *Parl. Debs*, vol. CXVI, col. 1161; Henriques, 'Victorian Poor Law', p. 367.

126. *PP*, 1834, vol. XXXVII, p. 1c. Southam was also a model Poor Law village, with a dispensary and compulsorily 'Independent Poor', see *Medical Gazette*, 27 Dec. 1827, pp. 56-7.

127. *PP*, 1834, vol. XXVIII, p. 78A.

128. *PP*, 1909, vol. XXXVII, pp. 237-8.

129. Anne Digby, 'The Labour Market and the Continuity of Social Policy after 1834: the Case of the Eastern Counties', *Economic History Review*, vol. XXVIII (1975), p. 73.

130. J.S. Davey to RC on Poor Laws, *PP*, 1909, vol. XXXIX, Qs. 3198-204.

131. *PP*, 1865, vol. XLVIII, p. 3.

132. Frederick Purdy, 'Extent of Pauperism in . . . Lancashire', *JSS*, vol. XXV (1862), p. 377; *L*, 11 May 1872, p. 655; *PP*, 1909, vol. XXXIX, p. 42; B.L. Hutchins, 'Statistics of Women's Life and Employment', *JRSS*, vol. LXXII (1909), p. 232.

133. *PP*, 1861, vol. LXI, pp. 33-4; *L*, 20 Apr. 1867, p. 495; Bosanquet, *Social Work*, pp. 2-3.

134. *PP*, 1895, vol. IX, Qs. 9577, 9653, 9694; Frederick Purdy, 'The Relative Pauperism of England, Scotland and Ireland', *JSS*, vol. XXV (1862); 'A Decade of the Scotch and Irish Poor Rates', *JSS*, vol. XXXIV (1871), p. 374.

135. *Medical Gazette*, 7 Feb. 1840, p. 761.

136. *L*, 11 Dec. 1909, p. 1767.

137. *L*, 10 Dec. 1836, p. 412; Richard Williams and G. Cornewall Lewis to SC on Medical Poor Relief, *PP*, 1844, vol. IX, Qs. 8404-6, 9784; *Medical Gazette*, 15 Apr. 1842, p. 155; *BMJ*, 24 Apr. 1886, p. 795.

138. *L*, 27 Apr. 1839, pp. 201-2.

139. *L*, 5 Nov. 1836, p. 235, 3 Oct. 1835, p. 49, 5 Dec. 1835, pp. 387-8, 19 Dec. 1835, p. 466.

140. *L*, 30 Jan. 1836, pp. 710-11, 18 Nov. 1837, p. 280, 4 May 1839, p. 222.

141. *PP*, 1844, vol. IX, Q. 9148.

142. *L*, 7 Apr. 1838, p. 56, 4 May 1839, p. 223.

143. *L*, 21 Dec. 1861, p. 610.

144. Rev. W.J. Coppard to SC on Medical Poor Relief, *PP*, 1844, vol. IX, Qs. 7283-4, 7301, 7306, 7382.

145. *L*, 1 Aug. 1868, p. 160, 28 Oct. 1871, p. 620, 26 Jan. 1867, p. 121.

146. *L*, 1 June 1872, p. 771.

147. *PP*, 1844, vol. IX, Qs. 2317-58.

148. *L*, 7 Oct. 1837, p. 60.

149. *L*, 12 Nov. 1836, p. 279; *PP*, 1844, vol. IX, Qs. 2341-3.

150. *L*, 22 Aug. 1846, p. 225.

151. *The Times*, 20 Oct. 1847.

152. R.T. Webb in *L*, 8 Jan. 1848, p. 54.

153. *L*, 15 Oct. 1836, p. 138, 4 Oct. 1851, p. 335, 11 Sept. 1858, p. 293, 3 Feb. 1872, p. 173. Bernard Shaw's remarks on 'Medical Poverty' in the preface to *The Doctor's Dilemma* are exaggerated, and refer to assistants and 'sixpennys' rather than GPs.

154. 'ATC' in *L*, 18 Sept. 1852, p. 274.

155. *L*, 12 Nov. 1836, p. 279, 10 Oct. 1840, p. 88; 'An Irish Angius on Herba', 8 Nov. 1851, p. 451.

156. E.g. typical cases in *L*, 21 Nov. 1818, p. 675 (badly managed childbirth); 30 May 1868, p. 704 (child given poisonous medicine).

157. *L*, 20 May 1882, p. 851.

158. *L*, 30 Jan. 1897, p. 331.

159. Minty, *Legal and Ethical Aspects*, pp. 10-13; for typical scandals about 'covering' an unqualified assistant, and the havoc wrought by incompetents, see *L*, 2 Jan. 1897, p. 55, 14 July 1894, p. 86.

160. *PP*, 1844, Qs. 2365-78.

161. *L*, 19 Sept. 1846, p. 332.

162. *L*, 10 Apr. 1875, pp. 518-19.

163. *L*, 2 May 1891, p. 1025.

164. *PP*, 1844, vol. IX, Qs. 2446-8.

165. *PP*, 1909, vol. XXXVII, p. 274.

166. *PP*, 1909, vol. XL, Qs. 34947-9.

167. SC on Medical Poor Relief, *PP*, 1844, vol. IX, Q. 9832.

168. *L*, 17 Feb. 1838, p. 751; *PP*, 1844, vol. IX, Qs. 9168-9, 9173; Rogers, *Reminiscences*, p. 80; *L*, 27 June 1868, p. 827.

169. *PP*, 1844, vol. IX, Qs. 3015-17, 3106; *PP*, 1909, vol. XXXIX, Q. 1932.

170. RC on Aged Poor, *PP*, 1895, vol. XIV, Qs. 4633, 4753, 4919.

171. *PP*, 1909, vol. XLI, Qs. 26182-4, 40461, 41761, vol. XXXVII, p. 29.

172. See previous note.

173. *L*, 1 June 1872, p. 772.

174. Rogers, *Reminiscences*, p. 83.

175. Preston-Thomas, *Work and Play*, preface by John Burns, p. vi.

176. *L*, 3 July 1858, p. 12.

177. R. Hodgkinson, 'Poor Law Medical Officers', *Journal of the History of Medicine*, vol. II (1956), p. 326; *L*, 15 Oct. 1883, p. 674.

178. *L*, 17 May 1873, p. 714; P.G. Craigie, 'English Poor Rate', *JRSS*, vol. LI (1888), pp. 465-6; *PP*, 1909, vol. XXXIX, pp. 48-9, Q. 1668.

179. *L*, 18 Nov. 1848, p. 560.

180. John Simon to SC on Medical Act, *PP*, 1878-9, vol. XII, Qs. 663-6; Edward Waters, Qs. 1509-55.

181. *L*, 6 Apr. 1833, p. 53.

182. See, e.g., Chadwick's statement to Social Science Congress in 1872, and the doctors' reaction, *L*, 1 June 1872, p. 776.

183. The numerous schemes agree in principle but vary in detail, e.g. *L*, 'Corvinus', 13 Feb. 1836, p. 803; John Tweedale, 12 Mar. 1836, p. 941; George Haygarth, 8 Jan. 1848, p. 52; H.W. Rumsey and Robert Ceely, 11 Mar. 1837, p. 858; H.W. Rumsey, *On Sanitary Legislation and Administration in England* (London, 1858).

184. *L*, 2 Jan. 1836, p. 543, 27 Feb. 1836, p. 871. Yeatman had been pressing for a medical panel fee for service system since at least 1831, cf. *L*, 30 Apr. 1831, pp. 152-7.

185. *L*, 4 May 1839, p. 223.

186. *Medical Times & Gazette*, 13 Feb. 1858, p. 173.

187. G.C. Lewis to SC on Medical Poor Relief, *PP*, 1844, vol. IX, Q. 9792; Hodgkinson, 'Poor Law Medical Officers', *Journal of the History of Medicine* (1956), pp. 314-29.

188. *L*, 6 Apr. 1872, p. 477, 1 June 1872, p. 776, 3 Aug. 1872, p. 160; see also the important article by Roy Macleod, 'The Frustration of State Medicine 1880-1899' in *Medical History*, vol. XI (1967).

189. *PP*, 1878-9, vol. XII, John Simon, Qs. 553-6.

190. Mr Howell, 'Lets have unity – and no distinction – lets all be called "doctors" – the public will sort out the best skilled "doctors" (cheers)' (*L*, 21 Jan. 1837, p. 600).

191. *L*, 27 May 1876, p. 783; SC on Medical Act, *PP*, 1878-9, vol. xii, Qs. 280-92, 1630; *BMJ*, 29 Jan. 1887, p. 225; *GMJ*, vol. LIII (1900), pp. 371-2.

193. *L*, 23 June 1860, p. 620, 6 Oct. 1860, p. 326.

194. *L*, 4 July 1896, p. 40.

195. *L*, 30 May 1835, p. 299.

196. *L*, 11 Jan. 1845, p. 42, 13 Nov. 1847, p. 528, 5 Mar. 1864, p. 285, 29 Feb. 1868, p. 300.

197. *L*, 16 Mar. 1872, p. 368, 21 Mar. 1885, p. 528, 7 July 1888, p. 26; H.W. Acland to SC on Medical Act, *PP*, 1878-9, vol. XII, Q. 218; Michael H. Cooper, *Rationing Health Care* (London, 1975), pp. 43-4; *Proceedings of the West London Medico-Chirurgical Society*, vol. III (1889), pp. 18-20.

198. *L*, 28 May 1864, p. 616, 7 July 1888, p. 26, 31 Jan. 1914, p. 346.

199. *L*, 4 Jan. 1845, pp. 21-2, 12 July 1845, p. 50.

200. *L*, 11 Oct. 1862, p. 395, 15 July 1865, p. 73.

201. *L*, 29 Oct. 1853, p. 425.

202. *L*, 17 Dec. 1898, p. 1611.

203. See, e.g., B.S. Rowntree, *Poverty: A Study of Town Life* (1902 ed.), p. 43.

204. *L*, 1 Nov. 1845, p. 492.

205. *L*, 3 Oct. 1840, p. 68.

206. *L*, 9 Feb. 1839, p. 737, 5 Dec. 1846, p. 624, 6 Feb. 1847, pp. 157-8; H.W. Acland, *PP*, 1878-9, vol. XII, Qs. 85, 87.

207. *L*, 16 Jan. 1858, p. 78.

208. *L*, 4 Jan. 1873, p. 29, 25 Dec. 1875, p. 919.

209. *L*, 12 July 1856, p. 58, 12 June 1875, p. 846.

210. *L*, 12 Nov. 1864, p. 301.

211. *Medical Gazette*, 25 June 1836, p. 488; Richard Faircloth, surgeon to Newmarket Union to SC on Medical Poor Relief, *PP*, 1844, vol. IX, Qs. 5698-735, H.W. Rumsey, ibid., Qs. 9078, 9086-90; *BMJ* (1898), p. 706.

212. Lee, 'Occupational Medicine' in F.N.L. Poynter (ed.), *Medicine and Science in the 1860s* (London, 1966), p. 165 (Cornwall); *L*, 6 Apr. 1878, p. 519 (Manchester iron-workers); 28 Mar. 1891, p. 751 (Durham). In 1882 the miners at the Llynvi Company pits in the Ogmore Valley struck when the management, in collusion with the doctors, appointed a doctor chosen by the management rather than continue the practice of the men selecting their own man. Apparently the strike failed (*BMJ*, 28 Oct. 1882, p. 852).

213. *L*, 6 June 1868, p. 735 (Southampton), 11 July 1868, p. 63, 8 Aug. 1868, p. 189 (Wednesbury).

214. *L*, 16 May 1868, p. 646, 17 Oct. 1868, pp. 519-20, 17 July 1869, p. 99, 21 July 1877, p. 109.

215. *BMJ*, 19 Oct. 1889, p. 900.

216. *BMJ*, 31 Aug. 1889, p. 502, 26 Oct. 1889, p. 959.

217. *Truth*, 26 Dec. 1895, p. 1570; *L*, 7 Jan. 1899, p. 53.

218. *L*, 8 Feb. 1862, p. 153.

219. *L*, 18 June 1864, p. 709; *BMJ*, 21 Sept. 1912, p. 748.

220. *L*, 11 May 1861, p. 468; *GMJ*, vol. XXXV (1891), pp. 443-4.

221. *BMJ*, 20 Feb. 1892, p. 404.

222. *BMJ*, 14 Dec. 1907, p. 1756.

223. *BMJ*, 20 Feb. 1892, p. 404, 28 Dec. 1907, p. 1860.

224. *PP*, 1834, vol. XXXVII, p. 25c.

225. *BMJ*, 9 Apr. 1892, p. 795, 24 Aug. 1907, p. 480.

226. *BMJ*, 31 Dec. 1881, p. 1078.

227. Patricia Branca, *Silent Sisterhood* (London, 1975), p. 27.

228. *L*, 12 Nov. 1831, p. 227.

229. *L*, 15 Sept. 1832, p. 764.

230. *L*, 12 Aug. 1854, p. 136; *BMJ*, 12 June 1869, p. 547.

231. George Howell, 'Cash Account', 1868 Diaries (Bishopsgate Institute, London); F.M. Leventhal, *Respectable Radical* (London, 1971), pp. 100-11. Howell noted in his diary at the end of 1867 that he hoped to 'lay by more cash . . . and only hope that we all have good health to carry out our desires'.

232. *L*, 11 Dec. 1875, p. 851.

233. *L*, 4 Aug. 1894, p. 282; G.L. Anderson, *Victorian Clerks* (Manchester, 1976), pp. 109, 185-6.

234. *L*, 26 Feb. 1842, p. 773 (Bath); 14 Jan. 1854, p. 46 (Plymouth).

235. *L*, 11 Jan. 1873, p. 67.

236. Henry Ashworth, 'Depression of Trade at Bolton', *JSS*, vol. V (1842), p. 78.

237. *L*, 5 Mar. 1864, p. 284.

238. *L*, 13 Aug. 1842, p. 692.

239. *L*, 22 Feb. 1845, pp. 216-17.

240. *L*, 19 June 1858, p. 610; *BMJ*, 25 Dec. 1869, pp. 682-3.

241. *PP*, 1878-9, vol. XII, Q. 1319.

242. *Medical Gazette*, 15 Sept. 1838, p. 986; *L*, 9 Mar. 1844, pp. 796-7, 27 Nov. 1847, p. 580.

243. *L*, 31 Dec. 1853, p. 625.

244. *Gazette of Health* (June 1817), p. 533; *L*, 20 Jan. 1838, p. 587, 13 Apr. 1839, p. 113; *Medical Times & Gazette*, 5 Nov. 1853, p. 480; *L*, 13 Jan. 1900, p. 143.

245. *L*, 29 July 1848, p. 131, 27 Jan. 1872, p. 120.

246. Minty, *Legal and Ethical Aspects*, p. 41.

247. *L*, 2 Oct. 1858, p. 365.

248. Gordon, 'The Army Surgeon', *St Andrews Medical Graduates' Association Transactions* (1872 and 1873), pp. 18-23; *L*, 20 June 1846, p. 694, 9 Nov. 1850, pp. 533-4.

249. Quoted in D.J. Phillips, 'Crime and Authority in the Black Country', D.Phil. thesis, (University of Oxford, 1974), p. 150.

250. *L*, 7 June 1856, pp. 642-3, 6 Mar. 1858, pp. 196-7.

251. *L*, 23 June 1860, p. 633, 7 July 1860, pp. 16-17, 28 May 1864, p. 608, 12 Jan. 1867, p. 53.

252. *L*, 14 May 1864, p. 569.

253. *L*, 6 Sept. 1890, p. 604.

254. *GMJ*, vol. XXXII (1889), pp. 2-9, 202-3, vol. XXXIV (1890), pp. 149-60; *L*, 9 Aug. 1890, p. 291.

255. *L*, 15 Oct. 1898, p. 1004.

256. Anthony Brett-James, *Life in Wellington's Army* (London, 1972), pp. 269-70; *GMJ*, vol. X (1878), pp. 408-9; *L*, 14 Jan. 1882, p. 82. L. Bickel (*Rise Up to Life. A Biography of Howard Walter Florey* . . . (Sydney, 1972), p. 61) remarks on the extensive folklore about the curative properties of moulds and implies that Florey must have known of this lore and must have been embarrassed by its associations with his work; L.J. Ludovici, *Fleming, Discoverer of Penicillin* (London, 1952), p. 133, quotes Fleming as saying, rather oddly, 'So far as I know there is nothing in the literature which would lead any worker to suspect that a substance with the chemical constitution of penicillin would have any value as an anti-bacterial agent. It had to happen by chance, and it was fortunate that the chance presented itself to me.'

257. John Tweedale, Lynn Regis, Norfolk, *L*, 1823, pp. 13-14, 1823-4, pp. 147-8; pp. 147-8; Tweedale writes that Dr Sutton and Mr Finch had successfully performed acupuncture before he tried it. He writes as if the practice was new but not very rare or little known (J. Webster, *London Medical and Physical Journal*, vol. LIV (1821), pp. 31-3). For further cases, see *L*, 31 Dec. 1825, p. 495, 30 Sept. 1826, p. 846, 22 Dec. 1827, p. 461.

258. The existing literature on the history of acupuncture in the West is poor and contradictory. J. Lanier, *Hirtoire, doctrine et pratique de l'acupuncture chinoise* (Paris, 1966) is unreliable. Acupuncture seems to have been little used in China itself in the nineteenth and early twentieth centuries: which prompts the irreverent speculation that Western medical missionaries might have taken it back there during this period. On the status of acupuncture in British medical esteem, see John Tatum Banks, 'Observations on Acupuncturations', *Edinburgh Medical and Surgical Journal*, vol. XXXV (1831), pp. 323-7; John Renton, Penicuik, *Edinburgh Medical and Surgical Journal*, vol. XXXIV (1830), pp. 100-3.

259. *L*, 28 June 1828, p. 409, 21 July 1832, p. 489. The mesmerism frauds can be followed in the *Lancet* from June 1838 to January 1839. See also George Rosen, 'Mesmerism and Surgery: A strange chapter in the history of Anesthesia', *Journal of the History of Medicine*, vol. I (1946).

260. *L*, 7 Jan. 1837, p. 539, 14 Jan. 1837, p. 559, 25 Aug. 1838, pp. 769-70, 5 Mar. 1842, p. 797.

261. *L*, 16 Oct. 1852, p. 362, 29 Sept. 1860, p. 324.

262. Fisher, *Lister*, p. 257; *L*, 29 Apr. 1871, p. 567.

263. A.E. Aust-Lawrence, *BMJ*, 16 Nov. 1889, pp. 1093-4; Jacques M. Quen, 'Acupuncture and Western Medicine', *Bulletin of the History of Medicine*, vol. XLIX (1975), p. 202; Felix Mann, *Acupuncture*, new ed. (London, 1971), p. viii.

264. *BMJ*, 28 Aug. 1858, p. 728.

265. *L*, 11 Apr. 1846, p. 424, 16 May 1846, p. 563, 26 Dec. 1846, p. 701; *Medical Times*, 27 July 1850, p. 107. Chiropodists were vivid charlatans and were very well known and popular. Among them was Mrs Seymour Hill, only 3 feet 10 inches high and of 'very plethoric habit'. She won universal esteem because of the 'very straightforward way in which she practised her calling' (*L*, 16 June 1860, p. 610). She never charged more than 5s. regardless of the wealth of the client. Napoleon III and the Empress twice brought her to France to cut their corns. Was she possibly the original for Miss Mowcher?

266. Mrs Clifton's recipe book – cutting from *Stamford Mercury* [1860s] (Ms Menzies Library, Australian National University).

267. *BMJ*, 25 Apr. 1905, p. 1023.

268. *L*, 25 July 1857, p. 95.

269. *L*, 9 Jan. 1858, p. 44, 3 Aug. 1861, p. 117.

270. *L*, 23 Jan. 1875, p. 139.

271. *L*, 12 Mar. 1859, p. 273.

272. *L*, 6 July 1861, p. 16, 3 Aug. 1861, p. 116.

273. *L*, 5 July 1862, p. 17.

274. *L*, 26 Nov. 1870, pp. 750-1.

275. *L*, 11 July 1868, p. 64.

276. Sophia Jex-Blake, *Medical Women – A Thesis and a History* (Edinburgh, 1886), pp. 95-6.

277. T.R. Forbes, 'Mortality Books of St Bride's', *Journal of the History of Medicine*, vol. XXVII (1972), p. 26.

278. E.g. St Leonard's Shoreditch, *L*, 1 July 1865, pp. 15-16, 29 July 1865, pp. 131 2, 7 Sept. 1861, pp. 235-6.

279. *L*, 26 Mar. 1870, p. 471; Craigie, 'English Poor Rate', *JRSS*, vol. LI (1888), pp. 464-5; *PP*, 1909, vol. XXXIX, Q. 2305.

280. Royston Lambert, *Sir John Simon*, pp. 518-46; Rogers, *Reminiscences*, pp. 100-1.

281. *JSS*, vol. XXXV (1873), p. 325.

282. *L*, 2 Mar. 1872, p. 305; B.L. Hutchens, 'Statistics', *JRSS*, vol. LXXII (1909), pp. 270-1.

283. J.S. Davy to RC on Poor Laws, *PP*, 1909, vol. XXXIX, Q. 2305.

284. *L*, 4 Aug. 1894, p. 287.

285. Norman Longmate, *The Workhouse* (London, 1974), pp. 263, 275.

286. *BMJ*, 16 June 1894, p. 1317, 6 Apr. 1895, p. 769; *PP*, 1895, vol. XIV, Qs. 5188-91, 10852, 12805.

287. Ibid., Q. 12805.

288. Ibid., Qs. 16032-4; *PP*, 1909, vol. XLII, pp. 33, 41-2; *L*, 10 Sept. 1892, p. 638 (Birmingham).

289. *L*, 4 Aug. 1894, p. 283; Dr McVail to RC on Poor Laws, *PP*, 1909, vol. XLII, pp. 33, 35.

290. Charles Goss, *L*, 19 Feb. 1887, p. 396, 8 Apr. 1893, pp. 812-13.

291. *L*, 21 July 1894, p. 149, 16 Aug. 1902, p. 463; RC on Poor Laws, *PP*, 1909, vol. XXXIX, Appendix VII, vol. XLI, Q. 38380 (Dr Niven on Manchester).

292. Ernest Hart, 'The Condition of our State Hospitals', *Fortnightly Review*, vol. III (1866), p. 222; *L*, 20 June 1891, p. 1412.

293. R. Hodgkinson, 'Poor Law Medical Officers', *Journal of the History of Medicine*, vol. XI (1956), p. 323; *PP*, 1909, vol. XI, Q. 22991, vol. XLII, p. 27; *L*, 24 Feb. 1872, p. 271; B.W. Richardson in *St Andrews Medical Graduates' Association Transactions* (1869), pp. 18-19.

294. *PP*, 1909, vol. XXXIX, Q. 9316.

295. *L*, 26 Jan. 1895, p. 236; *BMJ*, 30 Jan. 1886, p. 226.

296. *BMJ*, 20 Jan. 1894, p. 165.

297. *PP*, 1909, vol. XXXVII, pp. 240-1; *L*, 24 Aug. 1901, pp. 535-6.

298. *L*, 26 Dec. 1896, p. 1844, 23 June 1866, p. 694 (Rotherhithe), 22 Aug. 1868, p. 258 (Devonport), 11 Apr. 1868, p. 489 (Wigan); *BMJ*, 17 July 1869, p. 65 (Tavistock).

299. Rogers, *Reminiscences*, pp. 50-1; Louisa Twining, *Recollections of Life And Work* (London, 1893), pp. 121-5; Sir Edward Cook, *The Life of Florence Nightingale*, 2 vols. (London, 1914), vol. II, pp. 123-43.

300. *L*, 13 Apr. 1895, p. 945, 10 Apr. 1897, p. 1034.

301. *L*, 28 Jan. 1899, p. 251.

302. *L*, 14 Sept, 1901, p. 756.

303. *BMJ*, 16 Jan. 1892, p. 150, 21 Oct. 1905, p. 1059.

304. *L*, 18 Dec. 1886, p. 1185.

305. *PP*, 1895, vol. XV, p. 956, 1909, vol. XXXVII, pp. 164, 235-6.

306. *L*, 24 Feb. 1866, p. 218; *Medical Times & Gazette*, 5 Jan. 1861, p. 21.

307. Twining, *Recollections*, pp. 124-5.

308. Robert Hedley to RC on Aged Poor, *PP*, 1895, vol. XIV, Qs. 1614-15.

309. J.H. Bridges to SC on Metropolitan Hospitals, *PP*, 1890-1, vol. XIII, Q. 23301; *PP*, 1895, vol. XIV, Qs. 14615-16.

310. Ibid., Qs. 2407-12.

311. *PP*, 1909, vol. XI, Q. 23713.

312. Preston-Thomas, *Work and Play*, p. 211.

313. *L*, 8 Jan. 1842, p. 517.

314. *L*, 20 Jan. 1866, p. 75.

315. Longmate, *Workhouse*, pp. 143-4; Preston-Thomas, *Work and Play*, p. 238.

316. *L*, 1 July 1865, pp. 18-25, 16 Feb. 1867, p. 220, 14 Aug. 1909, pp. 447-8.

317. *L*, 23 Apr. 1870, pp. 587-8, 14 May 1870, p. 712, 4 June 1870, pp. 815-17.

318. Dr Edward Smith, *L*, 1 Feb. 1868, p. 168.

319. Baldwyn Fleming to RC on Poor Laws, *PP*, 1909, vol. XXXIX, Qs. 889-93.

320. Rogers, *Reminiscences*, pp. 6-7, 21, 75-88; *L*, 6 June 1868, p. 731, 17, 31 July 1869, p. 100, p. 130.

321. *L*, 29 Oct. 1881, p. 767.

322. *BMJ*, 15 Oct. 1887, p. 855, 24 Dec. 1881, p. 1039; *L* 10 Sept. 1859, p. 269, 16 July 1898, p. 161.

323. *L*, 3 Feb. 1872, p. 163; *BMJ*, 25 Oct. 1890, p. 969.

324. *L*, 17 Apr. 1875, p. 554.

325. Rogers, *Reminiscences*, p. 110.

326. Quoted in Longmate, *Workhouse*, p. 200.

327. *L*, 6 Aug. 1895, p. 897.

328. *L*, 26 Jan. 1895, p. 257, 20 Apr. 1895, p. 1020.

329. *BMJ*, 15 Feb. 1896, p. 357, 439; *L*, 8 Aug. 1868, p. 201.

330. *L*, 28 Feb. 1885, p. 395.

331. Preston-Thomas, *Work and Play*, p. 208.

332. *PP*, 1909, vol. XXXVII, p. 164.

333. Thomas Mackay, *The Reminiscences of Albert Pell* (London, 1908), pp. 289-93, 356-8; RC on Aged Poor, *PP*, 1895, vol. XV, Qs. 4224-31, 15762-16001, and Appendix IX, pp. 988-91; *L*, 22 Dec. 1883, p. 1098.

334. *PP*, 1895, vol. XIV, Qs. 2623-62; [Dame Henrietta Barnett], *Canon Barnett* (London, 1921), pp. 667-9.

335. *PP*, 1895, vol. XV, Qs. 9920-1, 10051-78, 13875.

336. *L*, 22 Dec. 1883, p. 1098.

337. *Charity Organization Reporter*, 16 Nov. 1876, p. 159, 23 Nov. 1876, pp. 163-4.

338. *Truth*, 14 Feb. 1895, p. 395.

339. Preston-Thomas, *Work and Play*, p. 237.

340. C.M. Fisher, *Life in Thomas Hardy's Dorchester 1888-1908* (St Peter Port, 1965), p. 16.

341. *L*, 18 Nov. 1865, p. 575; 56 & 57 Vict., ch. 73; Preston-Thomas, *Work and Play*, p. 235.

342. George Lansbury to RC on Aged Poor, *PP*, 1895, vol. XV, Qs. 13703-48.

343. Ibid., Qs. 10605-7.

344. Ibid.

345. *L*, 4 Sept. 1909, p. 76.

6 NEW PERSPECTIVES AND NEW PROBLEMS

Later-nineteenth-century commentators professed great esteem for the medical profession and its works; some contemporary critics display a scepticism amounting to contempt. The present crisis in health-care costs, the wavering of confidence in clinical procedures and the rivalry for status and money between the medical profession and the burgeoning new caring professions have made today's laymen-taxpayers less trusting than their fathers. The new social historians of medicine have been profoundly affected by this crisis, as have health economists and teachers of social medicine. Certainly the crisis has prompted many of my questions and speculations in this book.

Antisepsis and innovations in orthopaedics in the 1860s and 1870s — quite apart from the earlier discoveries in anaesthesia — rightly impressed laymen as great beneficent advances in the progress of mankind. Nowadays, however, laymen query brilliant technical accomplishments, heart transplants, some forms of brain surgery, for instance, on the grounds that they enhance the doctor's reputation and income rather than the patient's continuing existence, while their enormous costs in manpower, machines and money compete with morally better ways of allocating these resources. The 'social standing' of doctors is no longer sacrosanct either, as they come to be seen to be living very well at the taxpayers' expense and their claims to esoteric expertise are challenged by informed and increasingly sceptical patients who assert their equal right to think and speak both in the consulting-room and in local government health committees.

Critical appraisals such as these were seldom if ever made within the historical period which this book covers. In 1879 W.E. Gladstone, speaking as Lord Rector of Glasgow University, congratulated the doctors on their recent technical accomplishments and their new 'social standing' on an 'equality with the other cultivated or leisured classes'.[1] The scholarly journalist T.H.S. Escott, in his chapter on 'invalid life' in *Social Transformations of the Victorian Age* (1897), cited sanitary and hospital improvement and the 'general course of medical progress' as among the most 'blessed' of the transformations. His proof was the fall in the over-all mortality rate of the United Kingdom from 23 per 1,000 in 1855 to 18 per 1,000 in 1895. Escott credited the Prince Consort, Florence Nightingale and the doctors with initiating and carrying

414

through this large saving of life.[2] His view was a common one by the 1890s and it was to be endorsed and elaborated through the first half of this century, with its ablest exponents, G.T. Griffith and M.C. Buer, publishing in the mid-1920s.[3]

In 1976 the Professor of Social Medicine at Birmingham University, Thomas McKeown, magisterially swept such claims aside. In his *Modern Rise of Population*, the summation of a series of investigations lasting over twenty years, McKeown argued that medical intervention had little to do with the lowering of the death rate. This decline resulted from a reduction of deaths from infectious diseases and, McKeown suggested, a lessening of infanticide and starvation. He described authoritatively how the fall in the death rate from airborne diseases derived substantially from changes in their character and the relation of the organisms to their hosts. The death rate from water- and vector-borne diseases declined, he maintained, as a result of sanitary improvement. (I would add here, for adults at least.) In none of these developments, excepting the decline of smallpox, did medical procedures play a decisive role. McKeown was also disposed to discount for the first half of the century, as I have done for the decades before the 1870s, the effects of hygienic measures in water supply and food-handling. He finally plumped for improvement in nutrition as the grand cause of the reduction of mortality, although he did not demonstrate how this change came about; his very general claims about increases in improvements in agriculture and food supply all relate to the period before 1820s.[4] Like him, I think, bearing in mind the many studies of social conditions in poor countries, that more nearly adequate nutrition is of fundamental importance in helping people to survive, in increasing host-resistance to disease and probably in increasing fertility but, as I suggested in Chapter 3, we still know far too little about food supplies, the quality of food, methods of preparing it, and amounts eaten by various classes and various individuals within families through time. None the less, improvements in the physical environment of the people, in food and drink, in shelter, in working conditions, seem to have played the crucial role in nineteenth-century Britain. The rise of real wages after 1850, declining expenditure on alcoholic drinks from the mid-1870s and increasing food supplies probably lie at the core of this development. Here, as elsewhere, the next essential steps in research include comparisons with the experience of other European countries, and detailed 'health histories' of particular villages and town parishes, using census returns, parish registers, doctors', hospital, school, friendly society and trade union records and Poor Law union reports, by extension from the family history research recently published by Michael Anderson on Preston and Alan Armstrong on York.[5] The comparison of a Catholic Irish parish with a neighbouring Protestant English or Scottish one would be a good way of beginning.

Why were Gladstone, Escott and their contemporaries so deceived? The title and content of Escott's chapter are instructive. Although he quotes mortality rates and sanitary reform as proof of improvement, the substance of his chapter concerns the amelioration of the condition of the sick, at home, in hospitals and in workhouse infirmaries. The 'blessed' transformation comprises an extension to more people in more elaborate and effective ways, of the 'gracious work' of tending the sick. He implicitly admits that doctors could not cure, but only palliate.

Yet this was the key role of the doctor. In an age when sudden illness, disability and death threatened people at every stage of life doctors were necessary sorcerers who supplied an interpretation to otherwise meaningless afflictions. As Escott noted, doctors were taking over from the priests. They listened, diagnosed, palliated symptoms and mitigated discomfort where they could, and cured when Providence helped. The sufferer had his role as sick person confirmed. He could exhibit his individual plight to an expert auditor and observer; obtain an explanation – rephrased in mystical words – of the condition he described in simple general language to the doctor, and a prognosis, a divination of the likely future course of his malady. This prognosis was accompanied by rituals, the inspection of faeces and urine, blood-letting, diet, nasty medicines and anti-toxins, designed to reinforce the prognosis and ensure the predicted outcome.

The patient's command of the doctor's attention and his procedures depended upon his rank and ability to pay. In some cases the doctor's readiness to meet the patients' or relatives' demands resulted in his intervening too drastically, as I showed earlier with maternity attendance and infant teething cases. The upper classes could display pain to hold the doctor's interest; the lower classes, hardihood.

In this context mortality rates, whether quoted by McKeown or Escott, are largely irrelevant to understanding the interplay between patients and doctors. The fact that patients sought comfort from doctors throughout the century at ever-increasing costs in money and, in many cases, self-abasement, and afforded doctors an ever-increasing share of the national wealth and ever-rising status, suggests that in future research we should look more closely at patient-doctor relationships, and morbidity rates.

The profession's accretion of social power may also have been crucial in holding steady mortality rates, even if doctors achieved little reduction of them. In an age of increasing population in rapidly growing ill-managed, under-financed, ill-planned towns the respect that Southwood Smith, John Snow, William Farr, John Simon, J.B. Russell and others enjoyed enabled them to collaborate, in local government especially, with politicians and publicists in shaming and bullying local councillors and parliamentarians into allocating taxes to sanitary improvement. The doctors' pressure helped ensure that towns never lagged to the point of disaster in providing cleansing, drainage and other health services, as did the growing towns of Eastern Europe or China in the same period. Each major outbreak of infectious disease (always excepting influenza) enabled medical improvers and their allies to demonstrate both the vulnerability of all classes to the diseases harboured by the poor, and the costs of avoidable disease and dirt burdening the tax-paying classes. The cankers of filth and public extravagance, if left unremedied, would ultimately cause a breakdown of the state. George Godwin, the architectural journalist-reformer and the author of the significantly titled *Town Swamps and Social Bridges* (1859), John Simon, Charles Kingsley and Lord Shaftesbury made filth morally, politically and, finally, aesthetically intolerable.

It is a sad irony that after the 1870s the doctors' success in holding mortality rates through sanitary reform, allied with their increasing intimacy with private patients and the acceptance of germ-specific disease theory, should have redirected their energies away from environmental health provisions to person-to-person clinical treatment. By 1892-3 the Public Health Section of the BMA annual meeting was relegated to the shabbiest hall. The 17 subjects listed for discussion in the section, meat inspection, coroners' inquests, isolation of measles, ventilation of sewers, for example, were all well worn. Innovative men looked elsewhere, to the new bacteriology, abdominal surgery and gynaecology, not to that old subject Dr Rumsey had called 'state medicine' and Dr Farr, 'Hygeiology'. Nutrition was not discussed and investigation of the social conditions of various kinds of patients, for example, was not on the Public Health Section agenda, nor was it prominent on the agendas of other sections.[6] Such investigations would henceforth be conducted by laymen, led by Seebohm Rowntree, the Webbs and Lady Bell. By the twentieth century news of sanitary progress had all but disappeared from the *Lancet* and the *BMJ*. Forty years earlier it had formed a main part of every issue. By 1900 the journals were filled with highly technical reports of specialised clinical analyses and procedures.

Doctors had won full freedom to prescribe and manage treatments, both among their private patients and their dispensary and hospital inmates, regardless of the social and financial costs of the resources they used. They had abandoned Farr's larger vision of mixed councils of doctors and laymen managing the full range of health resources, food standards, building regulations and the provision of a state-salaried medical service providing treatment on a basis of individual patient need in schools, workplaces and neighbourhoods.[7] When the BMA and the doctors rejected this vision, with the tacit approval of the ratepayers who feared its costliness, the British people lost the best opportunity to build a rational and more equitable distribution of medical care; a system which might have been primarily preservative rather than reparative, and which might more effectively have decided priorities and contained costs. Something like this system is now slowly emerging in Britain and other Western countries, albeit harbouring gross inequalities of service and disregard of needs. The cost of health services is now such a drain on national economies everywhere that governments are being forced to act to limit medical incomes and compel patients to bear more of the costs of their treatment.

On the other hand, the popular distrust of 'centralisation' and 'medical despotism' did save Britain from the bureaucracy of 'medical police' that afflicted Prussia and France. It is not difficult to imagine Edwin Chadwick and similar high-minded functionaries compelling people to carry health record or national insurance cards and developing the compulsory notification of disease into a punitive system. The Contagious Diseases Acts are an ominous indication of what determined doctors, economists, military men and illiberal politicians could achieve when they combined for the health of the Empire.[8] Underlying such legislation, as it underlies medical Utopias like B.W. Richardson's *Hygeia*, is the belief that individuals and the state must conform to laws of nature, the violation of which is sin, expressed as illness, or pollution.[9] 'Hereditary' illnesses, especially the disabilities issuing from venereal diseases, were salient examples of preventible sin; in this notion lies one of the origins of the eugenics movement. In this light Samuel Butler's *Erewhon* becomes a more disturbing parable. Richardson, Chadwick and the Erewhonians were all prone to solving disease and poverty problems by 'forbidding' them.

Throughout the century orthodox medicine gradually overran and vanquished folk medicine. Many of the procedures in folk and quack medicine, as I have shown, were as destructive and costly as orthodox interventions. But the submergence of home herbal treatments was a loss.

This area of folk medicine, resting on shared understanding of the signature or properties of the herb, and private hope, spent little time on diagnosis and enjoined sensible procedures, rest, warmth and adequate diet. As Joseph Whatmore, a medical herbalist of Ashton-under-Lyne, explained in 1914:

> There is a very simple way among people generally, and I suppose the same applies to the most learned in the medical profession. Take, say, scarlatina or measles; surely mostly every mother knows pretty well what the symptoms that suggest scarlatina are. Say that these symptoms appear — namely, heat in the surface skin, running from the eyes or the nose, . . . all the simple symptoms which have only to be once seen to be known again; then they give their little simple remedies such as Yarrow tea . . . [to cause sweating] with the result that in . . . a few hours their children are invariably a great deal better and on the way to recovery. These ideas are exchanged between these people . . . They make no mystery about it.

Whatmore claimed that such family medication was more prevalent in the north than in 'southern counties, more especially a cosmopolitan place like London'. The relative shortage of doctors in the north would have contributed too. Control by the profession came much more slowly and patchily. In the north, especially, the working people combined love of botanising with self-medication.

> There are thousands of mothers and fathers who are doctors to their own households, and they never think of calling in a medical man until they see a very extreme case and then it is rather because they are more frightened at what a coroner's jury may say . . . than because they have any want of faith in their remedies.[10]

Even in 1973, researchers reported finding that 16 per cent of sufferers with symptoms of illness in Britain took no action and 63 per cent made some attempt at self-care. Only 20 per cent of sufferers actually visited a doctor, presumably to seek diagnosis and mitigation of the symptoms. But one honest doctor reported in 1974 that he was unable to make any definite diagnosis in 43 per cent of the consultations for illness.[11] In the nineteenth century doctors probably did better: looser, inclusive definitions such as 'fever' or 'inflammation' could satisfy everybody.

Self-medication was cheaper and more immediate than orthodox medicine and, if it relieved or cured the sufferer no more effectively, it harmed him or her less. Blood-letting, heroic dosing and 'low diet' must have inhibited the natural recovery that occurs in most cases of minor illness. The change in orthodox prescribing which began in the mid-1850s from dosing according to the supposed normal efficacy of the drug and allowing for adulteration to dosing according to the presumed needs of the patient according to age, size and degree of illness, was a fundamental advance and must in the long run have preserved many lives.[12] In view of this it is sad that the popular persistence of self-dosing after the middle of the century should have taken the form of swallowing patent medicines pressed on ignorant buyers through mass advertising.

The economic consequences of the changing pattern of mortality and morbidity have hitherto attracted little attention from economic historians and I lack the expertise to move beyond offering some crude assertions and raising some questions for investigation. The pattern of mortality and the increase of life expectancy in the nineteenth century were ideally suited to rapid industrialisation and economic growth. The heavy infant mortality which prevailed throughout the century restrained the pressure of population, while it removed encumbrances and released mothers for productive labour. Moreover, the gain in life expectancy between 20 and 40 enlarged the labour force at the most productive phase of the life cycle. It is also worth recalling, especially as morbidity is at least as important as mortality in affecting productivity and the people's standard of living, that the period of Victorian prosperity after 1848 and up to 1889 coincided with freedom from virulent influenza outbreaks, except for a mild epidemic in 1866.

In part, these gains justified Edwin Chadwick and William Farr. Chadwick, as Professor Fein has pointed out, was the first political economist since Sir William Petty to use the economic value of man to justify improved health services. Chadwick saw human beings as unit-investments of capital in productive force. In 1842 he estimated the national loss of production due to premature illness and death as £14 million, equivalent, possibly, to about half the national income from 'domestic and personal' labour. Farr, in his *Vital Statistics*, progressed to calculating the value to the state of a life according to future accrued income; that is, setting off investment in early nurture and sanitation against later wages and taxes. He estimated that a Norfolk agricultural labourer was worth £5 at birth, £56 at 5, £117 at 10, £192 at 15, £234 at 20, a peak of £246 at 25, £241 at 30, and thereafter declining to £138 at 55 and £1 at 70, and thereafter at a rising cost to the community, until at 80 the old man was costing £41 a year.[13]

As Fein remarks, this investment-oriented approach positively discourages expenditure in areas that will not yield a higher return.[14] In this context, the punitive, when it was not simply neglectful, approach by Chadwick and his fellow political economists to the old and the chronically disabled becomes more comprehensible. Their approach led instead to creating very broad categories of population which might be coerced into health and productivity – like the 'able-bodied' poor, workhouse children and the inmates of lock hospitals. This coercive, maximising frame of reference inhibited analysis of specific projects: thereby it blocked understanding of what was really happening and hence diminished sympathy with the sick and the old.

The local and personal costs of ill health were probably greater than Chadwick and Farr imagined. In Mile End during March 1868 there were 93 cases of reported fever and 14 of smallpox which came upon the public charge. Dr Corner, a local practitioner, estimated that each would have required treatment for at least a month, at a minimum of 2*s*. 4*d*. a day, equalling £349. 10*s*. 8*d*. Sixteen children were removed to the workhouse because their parents had been removed to the Fever Hospital. They cost 7*s*. each per week for six weeks, equalling £33. 12*s*. 0*d*. 'Several' of them became orphans and therefore became chargeable for some years. Many of the 107 patients removed to the Fever Hospital emerged destitute, presumably from loss of their employment and from medical costs. Even if only half of them received a fortnight's relief after discharge (Corner had not bothered, apparently, to ascertain this), at 5*s*. per week per family, the total would be £25. Altogether the public loss on this month of sickness, excluding its long-term consequences, was a minimal £408. 2*s*. 8*d*. Dr Corner lamented that cheap preventive measures, such as compulsory vaccination and 'proper sanitary enforcement', had not been applied.[15]

Dr Alan Sorkin has claimed recently that an improvement in the morbidity rate, and in life expectancy from birth from 30 to 32.5 years in poor countries requires an increase of 0.8 per cent in output per worker to maintain *per capita* income, but he adds that the extra 2.5 years of productivity would greatly exceed the 0.8 per cent.[16] He is writing about removing the debilitating effects of malaria, which are said to reduce the sufferer's productivity by an estimated 30 per cent. (In Britain the ague, which commonly meant malaria, largely disappeared in the north and east Midlands between about 1780 and the 1820s.) In principle, the most productive investment was probably in sanitary reform. To illustrate this very crudely; about £10.3 millions was borrowed in England and Wales for this purpose between 1850 and

1871; over these decades the total national income of Great Britain rose by around 40 per cent from £523.3 million to £916.6 million, while the number of males and females employed rose by only 20 per cent from 9.3 million to 11.8 million.[17] Sorkin's work provokes questions about productivity in the nineteenth century among TB victims and sufferers from occupational lung diseases. The diminution in the incidence of TB, quite apart from its beneficent results for family income, must have had a considerable effect on national productivity. But again I lack the expertise and information to pursue this problem, and mention it as only another item for research.

My bleak picture of Poor Law medicine is likely to leave the reader with the notion that the British were callous and mean. Yet there is one set of calculations which suggests that British paupers did much better than their Continental brethren. In 1871, in the midst of the Goschen-Stansfeld austerity campaign, Ernest Seyd, a member of the London Statistical Society, asked 'why we, undoubtedly the most loyal, the most religious, the most moral, and the wealthiest people in the world, should at all be troubled with pauperism . . . let alone the most intense in Western Europe?'[18] Seyd completed Table 6.1 from A. Emminghaus, *Das Armenwesen und die Armengesetzgebung in europäischen Staten . . .* (1870), the returns of the Bureaux de Bienfaisance and the Poor Law Commission reports.

Table 6.1: Great Britain — 1855-68 — 1 Pauper per 20-22 Inhabitants, or 4 2/3% of the Population

Prussia	1849-61	1 pauper per 20-56 inhabitants	Germany
Saxony	1856-64	" " " 54.9-56.9 "	2¼%
Württemberg	1855-66	" " " 29.9-52.0 "	of
Bavaria	1855-67	" " " 38.9-56.8 "	population
France	1853-60	" " " 35.0-30.1 "	France, 3% of population

In France the destitute had no right to assistance, but local private relief was organised by the Bureaux de Bienfaisance. In Germany, the communes supported their poor out of local taxes on luxuries and court fines. Seyd counted as paupers all persons reported by his correspondents as having ever received alms, that is, he included both casual and permanent paupers. He then divided the total amounts reported as being spent on the poor by the reported totals of paupers. This result showed Great Britain spending £7. 5s. 0d. on each pauper, Germany £1. 8s. 0d. and France 10s.

Seyd was a monetary crank who blamed bimetallism for the high rate of British pauperism. His statistics are doubtful and they can bear interpretations other than his. The very intensity of pauperism in Great Britain might well have reflected a more realistic and generous definition of destitution and need. Moreover, the general order of Seyd's figures is supported by a table in Mulhall's *Dictionary of Statistics*, which shows that in the late 1880s private charitable expenditure in the United Kingdom, at £10,000,000 was double that of France.[19] Even allowing for the dubious provenance of these tallies, the absolute difference between the reported expenditures confirms what British travellers noticed — the harrowing, hopeless degradation of the French sick poor. Similarly, Seyd's tables for Germany show that the qualifications for relief had been tightened to squeeze out about one-third of the destitute, well before the same process was applied in Britain. This tightening occurred just as the surge in the German economy was getting under way. Of course, growth in the economy could have reduced the number of the destitute, but reduction by as much as a third in this manner seems implausible.

If we take the relative proportions of world manufacturing output in 1870 as a very rough guide, the United Kingdom, with 31 per cent of the total, was double that of Germany, with 13.2 per cent, and was triple that of France with 10.3 per cent.[20] Yet France paid 15 times less per head in poor relief and Germany nearly five times less. The absolute differences in scale, and in timing of development of the various sectors, and emigration are doubtless important, as is the relatively much larger agricultural component in the German and French economies. Their rural communities offered kinship support and provided a cover for destitution and underemployment. None the less, the apparent divergences in generosity and humanity between Britain and France and Germany remain.

Ironically, the very absence of a state system of poor relief in Germany and France probably made it easier to introduce into those countries the medical police, insurance and infant health measures of the 1890s. But this is a little-explored subject. It is striking that the indexes to standard economic and social histories of Europe in the nineteenth century sometimes contain 'poor relief (England)' and usually 'insurance' and 'social legislation (1890s)' for Germany and France, but none that I have looked at in English, French or German mentions 'charity' or 'poor relief' in those countries, let alone Scotland or Ireland.

It is also arguable that British ratepayers could have contributed more to the expenditure on public and pauper health. The average local rate in England fell from 3s. 10¾d. in 1816 to 3s. 4d. in 1868 and then rose to 3s. 8d. in 1892. The average poor-rate was reduced from 3s. 4½d. in 1803 to 1s. 1½d. in 1892. A significant part of the ratepayers' saving must have gone to medical practitioners for private illness management. By 1893 doctors, led by Dr C.V. Poore of the BMA, were prominent in the 'revolt of the ratepayers' against taxation for local improvements. Despite the ratepayers' allegations, the sanitary revolution and its benefits for the nation in productivity had been achieved relatively cheaply. To recall the figures I mentioned in Chapter 4: the total local debt of England in 1892 was about £200,000,000: the largest single item was water supply, at £38,000,000; followed by 'public improvements – mostly sanitary', at £29,000,000; and 'sewage' at £20,000,000. We can put these sums in perspective by remembering that when the nation was believed to be imperilled on two earlier occasions, when the economy was much smaller, the government was said to have outlaid £120,000,000 on losing the American Colonies and £600,000,000 on the war against France. At the turn of the twentieth century the government readily spent £270,000,000 on the Anglo-Boer War.[21]

The groundwork for a new pattern of national redistributive expenditure was laid by Sidney and Beatrice Webb in the minority report of the Royal Commission on the Poor Law and Unemployed in 1909. They and their colleagues produced the information which exposed the old Poor Law system of medical relief as morally and administratively intolerable. On the basis of this new historical understanding they set the moral priorities and the structural guidelines for future social legislation and administration – for a system which could liberate people from fear and humiliation – old-age pensions, insurance against sickness and unemployment, special schemes of medical and educational care for special categories of the disabled. Their proposals were the more easily accepted by the taxpayers because the latter were concerned about the physical condition of the nation's cannon-fodder; but so far as the betterment of the nation's lower classes is concerned, the important point is that the proposals survived and took effect. The medical profession's usual role in these developments was to hinder progress, both by thwarting or ignoring plans to promote general health, and by securing its own narrow interests in the areas of private care and hospital provision. Expenditure on illness management now has the same uncontrollable expanding dynamism as expenditure on instruments of war; it is not yet of the same order of magnitude, but it is not inconceivable that, with a growing middle-aged and geriatric valetudinarian element in both rich and poor nations, it could become such.

Meanwhile we dither, promoting tobacco and warning against it, subsidising refined sugar whilst knowing its dangers, mildly penalising drunken drivers whilst being dimly aware of the prodigious human and monetary costs of traffic accidents. It is salutary to recall that, though some of the Victorians' actions were misguided, like their fierce fumigation procedures, and others were proved less successful than they expected, like compulsory vaccination, they acted, and did in the long run save the lives of millions.

Notes

1. W.E. Gladstone, *Rectorial Address* (Glasgow, 1879), p. 242.
2. T.H.S. Escott, *Social Transformation of the Victorian Age* (London, 1897), pp. 388-97.
3. G. Talbot Griffith, *Population Problems of the Age of Malthus* (new ed. London, 1967); M.C. Buer, *Health, Wealth, and Population in the Early Days of the Industrial Revolution* (new ed. London 1968).
4. Thomas McKeown, *The Modern Rise of Population* (London, 1976).
5. Michael Anderson, *Family Structure in Nineteenth Century Lancashire* (Cambridge, 1971); Alan Armstrong, *Stability and Change in an English Country Town* (Cambridge, 1974).
6. *BMJ*, 6 Aug. 1892, p. 301.
7. *British Annals of Medicine*, 16 June 1837, p. 758; Lee, 'Occupational Medicine' in F.N.L. Poynter (ed.), *Science and Medicine in the 1860s* (London, 1966), pp. 166-7.
8. F.B. Smith, 'Ethics and Disease in the later nineteenth century: the Contagious Diseases Acts', *Historical Studies*, vol. 15 (1971).
9. For Hygeia, see *Medical Times & Gazette*. 16 Oct. 1875, pp. 435-40, or *Transactions of the Social Science Association*, 1875. One of Chadwick's fullest expositions of his aims is in *JSS*, XXVII (1864), pp. 492-504.
10. See R.M. Titmuss in Poynter (ed.), *Medicine and Culture* (London, 1969), pp. 248-9; SC on Patent Medicine, *PP*, 1914, vol. IX, Qs. 11508, 11536, 11548.
11. Michael H. Cooper, *Rationing Health Care* (London, 1975), pp. 12-13.
12. Richard Oliver, *L*, 22 Aug. 1857, p. 195.
13. Farr, *Vital Statistics*, p. 566.
14. Rashi Fein, 'On Measuring Economic Benefits Of Health Programmes' in G. McLachlan and Thomas McKeown (eds.), *Medical History and Medical Care* (London, 1971) pp. 185-93.
15. *L*, 21 Nov. 1868, p. 675.
16. Alan L. Sorkin, *Health Economics* (Lexington, Mass., 1975), p. 124.
17. *L*, 18 May 1872, p. 686, quoting report of LGB; Phyllis Deane and W.A. Cole, *British Economic Growth 1688-1959* (Cambridge, 1964), p. 166.
18. Ernest Seyd, 'On Currency Laws and their Effects on Pauperism', *JSS*, vol. XXXIV (1871), pp. 8-15.
19. Michael G. Mulhall, *The Dictionary of Statistics* (London, 1892), pp. 111-13.
20. B.R. Mitchell, *European Historical Statistics 1750-1970* (London, 1975),

p.781; W.A. Cole and Phyllis Deane, 'The Growth of National Incomes' in *Cambridge Economic History of Europe*, Part I (Cambridge, 1965), pp.25-7.

21. H.H. Fowler, President of Local Government Board, *BMJ*, 30 Sept. 1893, p.752; Asa Briggs, 'The Political Scene' in Simon Nowell-Smith (ed.), *Edwardian England 1901-1914* (London, 1964), p.56.

BIBLIOGRAPHY

Parliamentary Reports and Papers

All papers are from the House of Commons series, unless otherwise stated.

Report from the Select Committee on Contagious Fever in London, 1818, vol. VII

Royal Commission on the Poor Laws, 1834, vols. XXVIII-XXXVII

Report of the Poor Law Commissioners on the Further Amendment of the Poor Laws, 1840, vol. XVII

Report from the Select Committee on Medical Poor Relief, 1844, vol. IX

Reports of Inspectors of Factories, 1846, vol. XX; 1852-3, vol. XL; 1868-9, vol. XIV

Report from the Select Committee on Medical Registration, 1847, vol. IX

Report from the Select Committee on the Pharmacy Bill, 1852, vol. XIII

Report from the Select Committee on Adulteration of Food, Drinks, and Drugs, 1854-5, vol. VIII

First Report of the Select Committee appointed to enquire into the Circumstances connected with the Employment of Women & Children in the Bleaching & Dyeing Establishments in England, Scotland & Ireland etc.

Second Report from the Select Committee on Bleaching & Dyeing Works etc., 1857, session II, vol. XI

Report from the Select Committee (House of Lords) on Sale of Poisons, etc. Bill, 1857, session II, vol. XII

Reports of Children's Employment Commission, 1863, vol. XVIII; 1864, vol. XXVII; 1865, vol. XX; 1866, vol. XXIV; 1867, vol. XVI

Special Report from the Select Committee on the Chemists' and Druggists' Bill, 1865, vol. XII

First Report of the Royal Sanitary Commission, 1868-9, vol. XXXII

Report from the Select Committee on the Adulteration of Food Act 1872, 1874, vol. VI

Report on the Outbreak of Enteric Fever in Marylebone and the Adjoining Parts of London, by J. Netten Radcliffe and W.H. Power, 1874, vol. XXXI, Part I

Report from the Select Committee on the Sale of Food and Drugs Act (1875) Amendment Bill, 1878-9, vol. X

Special Report from the Select Committee on the Medical Act (1858) Amendment [No. 3] Bill [Lords], 1878-9, vol. XII

Report of the Commissioners appointed to inquire respecting Small Pox and Fever Hospitals, 1882, vol. XXIX

Report from House of Lords on Metropolitan Hospitals & Provident & other public Dispensaries & Charitable Institutions for Sick Poor, 1890, vol. XVI; 1892, vol. XIII

Report from the Select Committee on Midwives' Registration, 1892, vol. XIV

First Report from the Select Committee on Distress from Want of Employment, 1895, vol. VIII

Report of the Royal Commission on the Aged Poor, 1895, vols. XIV, XV

Reports from the Select Committee on Food Products Adulteration, 1895, vol. X; 1896, vol. IX

Report of the Physical Deterioration Committee, 1904, vol. XXXII

Report of the Departmental Committee on . . . the Midwives' Act 1902, 1909, vol. XXXIII

Royal Commission on the Poor Law, 1909, vols. XXXVII-XLV

Report from the Select Committee on Patent Medicines, 1914, vol. IX

Periodicals

Anderson's Quarterly Journal of Medicine and Surgery
British and Foreign Medical Review
British Annals of Medicine
British Medical Journal
Charity Organization Reporter
Child-Study
Dublin Hospital Reports
Dublin Journal of Medical and Chemical Science
Edinburgh Medical and Surgical Journal
Gazette of Health
Glasgow Medical Journal
Guy's Hospital Reports
Household Words
Journal of London [later Royal] Statistical Society
Journal of Public Health and Sanitary Review
Lancet
Liverpool Medical and Surgical Reports

Liverpool Medico-Chirurgical Journal (later *Liverpool Medical and Chirurgical Journal*)
London Journal of Medicine
Medical and Physical Journal
Medical Chronicle
Medical Gazette (also *Medical Times and Gazette*)
Medical Intelligencer
Medical Press and Circular
Medico-Chirurgical Transactions
Memoirs of the Medical Society of London
Middlesex Hospital Reports
Once a Week
Opthalmic Hospital Reports
Pall Mall Gazette
Proceedings of the Brighton & Sussex Medico-Chirurgical Society
Proceedings of the West London Medico-Chirurgical Society
Quarterly Journal of Foreign Medicine and Surgery
St Andrews Medical Graduates' Association Transactions
St Bartholomew's Hospital Reports
St Thomas's Hospital Reports
Sanitation in the West
Sheffield Medical Journal
Transactions of the Clinical Society of London
Transactions of the Epidemiological Society of London
Transactions of the National Association for the Promotion of Social Science
Truth
West London Medical Journal
Westminster Hospital Reports
Westminster Review

Contemporary Articles and Monographs

All were published in London, unless otherwise stated.

Anon. *The Ladies Friend*. New ed. (n.d.) [c. 1800]
Anon. *Plain Observations on the Management of Children during the First Month, addressed particularly to Mothers*. 1828
Anon. *The Medical Profession in England*. 1834
Anon. *The Female Instructor*. 1841
Anon. *The Provident System of Medical Relief*. 1872
Andrew, Thomas. *A Cyclopedia of Domestic Medicine and Surgery*. 1842

Archer, Thomas. *The Terrible Sights Of London and Labours of Love in the midst of them.* (n.d.) [1870?]

Armstrong, John. *The Young Woman's Guide.* Newcastle-upon-Tyne [c. 1830]

Barlow, George Hilaro. *A Manual of the Practice Of Medicine.* 1861

Beeton, Mrs Isabella. *Book of Household Management* 1861. Reprinted Melbourne, 1977

Bosanquet, Helen. *Social Work in London 1869-1912.* 1914. Reprinted Brighton, 1973

Buchan, William. *Domestic Medicine.* 17th ed. Edinburgh, 1802

Buckton, Catherine M. *Food and Home Cookery.* 1883

Calkins, Alonzo. *Opium and The Opium-Appetite.* Philadelphia, 1871

[Chadwick, Edwin.] *The Poor Law Report of 1834.* S.G. and O.A. Checkland (eds.). Harmondsworth, 1974

Chadwick, Edwin. *Report on The Sanitary Condition Of The Labouring Population Of Gt. Britain* [1842], M.W. Flinn (ed.). Edinburgh, 1965

Chadwick, Edwin. *National Health . . .* B.W. Richardson (ed.). 1890

Chavasse, Pye Henry. *Counsel To A Mother.* 1869

Cheadle, W.B. *Artificial Feeding and Food Disorders of Infants.* 1889

Churchill, Fleetwood (ed.). *Essays on the Puerperal Fever and other diseases peculiar to women.* 1849

Clarke, Allen. *Effects of the Factory System.* 1899

Clayton, Edwy Godwin. *Arthur Hill Hassall.* 1908

Cooper, Henry. 'On the Cholera Mortality in Hull during 1849'. *Journal of the Statistical Society*, vol. XVI (1853)

Copley, Esther. *Catechism of Domestic Economy.* 1851

Creighton, Charles. *A History of Epidemics in Britain.* 2 vols [1891-4]. New ed. 1965

Drake, Mrs Barbara. 'A Study of Infant Life in Westminster'. *JRSS*, vol. LXXI (1908)

[Drysdale, George.] *The Elements of Social Science . . .* 26th ed. 1887

Escott, T.H.S. *Social Transformations of the Victorian Age.* 1897

Evans, George Washington. *The Antiseptic Treatment . . .* Reading, n.d. [c. 1870]

Farquharson, Robert. *School Hygiene and diseases incidental to school life.* 1885

Ferguson, Robert (ed.). *Gooch on some of the Most Important Diseases peculiar to Women.* 1859

Fox, William. *The Working Man's Model Family Botanic Guide; or, Every Man His Own Doctor.* 19th ed. Sheffield, 1909 (First published 1857. There were at least eleven editions before 1887.)

Gavin, Hector. *Sanitary Ramblings*. [1848] Reprinted 1971

Godwin, George. *Town Swamps and Social Bridges*. 1859. Reprinted Leicester, 1972

Graham, Thomas J. *On The Diseases Peculiar To Females*. 1834

Green, Joseph Henry. *Suggestions respecting the intended plan of Medical Reform*. 1874

Haden, Charles Thomas. *Practical Observations on the Management And Diseases of Children*. 1827

Hale, Mrs Sarah. *The New Household Receipt-Book*. 1834

Hanna, William. *Studies In Small-Pox And Vaccination*. Bristol, 1913

Hassall, A.H. *Adulteration Detected*. 1857

Hawkins, F. Bisset. *Comparative Statistics of the 19th Century*. [London, 1829] Reprinted 1973

Hollingshead, John. *Underground London*. 1862

Johnson, Edward. *Life, Health, and Disease*. 1861

Johnson, Walter. *The Domestic Management Of Children in health and disease . . .* 1858

Kanthack, Emilia. *The Preservation of Infant Life*. 1907

Newman, George. *The Health Of The State*. 1907

Notter, J. Lane and Firth, R.H. *Practical Domestic Hygiene*. New ed. 1902

Parkes, Mrs William. *Domestic Duties*. [fourth ed.] 1837

Phelps Brown, O. *The Complete Herbalist or the People Their Own Physicians*. 1867

Preston-Thomas, Herbert. *The Work and Play of a Government Inspector*. 1909

Ratcliffe, H. *Observations on the Rate of Mortality & Sickness existing amongst Friendly Societies*. [Manchester, 1850] Reprinted 1974

Richardson, Benjamin W. *Clinical Essays*. 1862

Richardson, Benjamin W. *Vita Medica: Chapters of Medical Life and Work*. 1897

Rogers, Joseph. *Reminiscences of a Workhouse Medical Officer*. 1888

Rowntree, B.S. *Poverty: a study of town life*. 1902

Savory, John. *A Companion to the Medicine Chest, and Compendium of Domestic Medicine*. 1840

Scharlieb, Mary. *The Hope Of the Future*. 1916

Schuster, Edgar. *Eugenics*. N.d. [1912-13]

Shaw, Charles. *Replies . . . to Lord Ashley, M.P.* 1843

Simon, Sir John. *English Sanitary Institutions*. 1890. Reprinted New York, 1970

Skinner, John. *Journal Of A Somerset Rector 1803-1834*. Howard and Peter Coombs (eds.). Bath, 1971

Skrimshire, Frederick. *The Village Pastor's Medical and Surgical Guide*. 1838

Smith, Edward. *Foods*. Sixth ed. 1879

Snow, John. *Snow on Cholera, with a Biographical Memoir by B.W. Richardson*. New York, 1936

Squire, Rose E. *Thirty Years In The Public Service*. 1927

Stewart, Alexander P. and Jenkins, Edward. *The Medical And Legal Aspects of Sanitary Reform*. [1867] New ed. Leicester, 1969

Sykes, John. *Public Health Problems*. 1892

Thomson, Spencer. *A Dictionary of Domestic Medicine*. 1853

Thorne, R. Thorne. *The Progress of Preventive Medicine during the Victorian Era*. 1888

Twining, Louisa. *Recollections of Life and Work*. 1893

Webb, Sidney and Beatrice. *The State And The Doctor*. 1910

Webb, Sidney and Beatrice. *English Poor Law History*, 2 vols. 1929. Reprinted 1963

White, Arnold. *Efficiency and Empire* [1901] New ed., G.R. Searle (ed.). Brighton, 1973

Willoughby, Edward F. *Hygiene: its principles as applied to public health*. 1888

Wood, Catherine J. *Cottage Lectures on Home Nursing*. 1893

In order to save space I have omitted secondary studies. They are comprehensively listed in H.J. Hanham's *Bibliography of British History 1851-1914* (Oxford, 1976), under 'Social Welfare' and 'Medicine'.

LIST OF CORRECTIONS

The Publishers regret that technical reasons prevented the inclusion of the following amendments in this paperback edition:

P22	line 8:	*for* Snow *read* Locock
P46	line 7:	*for* charring *read* charing
P57	line 23:	*for* that *read* than
P59	9 lines up:	*for* L[ecock] *read* L[ocock]
P65		Heading of Table 2.1 should read 'Death Rate under one year (per 1,000 live births) England and Wales, 1839–1912
P74	line 9:	*for* drachyton *read* diachylon
P75	line 24:	*for* juniperas *read* juniperus
P109	line 26:	*for* sqalling *read* squalling
P110	line 12 up:	close of bracket should occur after 'cured'
P152	line 10 up:	*for* 10.00 p.m. *read* 10.00 a.m.
P200	line 15:	*for* move *read* any move
P231	line 1:	*for* 10 per cent *read* 100 per cent
P231		line under Table 4.3 should read 'p. 348'
P271	line 10 up:	*for* and Edinburgh *read* Edinburgh
P287	line 12 up:	*for* Mycabacterium *read* Mycobacterium
P287	last line:	*for* light *read* night
P289	lines 11–12	the reference to Ireland in brackets should be deleted
P290	line 13:	*for* Dr J. Andrew's *read* Dr J. Andrew
P290	line 4 up:	*for* Livy *read* Levy
P292	line 20:	*for* professions *read* profession
P292	line 24:	*for* Deléphine *read* Delépine
P316	line 26:	*for* must *read* much
P331	line 8 up:	*for* stricture *read* structure
P332	line 22:	*for* Opthalmic *read* Ophthalmic
P339	line 23:	*for* Dr J. A. Coffin *read* Dr A. I. Coffin
P379	line 6:	brackets should be closed after 'Wakley'
P410	note 258:	*for* Hirtoire *read* Histoire
P415	line 24:	*for* before 1820s *read* before the 1820s
P422	Table 6.1:	heading of Table should be read as the first entry

INDEX

Abortion, 73–8
Ackerley, Captn., 339
Acland, T. D., 170
Acton, William, 70, 72, 294, 295, 297, 302
Acupuncture, 378–9, 410 ns, 257–8
Adams, Miss Bertha, 261
Adulteration of food and drugs: bread, 208–10; Beer & spirits, 210–12; butter, 212, 214; chloroform, 21; milk, 212–14; pickles, 210; tea, 210; opium, 98; workhouse food, 393
Adults: diet, 214–15; food & drink, 203–10 passim
Aged people, 316–20, 323, 382–4, 389–401, 402 n.1
Agricultural labourers: living conditions, 173–5
Alison, William Pulteney, 149, 234
Anaesthesia, 18–22, 59–60, 272–3, 328, 414
Anarcha, 9
Anderson, Michael, 416
Andrews, James, 290
Ansell, Charles, 316
Antisepis,18, 39–40, 271, 272–5, 276, 414
Anti-vaccination league, 166–7
Apothecaries, Society of, 23, 45
Appleton, R., 86
Armstrong, Alan, 416
Armstrong, J., 275
Arnold, A. P., 180
Arnott, Neil, 232, 235
Artizans Dwellings Act 1875, 224, 225
Ashby, Henry, 87
Ashwell, Samuel, 20
Asepsis, 275

Association, Ladies, for the Diffusion of Sanitary Knowledge, 218
Axham, Frederick, 287

Baby farming, 78–80
Baines, Mrs M. A., 218
Baker, Brown Isaac, 19, 299
Baker, Brown J. FRCS, 31
Bakewell, Dr Hall, 137, 138, 160, 161
Ballard, Dr E., 246
Bally, William, 234
Barclay, Ness, 84
Barclay, Whyte, 325
Barber, Dr Herbert, 85, 86, 87
Barber, H. A., 287
Barlow, G. H., 108, 243, 326
Barnardo, Dr Thomas, 237
Barnett, Rev. Samuel, 225, 397
Barr, Sir James, 121
Beecham, Thomas, 344–5
Beddoe, Dr John, 389
Beeton, Mrs I., 89, 108, 112
Benham, Dr F., 282
Beveridge, Dr R., 240
Birth rate: fall in, 118–9; of various social classes, 120
Blackmore, E., 139
Blackwell, Elizabeth, 41, 381
Blane, Gilbert, 145
Blindness, 332
Blizard, William, 263
Bloomfield, Bishop Charles, 230
Blood letting: childbirth, 17, 20, 26; cupping, 111; ear infection, 184; fever causes, 139–40; influenza, 324; measles, 146; scarlet fever, 139; surgery, 274; whooping cough, 108
Boards of Guardians, 250, 717, 763–4

Boards of Health: Cheltenham, 233; Edinburgh, 233
bone-setters, 284–7
Bonny, Francis, 51–2, 103
Boot, Jesse, 344–5
Booth, Charles, 383, 384–5
Broadhurst, Alderman, 113
Bread, 208–10
Brierly, John, 335
Bright, Richard, 244
Bristowe, J. S., 279
British Medical Association 45, 115, 186, 188, 300–1, 346–9, 362–3, 364–5, 369, 417–18
Brodie, Benjamin, 263, 295, 296
Brown, Blakely, 38
Brown, Isaac Baker, 19, 299
Brown, Phelps, 327
Brown, R. G., 249
Brudenall, Carter, 181
Buchan, William, 82, 84, 90, 139
Buchanan, Dr, 236
Buckton, Catherine, 89
Budd, William, 234, 245, 246 247, 290
Budgett, J. B., 51
Buer, M. C., 449, 415
Bury, W., 396–7, 400
Butter, Rev. Henry, 70
Buxton, H. St. Clair, 184

Callender, G. W., 275
Callisthenics, 184
Campbell, James, 179
Cameron, Spottiswoode, 100, 170
Cancer, 326–330; deaths, 326–8, 329, 330; diagnosis, 327; lung cancer, 329; quack treatments, 333–5; treatments, 328

434